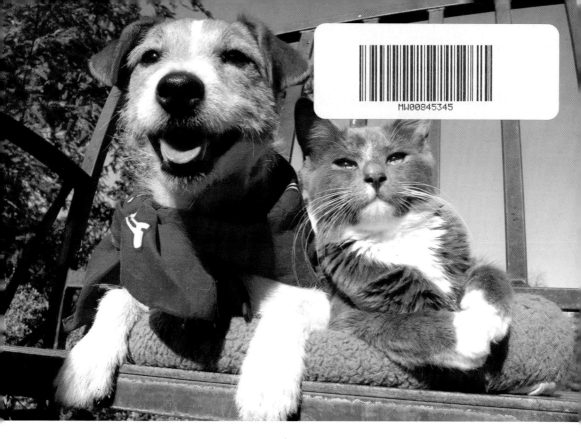

"This book is excellent. It's not just great training for veterinary students, but should be read by veterinarians, no matter how many years they've been in practice. The techniques in this book will help reduce patient stress, improve staff safety, and enhance professional satisfaction by improving our bond with our patients."

Laurie Bergman, VMD, Diplomate ACVB

"This book is a pictorial guide into the world of what to do and, as importantly, what not to do, to reduce dogs' and cats' fear of encounters with humans. If a picture is worth a thousand words, then this is a HUGE volume. The photographs show actual expressions of dogs and cats in real-life situations that anyone familiar with these animals will recognize. The methods of handling them are clearly shown, as are the results. This type of book is long overdue."

Bonnie V. Beaver, DVM, MS, Diplomate ACVB
Board-Certified Veterinary Behaviorist
Past President, *American Veterinary Medical Association*

"This book on low stress handling and restraint techniques is revolutionary. It is the mechanism by which veterinary hospitals can finally make the vital paradigm shift to animal-centered practices. These techniques allow those working in an animal hospital to consider the entire animal, not just its body parts. Ground-breaking!"

Ginny Price, MS, CVT
Animal Behavior Instructor
Saint Petersburg College
Veterinary Technology Program

"As a feline practitioner and advocate for respectful handling of our feline patients, I found this book by Dr. Sophia Yin to be a tremendous asset to all of us who work with cats. There is a huge need to reduce the stress of veterinary visits for our feline patients especially so that we can do the best for them both physically and emotionally. The old adage is so true— clients don't care how much we know until we show them how much we care—both for them and for their beloved pets. Dr. Yin gives great examples of how to handle anxious pets so that they are more relaxed, allowing for a more relaxed work environment for all and less injuries. Several techniques are unique, and are based on her own work with veterinary patients. With my passion for behavior, I found the entire book fascinating and a great asset for canine patients as well. The book is science-based, yet easy to read and full of great pictures, videos and suggestions for how to handle pets in different situations at the clinic. Understanding dogs and cats and why they behave as they do is brilliantly described and helps us see the world from their point of view. The information provided is also an excellent asset for staff training and education."

Ilona Rodan, DVM, Diplomate ABVP, Feline Practice
Cat Care Clinic and Behavior Consultations for Cats, Madison, Wisconsin

"I am a technician and attended Dr. Yin's handling seminar. I found it very informative and well presented, but wondered if a dog could really be won over within the first 5 to 10 minutes of an appointment while getting a history from the owner. Well, I cannot tell you how amazed, thrilled and excited I was to find that the techniques worked so well and so fast! I had two different appointments with canines that were known "caution" dogs and had bitten in the past. One actually greeted me from across the room with a snarling nonstop growl! I started the treat technique [chapter 14], and by the end of the 5 to 10 minutes I had both dogs accepting and looking for the treat which was now in my hand, and allowing me to pat them, with a much more relaxed "happy state." Both dogs were examined with an Elizabethan collar on. Although there was still some apprehension, there was no longer a struggle, no growling, no attempts to bite, no show of aggression—not even during the blood draw! We were able to remove the collar at the end of the appointments with both dogs still in a "happy state," still responding well to the treat technique. The growling dog was actually looking for attention! The owners were relieved and grateful that their pets had a good experience, as well as amazed at the difference in their pets' behavior. I wanted to thank you for such a wonderful training tool, along with all the other handling/behavior tools and information you presented. It will make a huge difference in my career, but more importantly, it will make a huge difference in the lives of owners and their pets who put off exams and medical treatment because of fear or aggression shown by the pet."

Dianna Larrabee, VT

Rarely do I use the word "revolutionary" when it comes to describing a textbook, but clearly this applies to "Low Stress......" Whether, like me, you've been handling dogs and cats for decades or are just entering the field, this book will give you insights and applications you can immediately put to use. Take some time to learn these approaches--it will be less stressful for people and animals, alike.

Kathy Meyer, VMD
President, *American Veterinary Society of Animal Behavior*

LOW STRESS
HANDLING, RESTRAINT AND BEHAVIOR MODIFICATION OF
DOGS & CATS

TECHNIQUES FOR DEVELOPING PATIENTS WHO LOVE THEIR VISITS

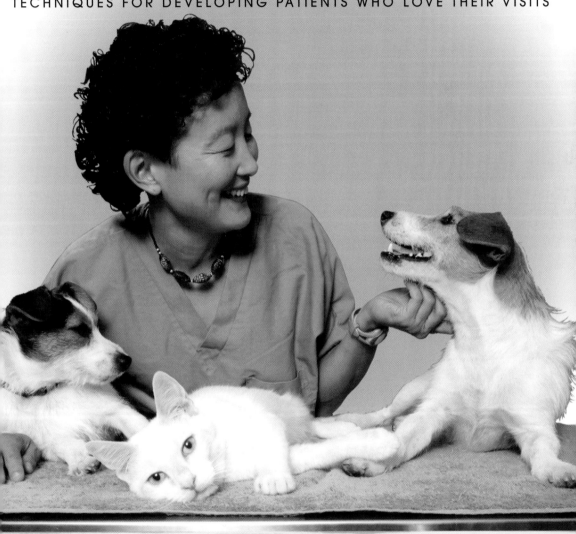

Sophia Yin, DVM, MS

Editors: Cheryl Kolus and Beth Adelman

Publishing Assistant: Amanda Huynh

Cover and Book Design: Diana Catherines

Cover Photo: Neil Michel, Axiom Photo Design

Photographers: Sophia Yin, Melissa Morris, Neil Michel

Illustrations: Miguel Garza

Flip book design: Mark Deamer

Production Coordinator: Sophia Yin, DVM, MS

Production Assistant: Melissa Morris

Video Editor: Sophia Yin, DVM, MS

Videographers: Melissa Morris, Sophia Yin

DVD Authoring: Dave Craig

Library of Congress Control Number: 2008911714

Printed in the United States of America

For access to the readers-only resources, register at www.nerdbook.com/lowstresshandling

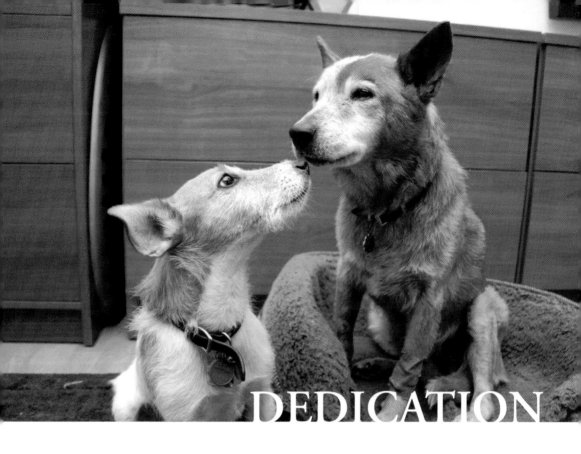

DEDICATION

To all of the dogs and cats

who could have had a better

hospital experience.

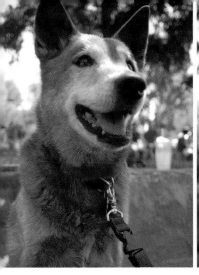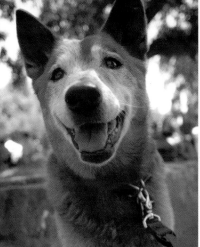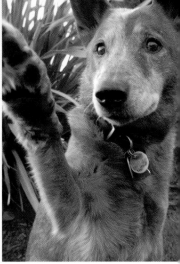

Acknowledgements

When I started this project many months ago, I wondered why no one had written a photo-illustrated book with a DVD on handling, restraint and behavior modification. Several months and 8 photo shoots into the project, the answer was clear: too hard, too time consuming and too many animals and people needed. Unfortunately, I had already decided I was going to do this, so I was stuck.

I'd like to thank the countless friends, colleagues, students, clients and innocent bystanders who somehow got wrangled into helping me with this project.

The following animals were wonderful models—sometimes of good behavior but also of all of the undesirable behaviors that occur regularly at the veterinary hospital or groomer's studio. We needed pets who weren't perfect to amplify any handling errors that were occurring.

Amadeus, Amelia, Ariel, Arnie, Autumn Leaves, Beep, Bella, Blackie, Blue, Buster, Calli, Cassidy, Charlie, Cheeto, Cody, Cole, Cowboy, Daisy, Dave, Dozer, Dervish, Duke, Elvis, Fluffy, Frank, Grey, Gus, Hallie, Hercules, Homer, Ivory, Jackie, Joey Fatwon, John Doe, Jonesy, Kelsey, Kimber, Kramer, Kujo, LittleMan, Lola, Maggie Moo, Maisy, Mama, Mattie, Max, Meggie, Mia, Milo, Mischa, Momi, Nellie, Oski, Panda, Pinot, Pixie, Piya, Podee, Rascal, Riley, Rocket, Rocky, Rosebud, Roxy, Roy, Rufus, Scooter, Scout, Shasta, Siam, Seigfried, Sierra, Sophie, Spike, Stellah, Summer Rain, Tanner, Teddy, Tibby, Tilly, Trixie, Ty, Vandal, Violet, Winter Sun, Zoe

I'm grateful to the human volunteers who helped demonstrated correct as well as incorrect methods of handling, and who tested out the instructions both the way they were meant to be read and the way the normal busy person reads directions. Our 50 or so photo shoots, which generated more than 20,000 photos, were sometimes long, sometime grueling and often humorous as we learned all of the little things that make handling go wrong. Most important, we learned that what one person does naturally, the other has to learn. This book is geared to the person who has to learn.

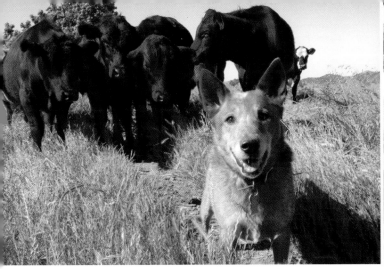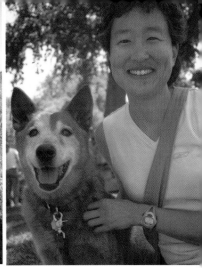

Alicia Tran, Amanda Huynh, Andy Lenius, DVM, Angelica Sierra, Bobbie Rios, Carlo Vitali, Chris Bui, Christopher Rosario, Diane Fabretti, , Gustavo Soberano, Iris Lo, Janet Edson, Janet Krovoza, Janine Hutchinson, Jared Julson, Jeannie Cruz, Jeremy Warren, Jim Douglas, Jonathon Ho, Kelly Moffat, Laurie Ho, Manuel, Meaghan Ripley, Melissa Morris, Michelle Lee, Miranda Blankenship, Rachel Terpstra, Raven Castillo, Roni Huerta, Sara C. Matos, Sara Taylor, Sarah-Kate Medelinskas, Shawnon Kaiser, Shereen Welling, Tiffany R. Setters, Val Ruszovan

A number of busy people helped in many other generous ways by reviewing various drafts of the manuscript, contributing photos, offering techniques and suggestions or generally providing support where needed.

Amanda Eick-Miller, Ashley Cameron, Brenda McCowan, Deanna Sanchez, Donna Dyer, Edward Price, Elaine Last, Erin Landeck, Frances Mooney, Ginny Price, Ilona Rodan, Jay McLean, Jenny Remensperger, John Capitanio, John Ukich, Kathy Meyer, Kelly Moffat, Laurie Bergman, Lisa Radosta, Lisa Wells, Mark Deamer, Monty Sloan, Pat Goodman, Ray Coppinger, Stephanie Ghirardo, Tonimarie Swann, Bob Walker, Lisa Wells, Jim Wilson.

Most of all, I'd like to thank Dr. Kelly Moffat for generously sharing her time and expertise, Melissa Morris, who was so adept at scheduling both animals and people to be in the right place at the right time, Amanda Huynh, who somehow successfully juggled all of the drafts and communications with the various designers and illustrators, and Zoe, my Australian Cattledog, who patiently put up with all of the volunteers and visitors and graced many of the clips with her cameo appearances. Zoe did not see this project to its end but she leaves her mark throughout the pages.

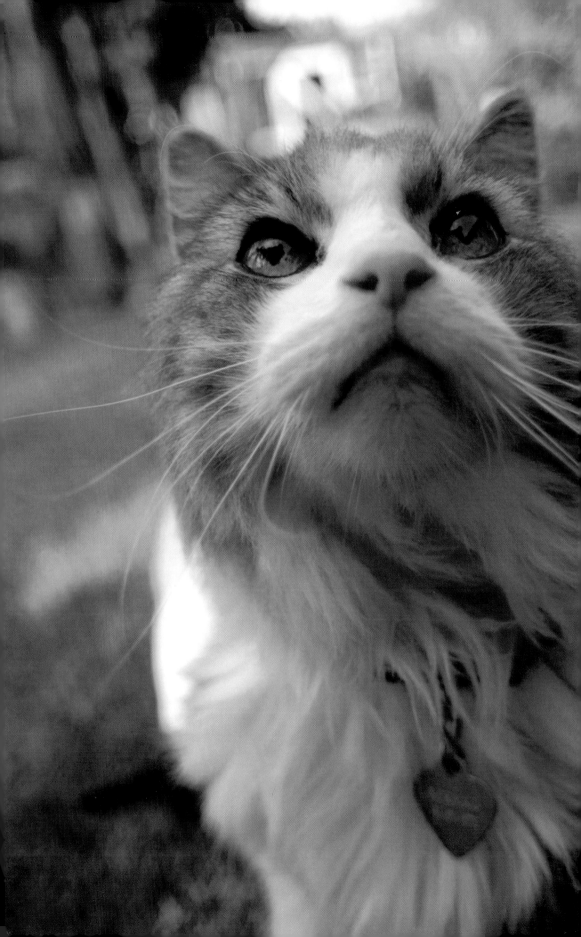

CONTENTS

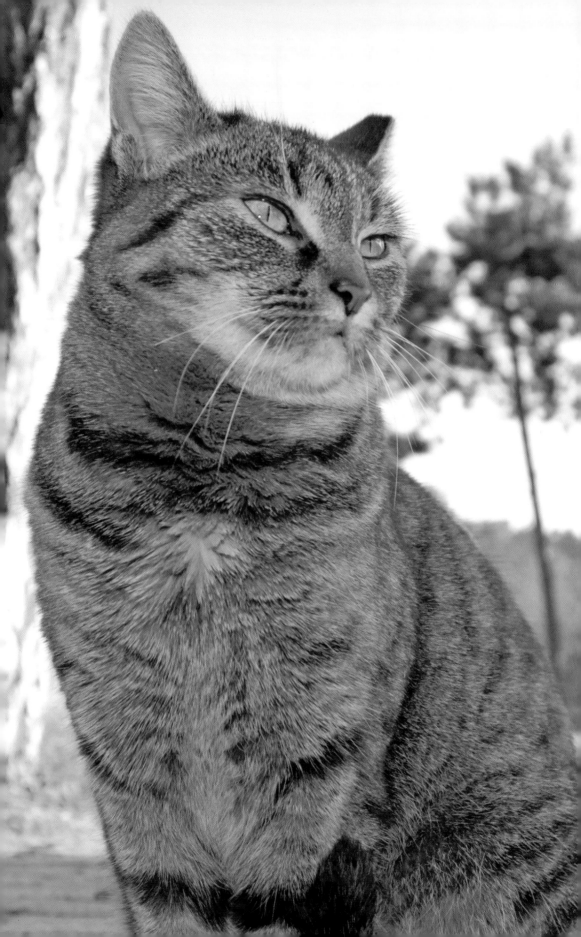

Bonnie V. Beaver, BS, DVM, MS, Diplomate ACVB, AVMA Past President

FOREWORD

It has taken the world a long time to really understand that a dog is not a wolf and that dominance is not the way to turn dogs into good dogs. Cats are also misunderstood. They are neither wild animals nor in need of domination. Even now, a lot of the pet-owning world still does not understand that concept. Usually, it is not their fault. They have received bad advice from the so-called "experts." The dog may have evolved from wolf ancestors, but even for wolves, careful observations show that it is seldom about dominant postures or behavior for controlling most situations. It is, instead, about pack leadership.

This book is a pictorial guide into the world of what to do and, as importantly, what not to do to reduce the fear of dog- or cat-human encounters. This is accomplished by increasing the trust of the animal in non-threatening ways. If a picture is worth a thousand words, then this is a HUGE volume. The photographs show actual expressions of dogs and cats in real life situations that anyone familiar with these animals will recognize. The methods of handling them are clearly shown, as are the results.

While every veterinarian who has a special interest in animal behavior will have slightly different approaches in how they positively handle the dog or cat, we all agree that it is time to get away from the "brute-a-cane" approach of solving all problems. It does not work, the animal's fear escalates, and people and animals get hurt. Things get worse every time the animal returns to a similar situation. By taking a little extra time to encourage positive behavior and reduce fear, it is possible to relieve stress in the pets, the owners, and the veterinary staff.

This type of book is long overdue. Everyone who reads it cannot help but think of how much positive impact it will have on the dogs and cats. Even if they are only affected by the information in one chapter, life will be better. That cannot be said about most books.

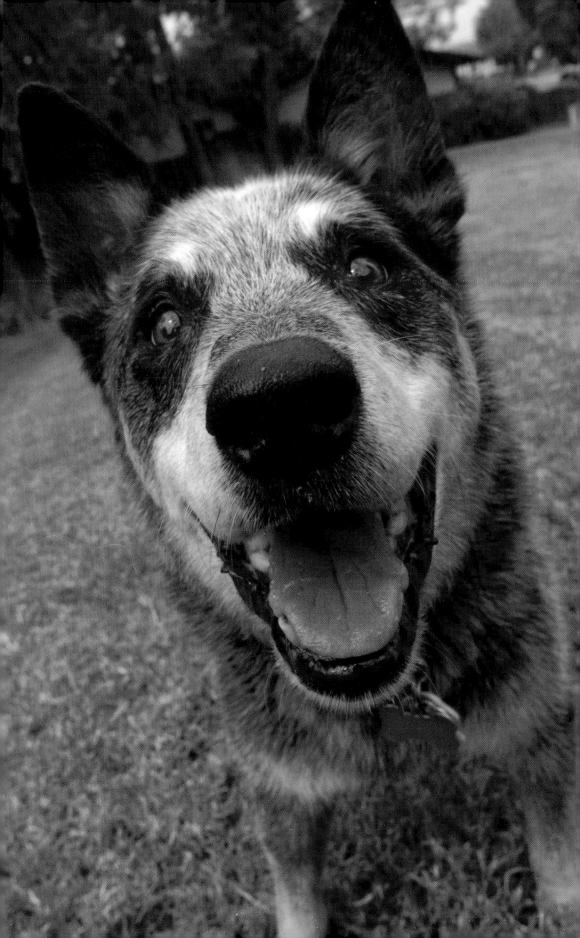

INTRODUCTION

It's man against a Miniature Poodle-Maltese mix as the popular dog trainer, Cesar Millan, pits his skills against a curly-haired football-sized dog that hates being groomed. He brushes the dog's face and head as the dog stands, seemingly willingly, except for the subtle twitch of his upper lip. "That's the beauty of becoming a pack leader," says Millan. "Because anything they used to dislike, they just learn to like, because they have no choice." The owner looks on, her face lit with the joy of what she sees as a miracle before her eyes. "So he learns that he can respect and trust this new human," continues Millan. "I just came into his life. I'm using 24-cent leash..." But then, as Millan stops to adjust the leash, the dog explodes with the emotion his earlier lip twitch had warned lay below. He screams and bares his teeth—holding his mouth wide open like a shield studded with sharp white stones. The puffy white alligator flails his head and bites the fingers of Millan's right hand. Millan calmly pulls his right hand away while holding the dog's neck and leash with his left hand. As he moves to reposition his right hand behind the dog's head, the dog—mouth agape in a tense threat, and feet up and clawing in full defense fight mode—bites Millan again.

Dog Whisperer with Cesar Millan, season 1, episode 4, "Josh and Boomer." Original air date September 16, 2004, National Geographic Channel.

My Caveman Days

From high school through my first years as a veterinarian, the Millan-like methods of forcing pets to bend to my will so that I could be the boss and teach them to behave guided my interactions with unruly animals in the veterinary hospital. I took this approach because it was what I had been taught by many different trainers starting 20 years ago.

> Pleasant visits to the veterinary office promote the establishment of trust and confidence in the pet as well as the client. Learning how to read our pet patients, communicate with them better and handle them more skillfully will
>
> 1. increase safety for the hospital staff;
>
> 2. increase our ability to treat patients and the willingness of owners to bring in their pets;
>
> 3. increase overall efficiency by developing patients who willingly comply with procedures;
>
> 4. build better relationships with both our clients and our patients.

More than two decades ago, my interest in behavior began out of necessity when my male Boxer, Max (Figures A and B), started showing aggression. He would growl and snap at anyone who tried to shoo him from the couch or move him out of their path, or even pet him when he was tired of being petted. The veterinarians I worked for said I might have to euthanize him down the road if I didn't fix his behavior. But they had no suggestions as to how I could fix his behavior or where I could get help. So I did the only thing I knew: I took Max to dog-training class when he was 3 years old.

At our first class, the instructor taught us the common method of teaching a dog to heel, and Max's behavior became markedly worse. As instructed, I hooked Max's long leather leash to the choke chain around his neck, and when he sniffed the grass instead of paying attention to me, I ran at full speed away from him. If he was still sniffing when the leash was almost fully extended, he would get a big yank that would have toppled a smaller dog. This quickly got Max's attention; by the third yank, he had learned to stay by my side. The instructor told me to continue this technique when Max ignored me. By the sixth yank, Max was aggressively growling and climbing up the leash after me to prevent the impending punishment.

Thus began a 7-year power struggle between Max and me. For the next 5 years, I searched everywhere for trainers who could help me with Max's aggressive behavior. I followed their instructions exactly. I learned to give a neck-wrenching yank while stationary by using my hips, much like martial artists use theirs when blocking, punching, or kicking. With this technique, I could usually keep Max in line by uttering a sharp "ah" or lightly jerking the leash to remind him of the pain that might occur if he disobeyed.

I went through 10 trainers, all with the philosophy that, like the alpha wolf, I had to remind Max of his lower rank by frequently standing over him and bullying him. I continued to follow their instructions diligently. Like a drill sergeant, I randomly made him perform behaviors in rapid succession, and I punished him when the behaviors weren't up to par. Although I also praised him for good behaviors, that was not particularly motivating for him, especially after being bullied or punished. Trainers also told me to throw Max, who weighed 76 pounds, on the ground and roll him on his back in an "alpha roll" when he disobeyed. I was even instructed to address Max's aggression by hitting him on the nose with a foam-covered wooden rod. When this made him more aggressive, I was told to hang him on a choke chain until he passed out, because it was important to win all aggressive encounters. The hanging didn't work. He passed out twice but was still ready to fight when confronted again.

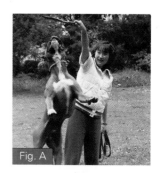
Fig. A

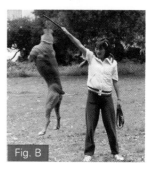
Fig. B

Max and I play with a stick. My 76-pound aggressive—but loveable—Boxer sparked my interest in behavior.

This progression of force was the general recommendation at that time for all dogs who defied their owners or showed aggression, regardless of the cause. If a dog was possessive of food or a toy, owners were told to use a choke chain, pinch collar or electronic collar correction. If a dog growled at another dog, even out of fear, owners were told to correct it. Everything was about forcing the dog to submit to the owner rather than changing the underlying emotional state that drove the behavior.

As a result of this thinking, I didn't start to trust Max until he was 10 years of age, when I found high-level obedience competition instructors who understood the science of learning and knew how to use positive reinforcement to shape behaviors. These trainers and methods focused on rewarding good behaviors and clearly teaching these good behaviors in a systematic, step-by-step fashion. Max's behavior improved and my understanding of him grew dramatically using these balanced techniques, but it was only a start. Although Max got his Companion Dog obedience title in three consecutive trials and always placed in the top 3 with high scores, Max and I never reached our full potential—in the obedience ring or at home. Without specialized training in behavior problems, even these top competition instructors could not specifically address aggression and its related behaviors. In fact, they still fell back on force when they deemed the dog stubborn or disagreeable, rather than understanding why the bad behaviors occurred.

TM

Gaining a New Understanding

After my experience with Max, the old training techniques seemed crude and barbaric. However, I still brought some of the old thinking into veterinary practice, because I had no better models to follow. I handled dogs skillfully, rewarded them with treats and other appropriate motivators for good behavior, and overall gave many dogs a good hospital experience. But I also warned owners that their unruly dogs needed to be disciplined. The dog should not be allowed to win such struggles; owners should put the dogs in their place. I restrained these tough–to–treat dogs more efficiently than a straight-jacket restrains a hyperactive child. Occasionally, I even scared a few puppies into struggling the way the Poodle mix Millan fought with did, and caused some to urinate or defecate out of fear. Because this was all I knew, I chalked up these results to owners failing to establish that they were the boss.

Despite some of my old tendencies, my experiences helped me recognize that more animals presenting to the hospital had behavior problems rather than medical problems and that these problems were leading to relinquishment and euthanasia. As a result, I decided to further my education in behavior. I knew I could often control behavior using force and treats, at least in dogs, but that perhaps there were better ways than the force methods to deal with problem pets. And clearly, punishment and force were a puny arsenal for dealing with difficult cats and species such as horses that are much larger than humans. I took an eclectic path of education that included not only graduate school, but several month-long natural horsemanship clinics, low-stress livestock herding clinics, electronic shock collar lessons, the Marin Dog Training Academy, Intermediate and Advanced Operant Conditioning Workshops (a.k.a. Chicken Training Camp) (Figure C), a 5-day Wolf Park symposium (Figure D), case observations with a veterinary behaviorist and as many volunteer opportunities as I could fit into my schedule.

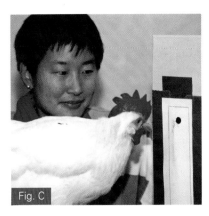

Fig. C

Marion and Bob Bailey Operant Conditioning and Behavior Analysis Workshop (a.k.a. Chicken Training Camp), Hot Springs, Arkansas: This chicken is learning that she should peck the black dot only when she sees the tiny red dot flash below it. (To see video, go to www.AskDrYin.com and watch Thinking Chickens.)

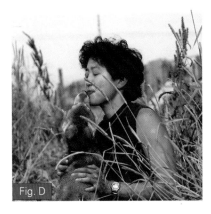

Fig. D

Wolf Park, Indiana (www.wolfpark.org): This wolf pup is friendly, but he would never make a good companion pet.

I combined this field experience with a master's degree in Animal Science at the University of California, Davis, with a focus on animal behavior. Here I conducted research on vocal communication in dogs and took coursework geared toward understanding how and why behaviors develop. I learned both how to implement behavior modification protocols and how to approach behavior problems methodically using the scientific method. And the experience I gained with a number of other species—including horses, goats, giraffes and porcupines—not only taught me a lot but was also a lot of fun (Figures E and F).

Armed with the science of learning and knowledge of the scientific method of asking questions, devising experiments and testing hypotheses about why behaviors are as they are, a new world opened for me. It was like I had been color-blind and now could see an entire spectrum. I observed the successes that colleagues experienced using positive reinforcement on dogs, birds and exotic animals. I also became aware of the adverse effects of force and the care needed when using it. With my newfound knowledge and skill, animals whom I had once viewed as stubborn now willingly behaved. What I had in the past mistaken for unruly behavior and a bid for dominance in the veterinary hospital, I now saw clearly as being due to fear and poor handling on the part of the humans involved. Prior to this education, my toolbox for handling animals was limited to a calm demeanor, an occasional treat and then Millan-like techniques used to wrangle the animal. Now I had the additional tools to address the underlying issues and enable me to get the tasks done—sometimes more quickly in the short run and always more quickly down the road.

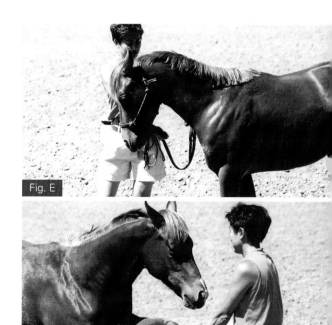

Fig. E

Fig. F

Training yearlings: Horses can be trained using a combination of natural horsemanship techniques and positive reinforcement with a bridging stimulus, such as a clicker. Natural horsemanship relies on immediately releasing pressure when the horse performs the correct behavior and then rewarding the horse with rest (a strong motivator in horses). It also focuses on using careful desensitization and, again, stopping to let the horse rest after good behavior. Adding a bridging stimulus to mark correct behavior, as well as adding other motivators or reinforcers, can help speed up training and ensure the horse is developing a positive association with you and the training situation. This yearling learned vertical flexions and to back up or move in different directions on cue while in vertical flexion. In just several sessions she learned how to do a turn on the forehand, turn on the rear and also move laterally on cue with a handler directing her from the ground. These exercises are important for strengthening overall communication between horse and human and provide handlers with the ability to signal to the horse exactly where the horse should stand during handling and procedures. This yearling also learned to remain calm and accept many types of handling that are important for everyday husbandry.

What's the Harm in Using Force?

You might wonder, "What's the harm in wrangling patients or using force, or teaching clients to manhandle the animals to establish who's boss?" One issue is that, like in the episode of Dog Whisperer depicted at the beginning of this Introduction, you—or worse, your client— could get bitten. In the average hospital, dog and cat bites as well as cat scratches are the most common cause of injury (Jeyaretnam et al. 2000). A survey of veterinarians from Minnesota and Wisconsin revealed that 92.3% had been bitten by dogs and 81% had been bitten by cats (August 1988). Additionally, in a study on risk factors for bite wounds to caregivers in a veterinary teaching hospital, Drobatz and Smith (2003) reported that at the University of Pennsylvania Veterinary Teaching Hospital, 80 to 115 bite wounds from dogs and cats were reported each year.

By restraining pets in a forceful, crude or unskilled manner, you could be breaking your promise to do no harm. Such handling can make pets behaviorally worse and even lead to aggression and, ultimately, euthanasia.

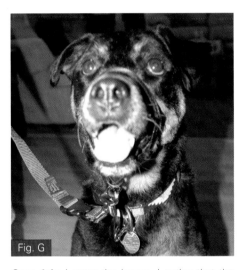

Fig. G

Besides creating a situation where animal caregivers could get injured, handling animals poorly or roughly can have even more serious implications. By handling animals in such a manner, veterinarians could be breaking the promise to "do no harm" on a daily basis. Restraining pets in a forceful or crude manner can make pets behaviorally worse to the point where they can no longer receive thorough veterinary care. It can even precipitate events that lead to heightened aggression at home and, ultimately, to euthanasia. These cases offer examples.

Case 1: As I enter the house, I notice that the graying Rottweiler is tense. She comes up but backs away, wondering if I had anything worthwhile to offer. I do. I have a bag filled with aromatic treats. The scent, followed by the sight of a few flying toward her, attracts her. She eats the treats and eventually sits for the ones I am holding in my hand. I respond by rewarding her repeatedly for her polite behavior.

"Gracie's a little apprehensive of visitors and really bad with other dogs," says her concerned owner. "At the hospital, she used to just shake and cower when they did anything to her. Recently I took her in because she seemed very arthritic. They took X-rays of her hips. After that she was so sore she couldn't walk for 3 days. Since then, she's been so aggressive at the hospital that they can't do anything with her. We can't get a muzzle on her anymore and the tranquilizers we give to her beforehand have no effect." (Figure G)

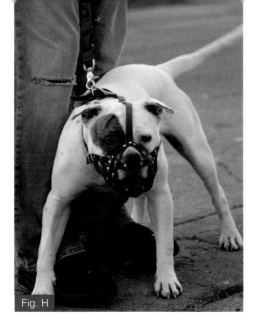

Fig. H

In the average hospital, dog and cat bites as well as cat scratches are the most common causes of injury (Jeyaretnam et al. 2000).

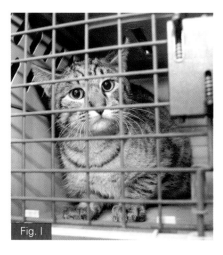

Fig. I

Case 2: A 10-month-old American Bulldog hurls herself to the end of the leash, growling and barking, her gaze aimed squarely at me as I stand casually talking to one of her owners who is standing right next to me. Her other owner, a 6-foot-plus weight-lifting enthusiast with the same build as the dog, is keeping her in check.

"Sierra's always been afraid of visitors but she used to cower and just try to stay away from them," he says. "After about 10 minutes in the same room with them, she would relax."

I look over at the barking, muscled mass of white. The telltale signs of fear are visible in spite of her loud efforts to mask them. Between barks and lunges, Sierra backs away and stands with a paw on her owner's foot, her ears flicking up and out to the side.

"She didn't actually become aggressive to people until a month ago after a bad episode at the veterinary hospital. She's never loved going to the vet's. Her tail was usually between her legs but she would hold still. That day, our other dog had lunged at her over a bone. Sierra fought back for the first time and got bitten. So she had to go in to get her wound repaired," explains the owner. "On this particular visit, she was still agitated from being bitten and tried to stay away from the veterinarian. She started growling and had to be muzzled and restrained by several technicians. Even muzzled, she fought them. Now she barks and growls at all visitors and at people on the street. All our friends who used to come over have to stay outside. They call her 'psycho dog.'" (Figure H)

Case 3: As the cat's eyes peered out from the carrier, I listened to the owners. "Skippy always hides when new people come over and has always been scared at the vet hospital. Because he's stressed by hospital visits, we hired someone to come over and trim his toenails. It was very stressful for him and for us. He hissed and hid after the event, and we couldn't touch him. Since then, he's been completely untreatable at the veterinary hospital, and he attacks the housekeeper and others who regularly work with us. He's bitten several people seriously, and they have had to go to the hospital." (Figure I)

Veterinarians and other animal-care professionals see these types of cases every day, and we do what we can to provide the best services given the behavioral challenges. Regardless, if we don't recognize and specifically address fear and unruly behaviors before they develop into aggression, we are likely sending pets home with worse behavior than when they came in. We might also be leaving the owner without a clue that progression of the behavior can often be halted early on, while ignoring the signs could lead to our inability to treat the pet later. You might think that such problems are beyond the scope of general practice; however, a few simple modifications in how we regularly handle our patients, along with the use of two basic counterconditioning techniques (both in the hospital and for clients to practice at home), can dramatically improve the pet's behavior and experience.

A Smarter Alternative to Force

Some readers might still have doubts. They might wonder, "Why not use force if the animal just appears to be unruly?" For instance, some dogs look happy in the waiting room but struggle and mouth you only when you try to trim their nails or restrain them. If you're stronger than the dog, why not just hold her with a death grip so you can power through the procedure?

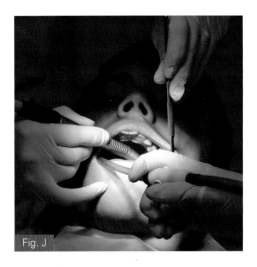

Fig. J

Our goal should be to help our patients enjoy their visits.

Because there are smarter ways.

To illustrate the point, consider this: Why do children misbehave at the dentist? (Figure J)

The answer is easy: They misbehave primarily because they are fearful. But if you thought they were misbehaving due to other reasons, would it be appropriate to strap them down or command them in a military voice to remain seated? How do children's dentists deal with the problem?

Pediatric dentists and others who work primarily with children have built a niche based on understanding the behavior of their young patients. Rather than forcefully holding the kids down, they provide the kids with a fun experience—from an inviting waiting room with cartoon murals, video games and staff who know how to talk and play with kids, to exam rooms with G-rated movies and kid-controlled remotes. They make a good first impression and maintain it throughout. (Figure K)

These dentists know that the oral health of the patient depends not only on their ability to diagnose and treat disease, but equally on their ability to gain the child's trust. In fact, a FAQ sheet from the American Association of Pediatric Dentists states:

Pleasant visits to the dental office promote the establishment of trust and confidence in your child that will last a lifetime. Our goal, along with our staff, is to help all children feel good about visiting the dentist and teach them how to care for their teeth. From our special office designs, to our communication style, our main concern is what is best for your child (www.aapd.org/pediatricin-formation/faq.asp).

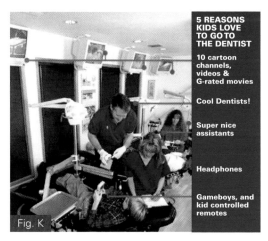

Fig. K

Ad courtesy of Dr. John M. Ukich, Pediatric Dental Center of North Idaho (www.dentalcareforkids.com).

While there are probably no veterinary clinics designed specifically for developing pets' confidence and trust, it's easy to make a few changes to the way we practice, with that goal in mind. The techniques are simple, the approach easy and the changes to the hospital relatively small. The benefits, on the other hand, are immense. Learning how to read our pet patients, communicate with them better and handle them more skillfully will

1. increase safety for the hospital staff;

2. increase our ability to treat patients and the willingness of owners to bring in their pets;

3. increase overall efficiency by developing patients who willingly comply with procedures;

4. build better relationships with both our clients and our patients.

Going From a Caveman Style of Animal Handling to a Low-stress Style

So how do we move from the caveman method of compliance ("I'll show them who's boss!") to a low-stress method ("You can trust me.")? First, we must understand that every action we make around an animal affects the animal's view of whether we are friendly, trustworthy or fearsome. We must also learn how to modify our actions and attitudes so that we can create the calm, happy, compliant patients that we desire.

To create this book, I spent the last year observing veterinarians, technicians and other animal-care professionals handling both dogs and cats. In doing

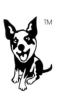

so, I collected many hours of video of different handling techniques. I've analyzed what works and why it works on a given animal and observed what handlers can get away with through sheer luck. I've watched caring, experienced technicians unknowingly cause their patients to become distressed and aggressive—even when working with the most socialized and well-handled pets. And I've seen others unconsciously performing small acts that were key to telling the patients they were in good hands. Combining these experiences with those gained in five years of lecturing to UC-Davis undergraduates and those gained in developing a scientifically tested professional dog training system (MannersMinder®, Premier Pet) has helped me devise a new type of handling book comprised of more than 1,500 photos and accompanied by videos illustrating key points. Key sections have been tested by both new and seasoned technicians, as well as complete novices.

The end result is a book that provides animal-care professionals with the behavioral knowledge to understand

1. why cats and dogs misbehave in hospital, grooming, shelter and kennel settings;

2. how these behaviors were formed;

3. how our actions and the environmental setting make these animals worse or better;

4. how to deal with problem behaviors in the hospital or work setting and how to help pet owners follow through at home.

> The photo illustrations and DVD have been carefully developed after viewing many technicians and examining the learning styles of animal handlers. In tests, 100% of people who only looked at the photos failed to imitate the photos correctly. Be sure to look at the photos, read the text and, when possible, watch the corresponding DVD clips.

References

American Veterinary Medical Association, Task Force on Canine Aggression and Human-Canine Interactions. 2001. A Community Approach to Dog Bite Prevention. *J Am Vet Med Assoc.* 218:1732-49.

August, J.R. 1988. Dog and Cat Bites. *J Am Vet Med Assoc.* 193:1394-98.

Drobatz, K.J., and G. Smith. 2003. Evaluation of Risk Factors for Bite Wounds Inflicted on Caregivers by Dogs and Cats in a Veterinary Teaching Hospital. *J Am Vet Med Assoc.* 223:312-16.

Jeyaretnam, J., H. Jones, and M. Phillip. 2000. Disease and Injury Among Veterinarians. *Australian Veterinary Journal.* 78:625-29.

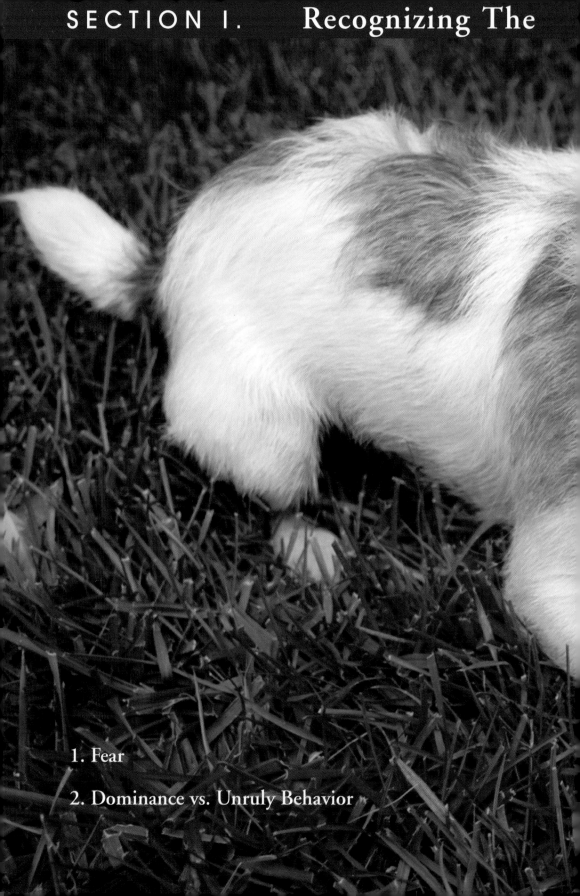

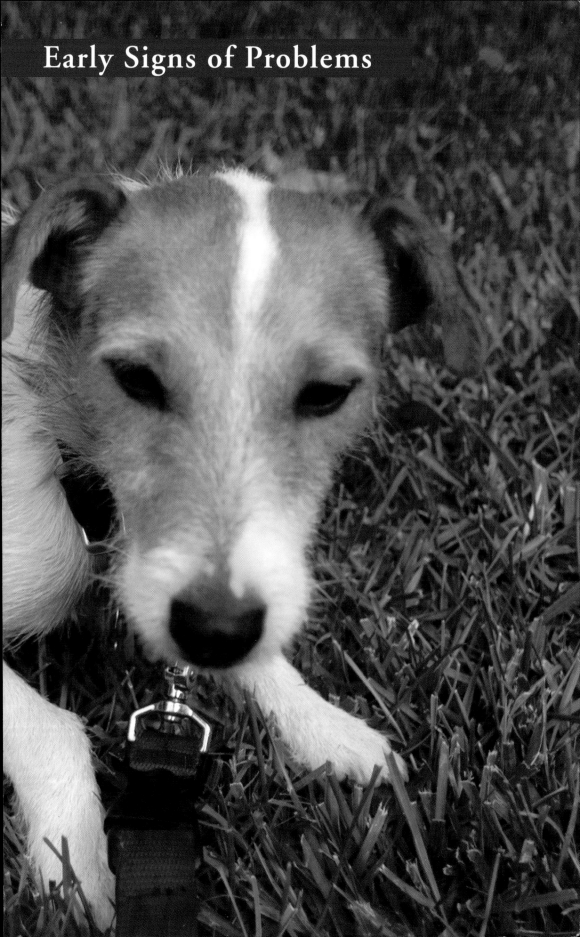

Early Signs of Problems

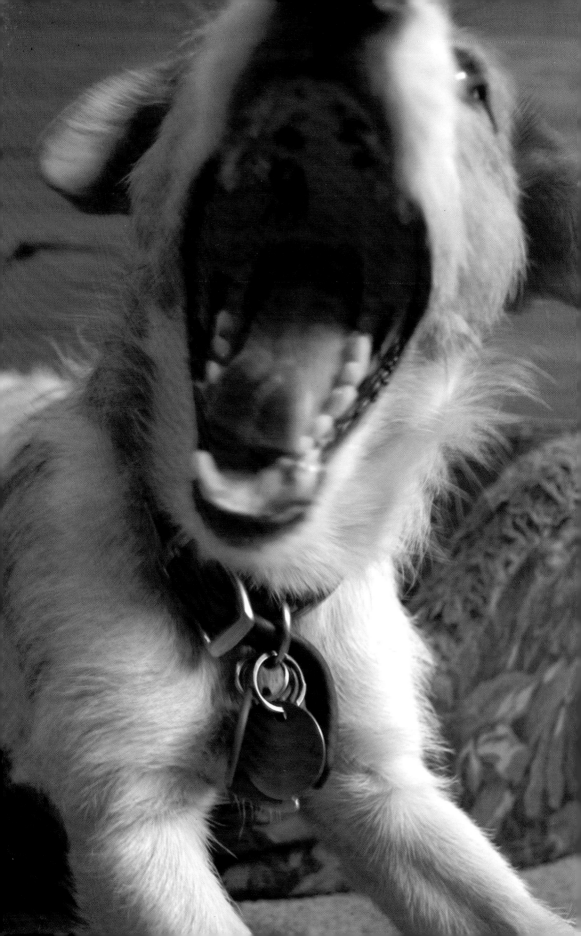

CHAPTER 1.
FEAR

With up to 90% of dog owners complaining that their dogs have behavior problems (Campbell 1986; Adams and Clark 1989; Vacalopoulos and Anderson 1993), and behavioral issues listed as the single reason for shelter relinquishments in 28% of dogs and 19% of cats (Salman et al. 2000), it's no wonder that so many of our dog and cat patients are difficult to handle. One might guess that the bad behavior is most commonly due to "cranky" cats or "dominant" dogs. But both in the hospital and out, the most common serious behavior problems are due to fear. In fact, fear is the number-one reason clients take their dog or cat to a veterinary behavior specialist (Denenberg et al. 2005). In dogs, fear frequently leads to fear-related aggression, and in cats the most common life-threatening manifestation is urination or defecation outside the litter box. Why are so many pets fearful? Fearfulness relates in part to the natural developmental stages that all animals go through.

1.1 Fear and Sensitive Periods for Socialization

All animals pass through a developmental stage early in life during which they accept everything around them and have no fear response. For altricial animals this is the **neonatal period**, and it lasts from birth until their eyes and ears open (Scott and Marston 1950; Serpell and Jagoe 1995), which in dogs occurs by about 2 weeks of age. During this phase, the sensory systems are immature and the animal's main goals in life are getting food and maintaining appropriate body temperature. Whoever provides them with food becomes their "parent"; consequently, animals can readily bond to other species if they are cross-fostered around this time. Because their sensory systems are so immature at this stage, neonatal puppies (and presumably kittens) are somewhat insulated from the world (Scott et al. 1951). A study by Scott (1958) showed that environmental stimuli and even traumatic experiences such as those causing pain do not appear to have lasting negative effects on puppies during the neonatal period.

> Because fear is the number one cause of aggression in the veterinary hospital, grooming shop and other pet care situations it's imperative that those dealing with pets be able to
>
> 1. understand the cause and basis of the fear;
>
> 2. recognize the overt as well as the subtle signs;
>
> 3. be aware of what people commonly do that worsens the fear and aggression.

Next comes the transition period, which only lasts about 1 week. During this phase, brainwave patterns start to mature, puppies no longer require anogenital stimulation by their mother to eliminate and puppies start play-fighting with their littermates (Serpell and Jagoe 1995).

The **socialization period**, the phase in which animals develop an attachment to parents, littermates and others in their group, starts at about 3 weeks of age in puppies and kittens. (Figure 1.1-A) For animals living with humans, they learn to accept humans, other pets and both their own and new environments as safe (Serpell and Jagoe 1995). For instance, a study by Freedman et al. (1961) found that Cocker Spaniel puppies handled for a week between 5-9 weeks of age were more socialized to humans than those handled for a week at an earlier or later age. These puppies also approached a passive handler more readily and were more easily trained to walk on a leash when tested at 14 weeks. Puppies who had not been handled were fearful even after many weeks of handling thereafter. Those handled at 7 weeks were the most well-socialized, and they reacted the best to being placed into a harness.

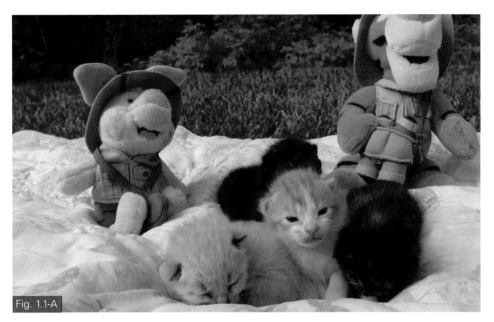

Fig. 1.1-A

Fig.1.1-A: At 3-4 weeks of age, these kittens can hear and see and are starting to ambulate. This marks the beginning of the sensitive period for socialization—the period during which kittens develop attachments to their parents, littermates and others in their group. In kittens, the socialization period is from 3-9 weeks (American Association of Feline Practitioners 2004).

Early during this socialization period (at about 3-5 weeks for dogs), animals may startle easily and react fearfully, but they recover quickly and can easily learn that the startling objects and people are safe. (Figures 1.1-B and 1.1-C) As the young animals mature, they become increasingly wary of strangers, unfamiliar animals and new objects and environments. (Figure 1.1-D) This developmental change corresponds with the animal's increased ability to ambulate. It's likely important for survival, as it helps prevent young animals from walking up to predators or into danger.

Undoubtedly, the exact timing of development varies by breed and for each individual. Additionally, some breeds and individuals might have a greater motivation to make social contact or be more curious and exploratory than others. Scott and Fuller (1965) concluded that the socialization period in dogs ran from about 3-12 weeks of age, with a peak sensitivity between 6 and 8 weeks. Regardless of the exact timing, continued periodic socialization through 6-8 months is probably important. Many dogs who are well-socialized at 12 weeks will regress without such reinforcement—possibly due to a fear period or heightened sensitivity to fear that might occur around 4-6 months of age (Serpell and Jagoe 1995).

The implication of these developmental stages is that pets should be introduced to many new people, objects, animals and environments early in life during the sensitive period for socialization, when their fear is relatively low and they can easily recover from fearful events. It is also a prime time for teaching them to accept being handled in many different ways. Early socialization helps these animals perceive unfamiliar

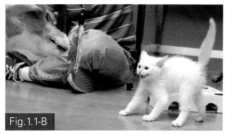

Fig.1.1-B: This kitten is startled when he first sees the dog.

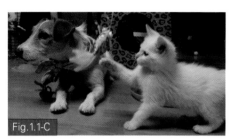

Fig.1.1-C: The kitten recovers quickly because he is early in his sensitive period for socialization.

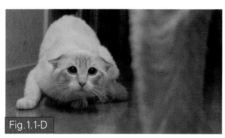

Fig.1.1-D: Here is an adult cat's response to the sight of a calm dog who is moving slowly. This cat was not socialized to dogs during his socialization period. He won't recover as quickly as the kitten did.

people and environments as non-threatening and enables pets to easily assimilate new people and animals into their homes. *(Video 1)* It also helps pets cope with potentially stressful events, such as schedule changes, the addition of new family members, moving to new environments and rough handling or other fear-inducing events.

1.2 Domestication vs. Tameness and Its Relation to Fear

The primary goal of early handling during the sensitive period for socialization is to tame animals; that is, to teach the pet not to run away in fear when humans approach. Animal behavior scientists measure an animal's willingness to approach humans by the animal's flight distance (Price 2002). Tame animals have zero flight distance, meaning that you can walk right up to them and they won't flee. Those who allow you to get within 11 feet but flee at 10 feet have a flight distance of 10 feet.

It's imperative to realize that domestication and tameness are not the same thing. While tameness occurs within the animal's lifetime, domestication is a process occurring over many generations by which a population or species of animals becomes adapted to living with humans in a captive environment (Price 1984; Price 1999). This adaptation involves both genetic changes that accumulate over many generations and environmentally induced events during the development of the animal that recur every generation. For instance, domestic dogs are well adapted to living with humans; wolves, on the other hand, are adapted to living on expanses of land vast enough to support enough prey for them to eat. In general, taming a wolf requires hand-rearing him as a pup, starting before 14 days of age. At Wolf Park, a wolf conservation park in Battleground, Indiana, researchers have found that even when raised with ample human contact and among wolves who are already tame, wolf puppies who are not hand-reared become extremely fearful of humans before 1 year of age (Klinghammer and

Goodmann 1985). (Figure 1.2-A) Dogs, on the other hand, require comparatively little handling to become tame and bond to people. Notice that as an overall survival strategy, the ability to live near or with humans has served dogs well. While there are more than 72 million pet dogs in the United States alone, wolves worldwide are on the endangered species list.

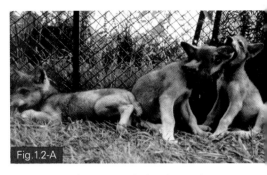

Fig.1.2-A: Wolf pups must be hand-reared starting before 14 days of age to develop into tame adolescent and adult wolves (Klinghammer and Goodmann 1985).

Animals can be domesticated but not tame, or they can be tame but not domesticated. For instance, dogs and cats who grow up in the wild or with no human handling or food provisioning when young are still domesticated, but because people can't get close to them, they are not tame. Birds such as the blue-footed booby of the Galapagos Islands, where animals have evolved free of predators, are not afraid of humans; thus, they are tame but not domesticated. Animals can also be tame but aggressive. For instance, many dogs have a zero flight distance from humans, so they're tame. But handle them in a manner they're not accustomed to or approach them in a way they perceive as threatening and they can become aggressive due to fear, territoriality or other reasons.

1.2.1 Is this species domesticated? Is the individual tame?

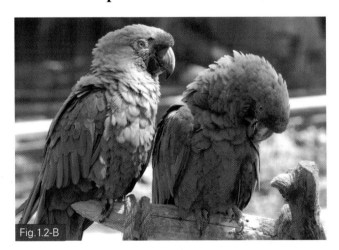

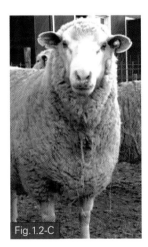

Fig.1.2-B: These parrots were raised in captivity, so they are tame. But parrots are not domesticated. They have not been raised for hundreds of generations with humans nor have humans specifically bred for many generations for tameness or other features that would improve their ability to live with humans. A captive parrot's genetic make-up is essentially the same as a wild parrot's.

Fig.1.2-C: This ewe (female sheep) is domesticated, but if you walk toward her she will run away. She is not tame.

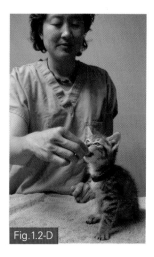

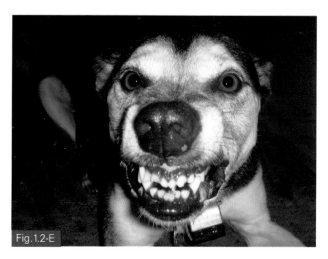

Fig.1.2-D: This kitten is both domesticated and tame.

Fig.1.2-E: Note that in scientific terms, tame is not synonymous with friendly or non-aggressive. This dog is both domesticated and tame, but she is aggressive to people who approach her when she's eating.

1.3 How Domestication Affects Tameness and Fear

Not surprisingly, domestication and tameness go hand-in-hand. To adapt to living in close proximity with humans, domesticated animals must be easier to tame and less emotionally reactive than their ancestral counterparts. If animals are in a constant state of fear because they view their environment as unsafe and the humans around them as threats or predators, then they are in a continuous state of high stress. The stress affects their immune systems, behavior and other physiologic functions (Price 2002)—for instance, their ability to mate and reproduce. This is one reason why non-domesticated species have difficulty breeding in zoos compared with their domesticated counterparts.

So how does domestication specifically affect tameness and an individual's ability to live with humans? A study by Dimitri Belyaev and his colleagues at the Institute of Cytology and Genetics at Novosibirsk, Siberia, sought answers to this question (Trut 1999). Researchers involved in the 40-year study started with commercial farm foxes and selectively bred them solely for tameness, to see if they could get a population that was as tame as the domesticated dog. All fox puppies were raised in the same manner, and the researchers scored them for tameness when they reached 7 to 8 months of age. In each generation, only the tamest were allowed to breed. The first generation of foxes was tamer than their parents but still fearful and dangerous to handle. By the 20th generation, 35% were tame. And by the 35th generation, 80% of the fox population was docile and eager to establish human contact. (Figure 1.3-A) These foxes whimpered to attract human attention, licked the experimenters' faces and even fought among themselves for access to the experimenters.

Overall, the domesticated foxes were tamer, less aggressive and less reactive to stressful stimuli. In addition, behaviorally and physiologically, they were paedomorphic or neotenous (they tended to retain juvenile traits). They had shorter skulls, many had floppy ears like those of puppies, and they behaved more like puppies. Canid pups generally bark and vocalize more than adults. They also more readily investigate new objects and individuals and form social bonds with unfamiliar individuals, even of different species. Similarly, the domesticated foxes readily sought attention from and bonded to the experimenters, despite relatively little handling and the fact that the experimenters were a different species. When tested in group enclosures, they competed for attention by snarling fiercely at each other. Even ones that escaped for several days eventually returned on their own.

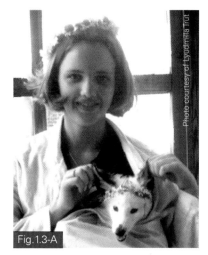

Fig.1.3-A: This domesticated fox resulted from generations of selection for tameness.

In addition to the overall tameness that selection for the trait brought, this population of fox puppies developed an expanded window for forming social bonds. Their eyes and ears opened several days earlier than their wild counterparts, marking the beginning of the sensitive period for social bonding. Their baseline corticosteroid levels, which presumably mark the closing of the sensitive period, also rose months later than those of the wild foxes. Having an expanded window for forming social bonds provides more time for them to bond with humans and other animal species living with humans, and to habituate to the odd objects, sounds and sights associated with human civilization. In the domesticated foxes, this window was 9 weeks, compared with 6 weeks in their unselected counterparts. The expansion was due primarily to a delay in the development of the fear response that follows the sensitive period for socialization.

The changes in tameness level and timing of the fear period in Belyaev's foxes correlated with differences in hormone and neurotransmitter levels. The delay in development of the fear response was linked to lower levels of corticosteroids, which are stress hormones. The levels rose later and remained at a lower level in the farm foxes, so that by the thirtieth generation, the levels were approximately one-fourth that of the wild animals. Additionally, the adrenal glands, which produce corticosteroids, released lower levels of corticosteroids when the farm foxes were subjected to emotional stress. Serotonin, a neurotransmitter in the brain that inhibits aggressive behavior, was higher in the domesticated foxes than in the wild ones.

Overall, the selection for tameness resulted in a fox who was tamer, less aggressive and less reactive to stressful stimuli, as well as a fox who went through an expanded sensitive period for socialization. Consequently, domestication imparted a number of changes that enabled these foxes to adapt to living with humans.

While domestication generally increases the ability of animals to become tame, it does not extinguish the fear response. The fear response still remains as an important trait that helps keep animals safe from danger. As a result, fear is a major issue that anyone dealing professionally with pets must address because it can lead to aggression and unruly behavior. But to deal effectively with fear day to day and remain safe, one first has to recognize it.

1.4 Recognizing Fear in Dogs

Fearful animals can have one of three responses: fleeing, freezing or fighting. Most people recognize overtly fearful dogs. (Figures 1.4-A and 1.4-B) These dogs adopt the same posture you would if you were walking on a soccer field and suddenly heard people yelling "heads up!" You would tense up, cover your head and duck down while leaning away from the possible threat. Simultaneously, you would turn your head away from the object to avoid being hit in the face, but you would probably still try to see where the ball was, so your eyes would look toward the object. A similar posture is shown by the dog in the photos below.

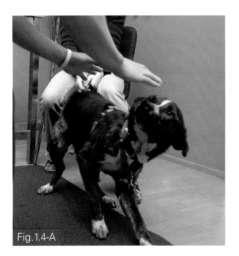
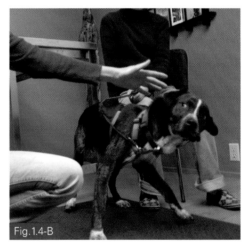

Fig.1.4-A

Fig.1.4-B

Fig.1.4-A, B: Fearful body posture: This dog is ducking to avoid being touched by a person. He is leaning away and cowering with his head and body low, and his entire body is tense. The dog's gaze is averted as if avoiding your eyes will keep you from seeing him, because a direct stare can be seen as a threat. His head is facing away from the person while his eyes are still trying to look in the direction of the hands. This causes the whites of his eyes to be exposed, a characteristic called "whale eye." His ears are also flat against his head and his tail is tucked under him. This pose is similar to one that you might take if you were trying to avoid getting hit by an object flying toward your head.

1.4.1a Dogs can show a cowering posture to different degrees.

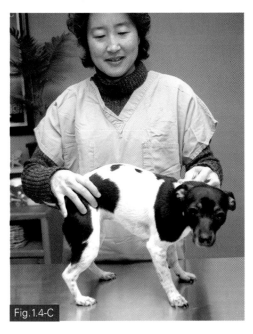

Fig.1.4-C: This dog is only cowering a little while standing. She is very tense though, which indicates nervousness.

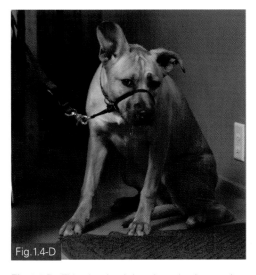

Fig.1.4-D: This dog is sitting, but she lowers her head as an unfamiliar person approaches.

Fearful vs. submissive posture.

Note that people sometimes incorrectly interpret a cowering posture as submissive and assume this behavior is good. They think it means the dog is telling them that he is willing to be subordinate to them. The cowering posture described above, however, occurs regardless of what's causing the fear. The cause could be another dog rushing up too quickly, a stranger looming over a shy dog, a sudden loud noise, a falling object or even the sight of something the dog is unfamiliar with, such as an umbrella. You'll learn in Chapter 2 that dominance and submission are established relationships between two or more individuals. Submissive postures are those intended to turn off aggression from other animals and signal that they will not fight. Submissive postures can be accompanied by muscle tension, trembling and other signs of fear if the potential for aggression is unknown or potentially harsh.

1.4.1b A furrowed brow and ears out to the sides or back are clues to the dog's emotional state.

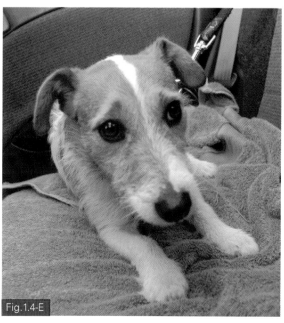

Fig.1.4-E

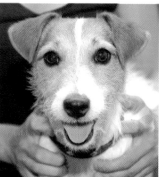

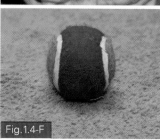

Fig.1.4-F

Fig.1.4-E: When scared, dogs hold their ears out to the side or back. But they can also hold their ears in these positions for other reasons. Do not rely on ears alone to determine the dog's state of mind. When they are fearful, their brows show varying degrees of furrowing. Here, my dog Jonesy is showing his fear of riding in cars.

Fig.1.4-F: When holding a ball in front of Jonesy, his ears perk forward.

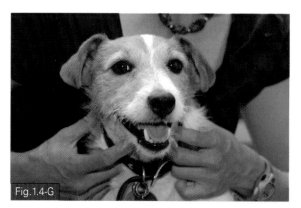

Fig.1.4-G

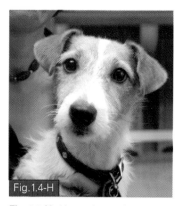

Fig.1.4-H

Fig.1.4-G: When he's enjoying being petted, as indicated by his rubbing against me, his ears go out and slightly back. Note that his brow is furrowed but he's not fearful. (Compared to Figure 1.4-E)

Fig.1.4-H: Here, Jonesy's ears are perked forward as he anticipates a treat.

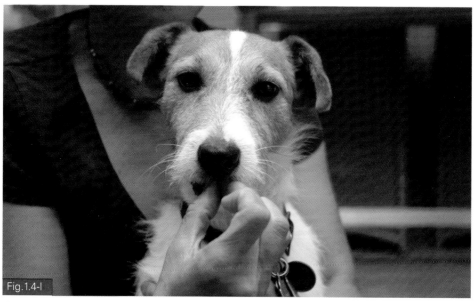

Fig.1.4-I: When he gets the treat and it's in his mouth or right in front of his nose, his ears go out slightly and back as his eyes try to focus on the tidbit near his nose. Note that his brow is not furrowed. (Compare again to Figure 1.4-E)

1.4.2 Dogs can also show more subtle behavioral indicators of fear and anxiety.

These are signs that owners and animal care professionals might miss early on. *(Videos 2 and 3)*

1.4.2a Hypervigilance.

Fearful dogs might glance in different directions frequently and for short periods in the same way that you might keep looking around for danger if you were caught walking alone in a bad neighborhood late at night and thought someone might be following you. Owners frequently think that their fearful dogs are just watching the scenery when they are actually scanning for danger. (Figures 1.4-J,K,L)

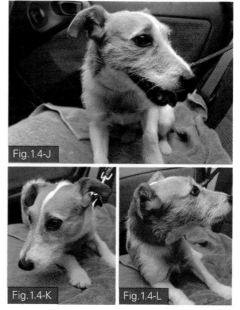

Fig.1.4-J, K, L: Jonesy is fearful of riding in cars even though he goes for rides 5 days a week and ends up in locations he enjoys. He's glancing around constantly, scanning for danger.

1.4.2b Lip-licking.

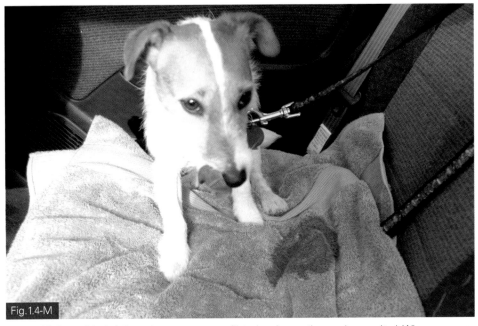

Fig.1.4-M: Dogs lick their lips when nervous, conflicted and sometimes when excited. When nervous, other signs of fear accompany the lip-licking.

1.4.2c Yawning and panting.

Anxious dogs yawn when they are not tired and pant when they are not hot or thirsty.

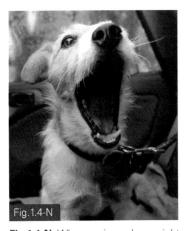

Fig.1.4-N: When anxious, dogs might yawn when they are not tired.

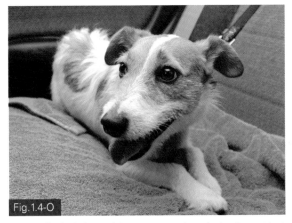

Fig.1.4-O: And they might pant even though they're not hot or thirsty.

1.4.2d Not eating.

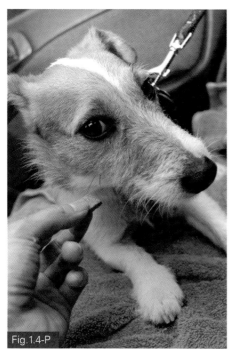

Fig.1.4-P

Fig.1.4-P: Dogs might stop eating when they are nervous or grab the food more aggressively.

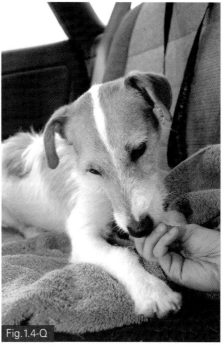

Fig.1.4-Q

Fig.1.4-Q: Now, several seconds later, Jonesy takes the treat that he refused earlier.

1.4.2e Salivating, urinating and defecating.

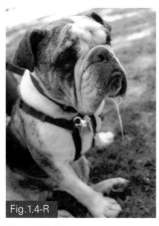

Fig.1.4-R

Fig.1.4-R: This dog is salivating in the absence of food.

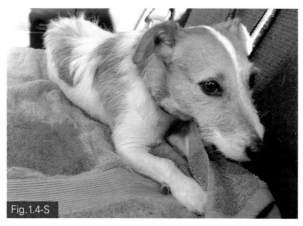

Fig.1.4-S

Fig.1.4-S: Urination and defecation might occur due to fear.

1.4.2f Acting sleepy.

One of the most important early signs of fear is that the dog acts sleepy or lethargic. Both of these dogs below have their eyes partially closed and are moving slowly. This tired demeanor can change from room to room or within seconds. When they are hypervigilant and moving in this lethargic manner, they appear to be looking around in slow motion.

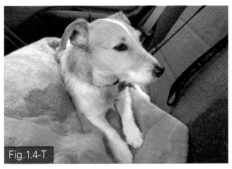

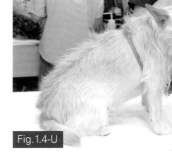

Fig.1.4-T: Jonesy looks sleepy.

Fig.1.4-U: This dog also appears to be sleepy.

1.4.2g Performing or responding to commands in a distracted manner.

When animals are fearful, they act distracted. Consequently, they may take longer to respond to commands that they perform quickly in a comfortable environment. In between commands they may look around (hypervigilance) or they may just move more slowly (acting sleepy). In any case, repeating the command in an increasingly angry or military tone may further increase their anxiety.

1.4.2h Offense is the best defense.

Dogs can easily learn that offense is their best defense and that they should attack when fearful, rather than flee or freeze—sometimes even before the object, person or dog has a chance to get close. (Figure 1.4-V) These dogs still show signs of anxiety and fear, such as averting their gaze, hiding and backing up. But the signs can be fleeting as they put up a strong front. They are likely to show clear signs of fear in other circumstances when out in public or at home, such that their owner characterizes their personality as fearful. *(Video 4)*

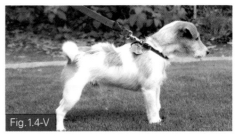

Fig.1.4-V: Jonesy adopts a highly aroused position when he sees objects—such as brooms—that startle and scare him. He's tense, leaning forward, tail and head held high, hackles up (piloerection). Ears are forward initially when the object is far enough away. As the object comes closer, he will show fear postures and back away.

Signs of Fear and Anxiety

- Cowering: head and body low, body leaning backward

- Muscles tense

- Trembling

- Head down, ears back or out to the sides and brows furrowed

- Panting, yawning, licking lips

- Salivation, urination, defecation

- Looks sleepy or moves in slow motion

- Performs commanded behaviors in a distracted manner

- Hypervigilant—scanning for danger

- Sweaty paws

- Shedding

- Shaking as if drying off from a bath

- Displacement behaviors such as itching when not pruritic, sniffing the ground when there are no new scents, looking distracted

1.5 What People Do to Worsen Fear and Elicit Aggression in Dogs

(Also refer to Chapters 8 and 9 in the text and on the DVD) *(Videos 5 and 6)*

Many humans can't understand why a dog would be afraid of them when they're obviously making friendly human gestures. If you look at it from a different perspective, however, the picture becomes clear. For instance, if you're afraid of spiders and your friend shoves a hairy tarantula in your face while reassuring you that it's friendly, would you feel safe? (Figures 1.5-A and 1.5-B)

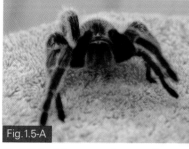

Fig.1.5-A: Many people are afraid of spiders and don't want to be near them even if they are harmless.

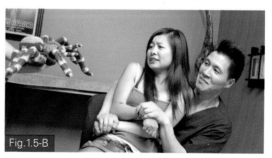

Fig.1.5-B: This woman is afraid of spiders, so she doesn't care whether a spider is friendly; she doesn't want it near her. In fact, she doesn't even like having a puppet spider near her face.

It's not likely you would want the spider near you. In fact, the only way you could get used to the spider is if you greeted it at your own pace. It would have to be on a table or in some other location where you could control your distance from it. Then, once you were ready, you could gradually approach for a closer look and even touch it. The same goes for dogs. If a dog is afraid of humans, he will not want humans approaching, staring at or otherwise directing their attention toward him.

1.5.1 Look at it from the dog's point of view.

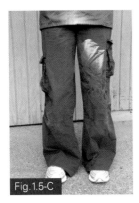 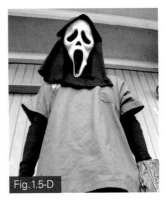 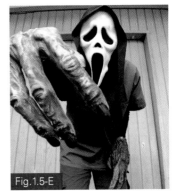

Fig.1.5-C: Fearful dogs may show minimal signs of fear when they are standing near you and they see primarily your legs.

Fig.1.5-D: But once they see your face staring down at them, you might suddenly look like a monster to them.

Fig.1.5-E: Avoid reaching for the dog. Reaching your hand out in what you consider a friendly gesture looks to the dog like you are reaching menacingly.

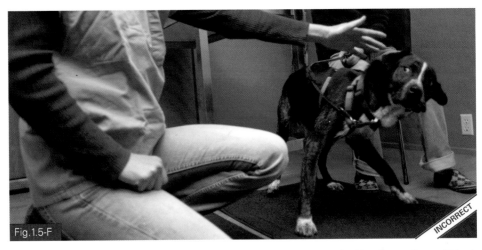

Fig.1.5-F, Incorrect: This dog backs away when the technician reaches for him. Some dogs will back away, others will bite. If you were afraid of spiders, you would not want one to reach out and try to touch you. You would prefer to approach at your own rate.

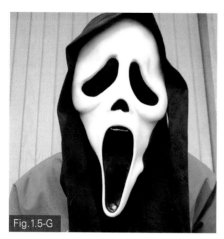

Fig.1.5-G

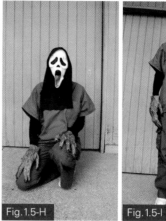

Fig.1.5-H

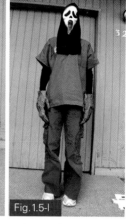

Fig.1.5-I

Fig.1.5-G: Avoid squatting close to the dog while facing him. Many people think you should get down to the dog's level. But if you do this while standing right next to the dog, suddenly your face is right in his face.

Fig.1.5-H, I: While it's true that you're less intimidating if you make yourself look small, to keep your face out of the dog's personal space, it is best to squat far away from the dog.

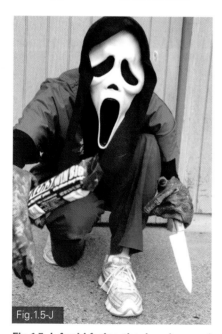

Fig.1.5-J

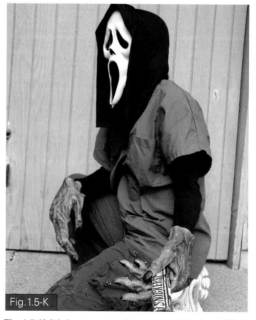

Fig.1.5-K

Fig.1.5-J: Avoid facing the dog. A general recommendation is that you countercondition the dog to your presence by offering treats. But if you do so by staring at the dog while reaching out with the treat, the dog may take the treat and then bite afterward. To the dog, you might be luring him in so that you can attack him.

Fig.1.5-K: It's best to stand or squat sideways. When giving treats to fearful dogs, just toss the treat while standing or kneeling sideways to the dog. Looking at and approaching the dog directly is threatening to him. Note that you may have to toss many treats in a row before the dog starts to trust you.
(refer to Chapter 14 to see examples)

1.5.2 Problems might occur after the initial greeting.

Often people manage to successfully get through the initial greeting with the fearful dog, but then they make a quick or inappropriate move that scares him into snapping or running away. This is again similar to the situation with the spider. Even when you're finally comfortable enough to examine and touch the tarantula, if it suddenly moves its mouthparts or waves one of its legs in the air, you might jump away out of fright. To you, these movements conjure images of the tarantula leaping and biting at you, whereas to the tarantula the movements are just a subconscious change in position or maybe even a signal of friendly intent.

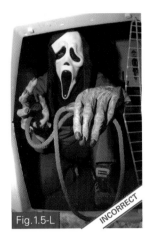

Fig.1.5-L

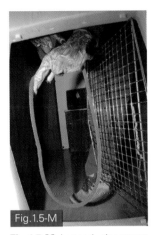

Fig.1.5-M

Fig.1.5-L, Incorrect: Avoid approaching head on. Facing the animal when he is cornered is especially threatening. It can cause dogs to attack.

Fig.1.5-M: Instead, place your body sideways and reach in. Or stand out of the way so that the dog sees primarily the leash and comes out on his own.

So the trick to ensuring that you don't frighten the dog even after the initial greeting is to gradually let him get used to you in different positions. Avoid leaning over him, reaching over his head or grabbing and hugging him, which makes him feel confined. Instead, move slowly and smoothly to give him a chance to back away. Most important, always be aware of the signals he's sending you with his body language.

1.5.3 What body language should you see?

The body language you'd like to see when greeting a dog is one that says this whole business is ho-hum, as when you're greeting a casual acquaintance. The dog should remain relaxed with his muscles loose rather than tense and stiff. His gaze should be steady and soft. His tail should either wag in a relaxed manner or hang loosely down, and he should never suddenly freeze. Beware of misinterpreting a tail wag. A wagging tail can be an indicator of high arousal or a dog in conflict regarding whether to approach or flee, rather than an indicator of a friendly, happy pet. In general, a wide, sweeping wag in a tail held somewhat even with the body is more likely to indicate that the dog is **friendly and relaxed.**

1.6 Recognizing Fear in Cats

As with dogs, cats who are fearful are tense. They make themselves small, lean back and lower their heads. The degree to which they do these things depends on how scared they are.

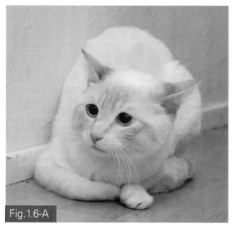 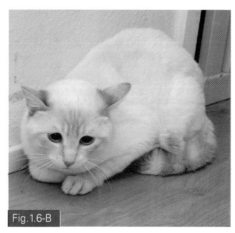

Fig.1.6-A, B: This cat is nervous in this environment, so she lies down against a wall and remains still. She may look relaxed and even sleepy at times. Often people mistakenly interpret this as a tired cat. Cats will also act hypervigilant when scared. Unlike dogs they may not glance quickly in different directions by moving their head. Rather, they tend to use their ears like a second pair of eyes. Their ears change direction frequently when they are being hypervigilant. And when they are agitated and losing patience, their tail starts to twitch.

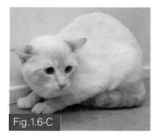 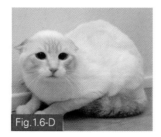 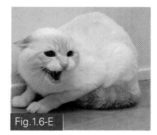

Fig.1.6-C, D, E: Here's the same cat, seen as a dog walks down the hall past her. As the dog approaches, she pulls herself into a smaller position, hugs the wall more and moves her ears down and then back. When the dog gets too close and she's unable to escape by running, she hisses (defensive aggression).

Cats can also make themselves look bigger when fearful.

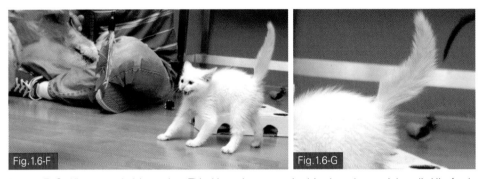

Fig.1.6-F, G: Kitten startled by a dog: This kitten has an arched back and a straight tail. His fur is piloerected along his back and his tail. His ears are back, he's leaning away and he's hissing.

1.7 What People Do to Worsen Fear and Elicit Aggression in Cats

(Also refer to Chapter 10)

In general all of the factors that worsen fear and elicit aggression in dogs do so in cats too. Thus take care to apply all the greeting principles for dogs to cats too. (Figure 1.7-A)

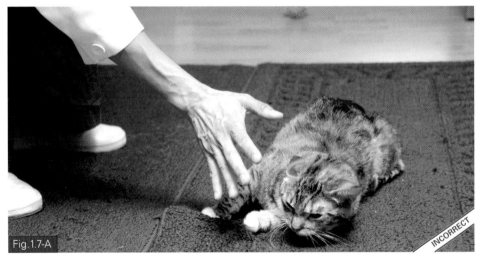

Fig.1.7-A, Incorrect: Avoid looming over, staring at and reaching for cats. This type of greeting can be as distressing to cats as it is to dogs. Also, avoid petting cats when their body posture indicates they do not find this comforting or rewarding. It's easy to accidentally greet and handle cats improperly because their fear response is often less obvious to the observer. In the early stages of fear cats tend to freeze silently or just walk away casually. But if these signs are missed and improper actions taken the cat may progress to a fractious, untreatable cat after multiple hospital visits.

TEST YOUR CANINE AND FELINE COMMON SENSE

Understanding dogs and cats requires that you take the time to observe the pet's behavior. Once you do, you might find that you know more than you think. Can you answer these questions?

1. How do you know when a cat or dog enjoys being petted?

2. Children who own friendly dogs are probably more likely to be bitten by their friend's dogs or unfamiliar dogs than those who don't own dogs. Do you know why?

3. How do you know when your cat or dog doesn't want to be petted?

4. Young boys are by far the most likely group of people to be bitten by dogs. Based on what you know about young boys and dogs, can you guess why?

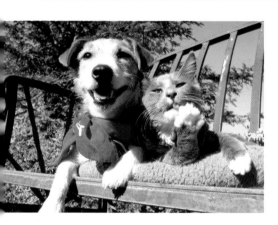

Answers:

1. He approaches you with a relaxed body posture. He might rub or lean against you. When you pet him, he stays relaxed and wags his tail. Or he raises his head so that it meets your hand. When you stop, he may rub against you again to solicit petting or push his head against your petting hand.

2. These children think all dogs are happy to see people. So they treat other dogs the way they treat their family dog, instead of greeting the unfamiliar dog politely and respecting his space.

3. He either doesn't respond to your petting or stiffens his body, or he walks away or shows a body posture indicating fear (ears back, leaning away). If these postures have no effect, he might growl or snap or hiss or bite. Cats often show a tail twitch.

4. As a group, young boys are loud, move quickly and tend to ignore the dog's signals. Often these kids also play games that trigger the dog to bite, such as rough-housing with the dog or jumping toward and away from dogs who are tied. (In fact, this is how you'd train a protection dog to bite.)

References

Adams, G.J., and W.T. Clark. 1989. The prevalence of behavioural problems in domestic dogs; a survey of 105 dog owners. *Australian Veterinary Practitioner* 19:135-37.

American Association of Feline Practitioners. 2004. *Feline Behavior Guidelines from the American Association of Feline Practitioners.* Feline_Behavior_Guidelines.pdf, http://www.aafponline.org/resources/guidelines/ (accessed June 1, 2008).

Campbell, W.E. 1986. The prevalence of behavioral problems in American dogs. *Modern Veterinary Practice* 67:28-31.

Denenberg, S., G. Landsberg, D. Horwitz, and K. Seksel. 2005. A comparison of cases referred to behaviorists in three different countries. In *Current issues and research in veterinary behavioral medicine: Papers presented at the 5th International Veterinary Behavior Meeting,* ed. D. Mills, E. Levine, G. Landsberg, D. Horwitz, M. Duxbury, P. Mertens, K. Meyer, L. Radosta Huntley, M. Reich, and J. Willard. 56-62. West Lafayette, Ind.: Purdue Univ. Press.

Freedman, D.G., J.A. King, and O. Elliot. 1961. Critical periods in the social development of dogs. *Science* 158:1645-1652.

Klinghammer, E., and P.A. Goodmann. 1985. *The management and socialization of captive wolves at Wolf Park.* Battle Ground, Ind.: North American Wildlife Park Foundation, Inc.

Price, E.O. 1984. Behavioral aspects of animal domestication. *The Quarterly Review of Biology* 59:1-32.

Price, E.O. 1999. Behavioral development in animals undergoing domestication. *Applied Animal Behaviour Science* 65:245-71.

Price, E.O. 2002. *Animal Domestication and Behavior.* New York: CABI Publishing.

Salman, M.D., J.C. New, P.H. Kass, and J.M. Scarlett. 2000. Behavioral reasons for relinquishment of dogs and cats to 12 shelters. *Journal of Applied Animal Welfare Science 3* (2):93-106.

Scott, J.P. 1958. Critical periods in the development of social behavior in puppies. *Psychosomatic Medicine* 20:42-54.

Scott, J.P., E. Fredericson, and J.L. Fuller. 1951. Experimental exploration of the critical period hypothesis. *Personality* 1:162-83.

Scott J.P., and J.L. Fuller. 1965. *Genetics and the social behavior of the dog.* Chicago: Univ. of Chicago Press.

Scott, J.P., and M. Marston. 1950. Critical periods affecting the development of normal and mal-adjustive social behavior in puppies. *Pedagogical Seminary and the Journal of Genetic Psychology* 77:25-60.

Serpell, J., and J.A. Jagoe. 1995. Early experience and the development of behavior. In *The domestic dog: Its evolution, behavior and interactions with people,* ed. J. Serpell. 80-102. Cambridge: Cambridge Univ. Press.

Trut, L.N. 1999. Early canid domestication: the farm-fox experiment. *American Scientist* 87:1959-97.

Vacalopoulos, A., and R.K. Anderson. 1993. Canine behavior problems reported by clients in a study of veterinary hospitals. *Applied Animal Behaviour Science* 37(1):84 (abstract only).

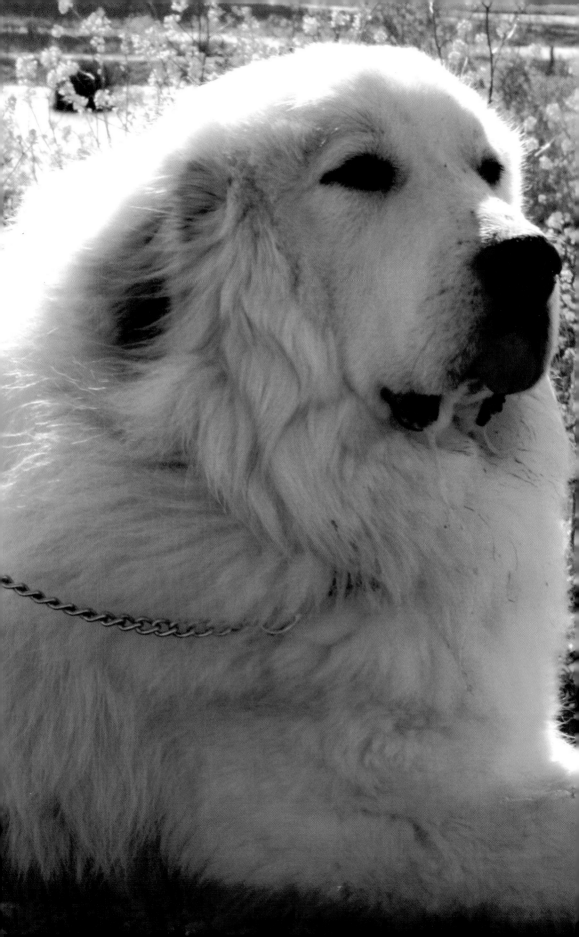

CHAPTER 2.
DOMINANCE
vs. Unruly Behavior

"We adopted Berkeley, a male Basenji, a few weeks ago from breed rescue," explains the concerned woman on the phone. "Since then we've noticed that he growls and barks at women and girls. He is usually good with me and has bonded well with my husband," she continues. "But sometimes he gets snarly and growls at me when I'm near him. The other night we had an incident. I got out of bed in the middle of the night, and when I approached the bed to get back in, he growled at me. I did what my friend told me, which was to grab him, put him on his back, put my face up to his and growl back at him. He bit me in the face. I had to go to the hospital to get stitches."

We have all heard advice that relates dog behavior to wolf behavior in the wild. "The alpha wolf always eats first; therefore you should always eat first so your dog knows you're the leader." "Always go through the door first because an alpha would go out ahead." "If your dog growls or barks inappropriately or otherwise misbehaves, put him in his place by doing an alpha roll, where you force him onto his back until he submits. This is what the alpha wolf does to his subordinates, and it's what you should do so your dog knows you're the boss."

But are these statements true, and should they be used with all dogs?

Virtually every veterinary behaviorist, applied animal behaviorist and animal trainer agrees: The solution to better behavior in pets involves teaching the animal that the humans handling her are predictable and trustworthy—in essence, good leaders. But does learning to lead mean you have to dominate the animal or mimic what you think wolves do in the wild? In the case of Berkeley, who turned out to have fear-related aggression toward women, the results were dangerous.

About 20 to 30 years ago, social dominance theory and ideas about wolf behavior in the wild were the primary models that guided how dogs were trained. Similar ideas prevailed in dealing with horses and other companion animals, too. For dogs, training focused on punishing bad behavior by using choke chains, pinch collars and electronic collars, because in the wild wolves were seen to gain higher rank through force. In horses, other devices such as stud chains are used in a similar manner.

Since then, our understanding of dog behavior in relation to wolf behavior, as well as our understanding of dominance and hierarchies in wild animals, has become clearer. Furthermore, the science of learning has provided a better understanding of why animals behave as they do and how their behaviors can be modified. Regardless of this new information, the old misinformation regarding dominance and wolf behavior and its applications to dogs abounds. To understand where dominance theory fits in with our updated knowledge of behavior and behavior modification, and to realize which behaviors it does and does not explain in our companion animals, one first has to have a good working knowledge of dominance theory.

2.1 Dominance Is a Relationship Between Two or More Individuals

While people commonly describe dominance as a trait of an animal, it is not a personality trait. Dominance is a relationship between individuals that is established by force, aggression and submission in order to determine who has priority access to multiple resources, such as food, preferred resting spots, or mates (Bernstein 1981; Drews 1993).

For instance, when bulls are introduced to one another, they immediately fight to establish rank. The highest ranked bull is the one who wins the encounters with all the other bulls, causing them to move away (Bouissou 1972). The highest ranked bull will then have priority access to females during mating season, food, and resting and grazing areas. (Figure 2.1-A) During mating season, the others will defer or move away from females in estrus if

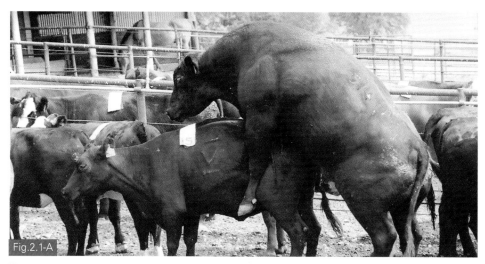

Fig.2.1-A: The highest ranking bull in a multi-male group has priority access to females during mating season.

Dominance is not a personality trait. Dominance is a relationship between individuals that is established by force, aggression and submission in order to determine who has priority access to multiple resources, such as food, preferred resting spots, or mates (Bernstein 1981; Drews 1993).

a higher ranked bull is near or approaching. They will, however, still attempt to sneak copulations with the estrus females when higher ranked males are not close enough to prevent such matings. As a result, in a pasture of several males and many females, the offspring will be sired by more than one bull, but the highest ranked bull will have the most matings.

Similarly, the dominant bull might chase subordinates away from a particular food source, or the subordinates might just defer automatically. But the subordinates might also sneak back to the food source when the dominant individual is not available to guard the resource. They might also be able to feed near the dominant bull if there's a barrier through which the dominant bull cannot easily reach the subordinates while they eat (Bouissou 1970, cited in Price 2002). In both cases, the subordinates are not trying to challenge the dominant bull for higher rank; they are simply using an alternate strategy for mating and obtaining other resources.

This is the general manner in which hierarchies work in animals who live in groups, including the relative of the domestic dog, the wolf. In wild wolf packs consisting of family units and in captive-raised wolf packs consisting of mixed individuals, the highest ranked—or alpha—female and male are generally the only pair who mates. The entire pack cooperates to help raise the offspring. The one mating pair per pack does not occur democratically; rather, both the alpha male and alpha female guard their mate from copulating with subordinates, and they also prevent subordinates from mating with one another. Overall, as with other wild group-living animals, wolves fight to establish higher rank so that they can have increased access to valuable resources, including mating opportunities. As long as they are present to guard the resource, they have priority access, but others can use alternate strategies for gaining resources.

2.2 Behavioral and Physical Traits Can Affect Dominance Rank

Unlike a personality, which by definition is a set of behavioral characteristics that stays the same across different contexts (Capitanio 1999), rank changes depending on the group to which an animal belongs. If four individuals who are dominant in their own social groups are all placed together, only one will be dominant in the new group (Capitanio, written communication 2008). Certain personality traits and physical traits do, however, improve the chances that an individual can attain higher rank within a group. In some cases, the characteristic advantages have to do with size and weaponry. For instance, numerous studies have found that in species that generally fight upon introduction—such as mice, cattle and pigs (Martinez et al. 1998; Barnett et al. 1993; Bouissou 1972)—the larger individual has the advantage and often becomes dominant over the smaller individuals (Bouissou 1972; Rushen 1988). (Figure 2.2-A)

Similarly, multiple physical factors can interact to affect dominance rank. For instance, a study in Friesian heifers (young cows who have not yet calved) looked at groupings of four newly introduced heifers. In each grouping there was one large heifer with horns, one small heifer with horns, one large heifer without horns and one small heifer without horns. All spontaneous interactions were recorded and the winners of each aggressive interaction noted. Not surprisingly, the large heifers

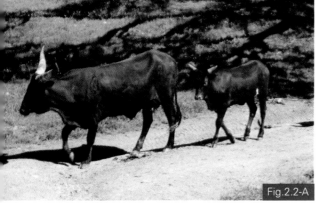

Fig.2.2-A: Factors such as size and weaponry influence an individual's ability to attain a high rank in a social group.

with horns tended to rank as number 1. The small heifers with horns and the large heifers without horns ranked similarly. The small heifers without horns ranked the lowest. The study showed that both size and weaponry interacted to give heifers the most advantage. A second experiment looked at heifers introduced in pairs to parse out the importance of horns versus size. The researchers found that when a large heifer with no horns was paired with a small heifer with horns, the heifers with horns gained higher rank 75% of the time. These results indicate that in cattle, both size and weaponry are important, but weapons are more important than size in successfully establishing higher rank.

Behavior can also affect dominance rank. In one study comparing aggression in different breeds of bulls, the bulls were introduced in groups of three (Wagnon et al. 1966). Each grouping consisted of one Hereford, one Shorthorn and one Angus bull. Despite their smaller size, the Angus bulls achieved the highest rank most of the time because they were the most aggressive. Being aggressive does not necessarily mean a higher rank, though. In the group-living song birds called great tits, more aggressive birds tend to attain higher rank when paired with an unfamiliar individual. When placed in a group, however, they don't always rank near the top. In fact, they might rank near the bottom because when they lose a fight, they tend to take longer to recover.

Social environment also plays a role in determining rank for some species. For instance, Capitanio (1985) reported that the rank a macaque monkey achieves when paired with one individual does not necessarily predict her ranking in a group with the same individuals. In Capitanio's study, he tested two groups of monkeys. Group 1 consisted of individuals artificially reared with an inanimate companion—a hobbyhorse (HH). Group 2 consisted of individuals artificially reared with a dog companion. Each individual of the HH group was paired with each of the other individuals in the HH group and a ranking of 1-6 was determined. Then all the HH macaques were placed into one large group and the ranks determined. The researchers found that each individual retained the same ranking. When the same procedure was performed with the six macaques raised by dogs, the results were different. The ranking determined by pairing all combinations of two individuals was different from the ranking when all six were placed in one big group. In both cases the hierarchy was stable, but the dog-raised macaques were able to develop alliances with other macaques and these alliances affected their group rankings. Thus, social behaviors other than aggression can influence rank in some species.

2.3 How the Dominance-Submissive Relationship Is Maintained

It is important to realize that an actual dominance-submissive relationship only exists when one individual consistently submits. Once a dominance-submissive relationship is established, it is reinforced through warning postures and ritualistic aggressive and submissive displays rather than full-blown fighting, although the ritualistic displays can be quite aggressive. The most stable relationships are those in which the submissive individual automatically defers to the dominant individual in the absence of any threatening postures by the dominant animal. For instance, the higher-ranked individual approaches a preferred resting spot directly and the subordinate moves away. Or the dominant individual approaches the subordinate to walk by and the subordinate averts his gaze.

Once a ranking is established, affiliative bonds can be forged among individuals in a group through non-aggressive gestures such as mutual grooming. (Figures 2.3-A and 2.3-B) This is one way that alliances are born. In less stable relationships or in those in which the dominant individual has an aggressive personality or is not confident about her ability to maintain higher rank, continued robust aggressive displays occur. The dominant animal might run across an enclosure to guard even low-value resources from the subordinate animal, or she might show prolonged displays of aggression that regularly incite a fear response from the subordinate.

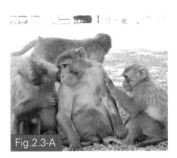 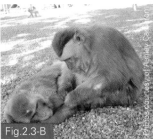

Fig.2.3-A, B: In the macaque social system, alliances are important for establishing and maintaining rank. Affiliative bonds can be forged among individuals in a group through non-aggressive gestures such as mutual grooming.

2.4 Dominance-Submissive Relationships Are Different Between Dogs and Wolves

(Video 1)

2.4.1 Dominance-submissive relationships do exist among some household pets.

With many of our household pets, including dogs and cats, dominance-submissive relationships between individuals may exist. But hierarchies are not necessarily linear, individuals can share similar ranks and clear hierarchies may not always exist. In some households, certain individuals clearly have priority access to resources and might use aggression to establish this priority. For instance, my 16-year-old female Australian Cattle Dog, Zoe, claims first access to food, sleeping areas and my attention. If these resources are available and she wants them, she will guard them from my lower-ranked dog, Jonesy, a 2-year-old male Jack Russell Terrier. (Figures 2.4-A,B,C) Sometimes she guards subtly with just a glance, and other times more aggressively with bared teeth and a snap or lunge. Jonesy always defers to her. But he will sneak around her to get to his destination or steal a food item when she's not looking. These resources are only an issue when Zoe wants them enough or has the ability to guard them from Jonesy. So, for instance, she rarely guards or takes his toys because she doesn't like to play with them. And when food or a stuffed Kong toy are already in Jonesy's possession, she lets him keep it, although she occasionally looms over him until he gives it up. In addition, we frequently have canine guests who stay for several days to several weeks. Zoe invariably establishes her top position regarding valued resources, whereas Jonesy and the guest usually share the same rank. That is, they share toys or steal toys and food equally.

2.4.2 Dogs have a tempered drive to attain high rank, compared with wolves.

So what's different about wolf and dog hierarchies? One difference is that dogs have a tempered drive to gain high rank, compared with the average wolf. At Wolf Park, where unrelated wolves live in small packs in captivity, researchers have noted that status is often gained opportunistically. Consequently, whereas dogs tend to show clear signs—or posturing—that they are vying for higher status, signs of imminent attacks in wolves are often subtle or even absent. Each interaction between wolves is a way for one wolf to test the other for weakness. As a result, the lowest-ranked wolf in the pack might attack the alpha wolf during play if he detects the alpha wolf is ill or weak. Thus, the lowest-ranked wolf could opportunistically attain the alpha position (Yin 2004; Klinghammer E., personal communication 1999). Wolf hierarchies and those of other wild animals, such as macaques, are so competitive that when an individual is removed from the group for as little as several hours to one day, he or she may have to reestablish rank upon reintroduction (Goodman P., written communication 2008). Dogs are generally much more relaxed about rank. They can easily be away from their group for weeks to months and then re-enter seamlessly.

It's not surprising that wolves have a more rigid ranking system and a greater desire to achieve dominance. In the wild, where wolf packs most often consist of parents and their offspring from one or more generations (although they can contain unrelated wolves), and in wolf packs raised in captivity (where wolves may or may not be related), generally only the highest ranking male and female mate and other group members help support the puppies. Note that

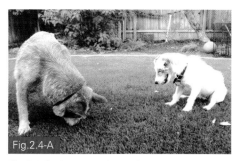

Fig.2.4-A: Jonesy waits patiently as Zoe searches for kibble that was tossed in the grass.

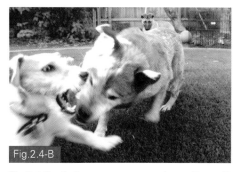

Fig.2.4-B: If Jonesy gets too close, Zoe will snap at him. Even though Jonesy always backs away, in situations where he has to dive away quickly, Jonesy barks and growls defensively while making his escape.

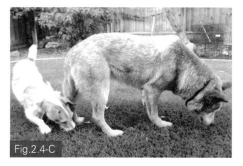

Fig.2.4-C: Jonesy still sneaks behind Zoe and steals food when she's not looking. By doing so, he is not testing his rank; rather, he's using an alternate strategy for obtaining treats.

because packs are generally comprised of parents and their offspring rather than competing individuals, wolf biologists rarely use the term "alpha" to describe the pack leaders (Mech 1999; Mech 2008). Dogs, on the other hand, often breed promiscuously; multiple females breed with multiple males. In fact, a study of feral dogs in Italy found that all the females reproduced, allowing the group to meet its full potential for population increase. No attempts were made by adult dogs to control the reproduction of other dogs (Boitani et al. 1995). Consequently, rank in dogs might not have as much of an effect on the individual's ability to pass on his or her genes.

This difference in social systems and the related differences in drive for high rank are most likely due in part to the process through which they evolved. Contrary to popular belief, dogs probably evolved through a process of self-domestication as scavengers, rather than as hunters, over the last 15,000 years (Coppinger and Coppinger 2002). (Figure 2.4-D) According to this theory of self-domestication, people moving into settlements accumulated trash around their living areas and in dumps. Wolves with low flight distances scavenged in the trash sites and weren't scared away when people approached, while those with greater flight distances fled when people approached from as far as a mile away. The ancestral wolves who had lower flight distances were able to survive and reproduce better in environments near humans than were other wolves. Over many generations, they changed genetically into a separate population that

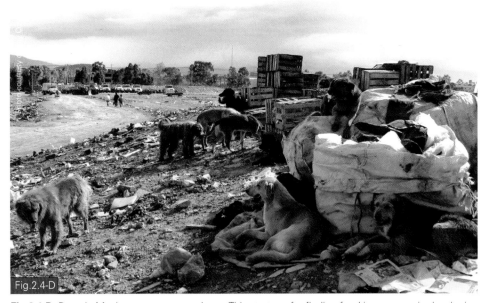

Fig.2.4-D: Dogs in Mexico scavenge at a dump. This strategy for finding food is common in developing countries where dogs typically survive by scavenging rather than hunting. Most of these dogs lived in people's houses at night and roamed the city during the day, so most were free-roaming dogs rather than feral dogs living without direct contact and direct feeding or sheltering by humans (Boitani et al. 1995). The phographer, Dr. Ray Coppinger, stated that although these dogs were owned by humans, they would not allow him to to pet them.

was easier to tame and could more easily live in close proximity to humans. As scavengers living off humans, they did not need to live in cohesive packs. Thus, unlike wolves, feral domestic dogs do not live in tightly knit family units that cooperate to hunt, rear young and protect communal territory—three factors that define canid packs (Mech 1970 cited in Boitani 1995). Rather, they live in what one might more appropriately call groups (Boitani 1995), with group size dependent on ecologic conditions. In some conditions, dogs often spend much time alone rather than with other group members (MacDonald and Carr 1995). The primary benefit of living in a group seems to be increased ability to defend a territory or resource, since feral dogs sometimes have to compete with wolves or other scavengers for food. Dogs also accept others into their group more willingly than do wolves.

A lower drive to attain high rank, compared to wolves, is also seen in the way dogs greet new individuals. For wild animals like wolves and many primates, the appearance of new individuals is generally seen as a threat. It is the norm for these animals to fight upon first greeting. While ritualistic posturing might be displayed during greetings and can decrease the likelihood of full-on fighting, aggression and injuries do occur. The aggression and posturing continues until a dominant–subordinate relationship is established.

Unlike wolves, socialized dogs are more likely to be friendly upon greeting. Just as humans greet with a handshake and an interest in getting to know each other, rather than an interest in attaining high rank, dogs typically greet just to determine whether the other individual will be friendly and playful. In fact, we want our dogs to be friendly with all other dogs so they can play at dog parks and get along in our human-based society. The domestic dog's sociability toward other dogs is likely due in part to neoteny, the retention of puppy-like traits. Like the foxes in the farm fox study (Chapter 1) that were bred solely for tameness and retained their juvenile physiological and behavioral traits, domesticated dogs also appear to be neotenous. They readily investigate new objects and form social bonds with unfamiliar individuals, even from other species, in the absence of specific taming techniques.

2.4.3 Dogs have a less ritualized communication system.

Along with a less rigid hierarchy and dominance-submissive relationships, dogs also have a less ritualized communication system. Wolves regularly display their status through ritualized postures and greetings. The alpha wolves are easy to recognize because they greet with head high and tail raised. Subordinates routinely approach the alpha wolves in a submissive manner—crouching with tail low, licking lips and rolling over to expose the belly (submissive roll). Note that the high-ranked wolves do not throw the subordinates into a roll; rather, the subordinates offer the submissive roll as a sign of their deference in the same way one might kneel or curtsy when greeting royalty. (Figure 2.4-E)

In contrast to wolves, dogs with established relationships do not routinely greet each other every morning in a manner that displays their rank. (Figures 2.4-F and 2.4-G) Additionally, the postures dogs are able to show vary somewhat by breed. Paedomorphic breeds (those resembling more juvenile stages of wolf development) like the Cavalier

King Charles Spaniel have a smaller communicative repertoire than breeds that more physically resemble the adult wolf (Goodwin et al. 1997).

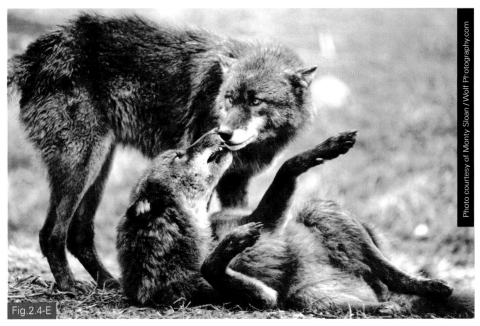

Fig.2.4-E: Wolves greeting: When wolves greet, subordinates exhibit submissive displays while the dominant wolves take a different stance. This reinforces their positions.

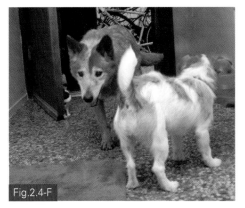
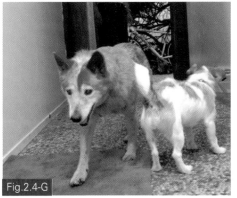

Fig.2.4-F, G: Dogs greeting: These two dogs live together. The Australian Cattle Dog is higher ranked. They barely acknowledge one another when they see each other first thing in the morning or during other reunions, such as here where Zoe arrives home.

For aggression to be defined as due to dominance, it must occur over multiple types of resources such as food, resting spots and attention from other individuals, and the aggressive animal should show signs of confidence rather then postures indicating conflict or fear. If an animal shows aggression only over items in one class, such as multiple food-like items or multiple toy-like objects, then the aggression is termed food-possession aggression or toy-possession aggression and is not related to rank.

2.5 How Dominance Theory Relates to Interactions Between Humans and Animals

While in some cases humans have problems with their pets because their pets are using aggression to guard multiple types of resources, in most cases our problem is that the pets are just unruly or misbehaving. For instance, dogs jumping on people are not vying for higher rank; they are simply jumping because they want attention and they often get it by doing so. When dogs jump on counters to steal food or cats jump up to investigate when you're not in sight, despite having been punished previously when you are present, they are using an alternate strategy for obtaining food and getting the chance to investigate. Their strategy is rewarded because they often do get the food and do get to investigate, at least for a short period. These unruly behaviors occur not because the animals are vying for rank but because the behaviors have been rewarded in the past. As such, a dominance-submission model is irrelevant for most of the behaviors we want our animals to perform, such as coming when called, walking calmly on leash or not jumping for attention.

2.5.1 Unruly behavior can lead to aggression.

Behavior does not have to be motivated by anger or aggressive intentions to lead to aggression. Frequently, normal puppy and adolescent behaviors that are rewarded can develop into aggression. For instance, puppies who are inadvertently rewarded with attention and play for nipping can turn into adult dogs who grab and bite when excited. In fact, because arousal and aggression are on a continuum, any overly aroused behaviors, such as lunging or barking, when rewarded enough in some dogs, can escalate to aggression. *(Video 2)*

2.6 Problems With Dominance Theory and the Use of Force

Even in the case of dominance-aggression or other situations where you think force can yield faster results, using force to address issues comes with many problems and unintended adverse effects (Yin 2004; AVSAB 2007). Just as you shouldn't administer a potent immuno-suppressive drug without informing the owners of the potentially fatal side-effects, force should not be used unless the veterinarian, behaviorist or trainer articulates the potential negative effects to the owner. It's also imperative that the person recommending the techniques has a plan of action in case adverse effects are seen. The American Veterinary Society of Animal Behavior (2007) feels so strongly about this that it states in its position statement and guidelines on the use of punishment that, "The standard of care for veterinarians specializing in behavior is that punishment [force or aversives] is not used as a first-line or early-use treatment for behavior problems" (AVSAB 2007). They also recommend that dominance theory not be used in most cases of companion animal problems (AVSAB in press). Some adverse effects of punishment are described below.

> "The standard of care for veterinarians specializing in behavior is that punishment is not used as a first-line or early-use treatment for behavior problems" (AVSAB Position Statement on Punishment, 2007).

2.6.1 Punishment must be strong enough to be effective.

First, the force or punishment (terms used synonymously here; see Chapter 5 for the scientific definitions of the terms) must be strong enough to suppress the behavior completely or else the animal will start performing the behavior more frequently again (Azrin 1960). One major mistake that owners make is starting with a level that's too low. As a result, one frequently must escalate the intensity to continue obtaining the same effect (Azrin et al. 1963). So the owner increases the intensity and the animal temporarily stops the behavior again. After a few punishments at this level, the pet becomes immune once more.

When starting with a level that's marginally low, you habituate the pet to the pain or lose the startle effect. (Figure 2.6-A) Often, you must keep escalating the intensity, until suddenly you're at a level that can be physically dangerous. For instance, electronic anti-bark collars can cause burn marks on dogs (AVSAB 2007). Choke chains can damage the trachea, increase intraocular pressure in dogs thus potentially worsening or contributing to glaucoma in susceptible breeds (Pauli et al. 2006), cause sudden collapse from non-cardiogenic pulmonary edema due to temporary upper airway obstruction (Drobatz et al. 1995) and cause nerve damage.

Even if you do achieve a high enough level of punishment, the effects might not last forever. Dominance rank is often short-lived in animal social groups. In wild animals, it typically lasts only several years or through one breeding season. This reign is relatively short

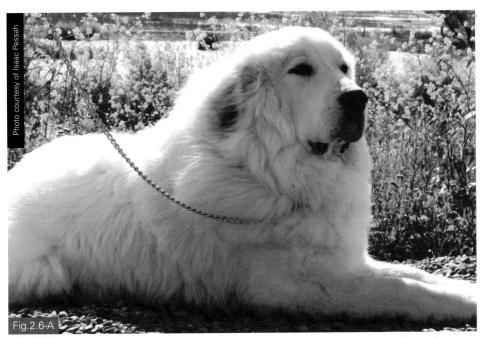

Photo courtesy of Isaac Pessah

Fig.2.6-A

Fig.2.6-A: I once tested a remote-controlled citronella collar on a chicken-chasing Great Pyrenees named Charlie. When Charlie ran up to the chicken coop in my yard and stared in, I set off the collar, which squirted a quick jet of unpleasant citrus-smelling spray past his nose. The first squirt startled him, causing him to shake his head and back off. Several seconds later, he went right back, which earned a second squirt. By the third squirt, the aversiveness was diminishing, and by the fourth or fifth, it no longer had any effect. When we trained the alternate behavior of having Charlie focus on his owner for treats, the dog learned within minutes to ignore the chickens, even when they were out of the coop.

because rank is repeatedly tested and can be maintained only as long as individuals are physically strong enough to win aggressive encounters. (Figure 2.6-B) Thus, depending on how well a human can continue to punish with enough force using this model and how aggressive the pet is, the human might not be able to retain rank. In a family, children and elderly individuals can rarely establish high rank through force.

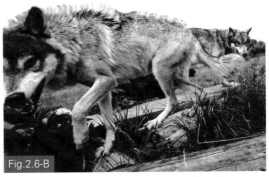

Fig.2.6-B

Fig.2.6-B: This young female wolf is growling at her mother. The tensions between the two had been mounting to the point where if one was not removed, it would likely eventually lead to a dominance fight.

2.6.2 The punishment could cause intense fear, which may generalize.

Another issue with punishment is that, while an appropriately high intensity or strong enough aversive can suppress behavior effectively, it can also cause the animal to become overly sensitive or fearful of the object, place or person associated with the aversive. This fear can then generalize to similar objects, contexts or people (Domjan 2003). (Figure 2.6-C)

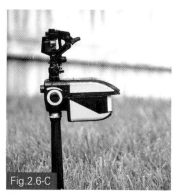

Fig.2.6-C

Fig.2.6-C: I tested a motion-activated sprinkler system called the Scarecrow, which is designed to keep unwanted animal intruders out of a designated area. When my dog Zoe walked within its range and it gave its characteristic "shwook-chuka-chuka" sound as it sprayed, she immediately ran inside to her crate and was so disturbed that she refused to go into the yard for several days, even for meals. Months later, she heard a similar sound in a different context and became so anxious that if she had been off leash, she would have run off and been unresponsive to my cues for her to come. Zoe is not usually scared by much, so I was surprised at her response to this product.

As a result of the two adverse effects just described, using punishment requires great skill and expertise in evaluating animals. To complicate matters, the evaluation must be based on the individual animal's perceptions, rather than our own. For instance, most people are likely to believe that prong collars and electronic collars are torturous, and citronella collars, spraying with water or scaring animals with a loud sound is always more humane. But it's the animal who decides which stimulus is more aversive. When I started training my dog Zoe years ago with the old training methods (see the Introduction for more details), I used a prong collar and a choke chain. She responded with no major lasting fearful behavior. When I trained her to come when called from long distances off leash using an electronic collar—set on a low pager or static level and turned off as soon as she started to come after being called—she was happy to come running right away. But when I tried the seemingly harmless burst of water, she suddenly developed an intense fear of similar sounds.

2.6.3 Punishment can cause aggression.

One dangerous side-effect is that punishment can cause aggression. This has been established since the 1960s based on studies with rats, cats, monkeys, hamsters and other animals as subjects (Azrin et al. 1968). When researchers applied a foot shock to animals, the animals attacked their cagemates aggressively. Pain-aggression reactions have been shown to occur in a wide variety of animals in response to many different aversive events. In fact, a recent study in dogs (Herron et al. 2008) found that confrontational techniques such as hitting or kicking the dog for undesirable behavior, growling at the dog, performing an "alpha roll," staring the dog down and enforcing a dominance down frequently elicited an aggressive response from the dog. The aggression can be redirected toward inanimate objects as well as other animals, including humans, and the punishment that incites it need not be physical. (Figure 2.6-D)

Note that because children and elderly people are the least likely to be able to execute punishment at a high enough level to suppress the behavior or with the correct timing, they are the most likely to be bitten when using force.

2.6.4 Punishment must occur while the animal is performing the undesirable behavior.

Timing is a challenge with all techniques, but it is particularly tough with those that involve punishment or aversives. One of the primary problems is that people tend to purposely use punishment long after the behavior has taken place, even though research has shown that punishment is not very effective when delayed (Camp et al. 1967). For instance, owners come home from work to find that their dog has raided the garbage can or chewed up the couch, and they lose their temper. While screaming in rage at their dog might make the owners feel better (positive

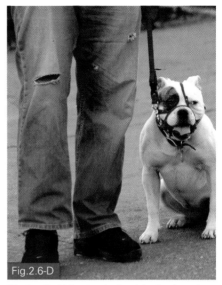

Fig.2.6-D

Fig.2.6-D: This dog is fearful of other dogs and barks at them. Her owners were told to use a choke chain correction and later a pinch collar correction when that didn't work. Then they escalated to the electronic collar. The dog became more aroused and redirected her aggression toward the owner, ripping holes in his pants.

reinforcement for them), thoughtful evaluation down the road often reveals that their rampage delivered the wrong message. If later they notice that the dog now slithers away or stays in bed instead of greeting them at the door, even when she hasn't created a mess, then the lesson she learned was that her owners are sometimes angry and out of control when they come home. Even if the dog slinks off only when there's an accident or overturned trashcan in the house, she still didn't get the message straight. Instead of learning that she shouldn't poop in the house or rummage through the rubbish, she may have just learned that poop is not permitted in the house or that trash on the floor is taboo. You can tell when she has the wrong idea because she'll crouch down fearfully or submissively, expecting punishment, even when she's not the culprit who created the mess. This incorrect learning can occur even when the delay in punishment is relatively short. Camp and his colleagues (1967) found that even a delay of 2 seconds is significantly less effective than punishment that occurs while the animal is performing the undesirable behavior. And a delay in punishment of 30 seconds is as ineffective as performing the punishment randomly with no relation to the undesirable behavior.

Punishment can still be difficult in cases where the owner plans to time the punishment correctly. Coordinating a physical punishment with enough speed to surprise the pet and enough force or intensity to get an effect is more difficult than just delivering a reward such as a treat.

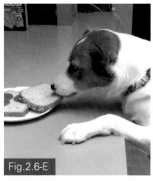

Fig.2.6-E

Fig.2.6-E: This dog chooses to steal food in spite of the fact that he has been reprimanded in the past. The immediate reward of eating the food outweighs the future possibility that someone may learn what has happened and punish him.

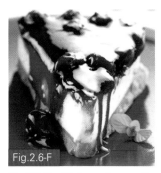

Fig.2.6-F

Fig.2.6-F: Dieters frequently splurge on desserts despite the high calorie count because the immediate reward outweighs the future possibility of gaining weight.

2.6.5 Immediate rewards may outweigh the future possibility of punishment.

Even when pets do understand what the punishment is for, the immediate rewards of doing something "bad" often outweigh the future possibility of punishment. (Figure 2.6-E) Indeed, in their punishment experiments Camp et al. (1967) found a decrease in suppression of undesirable behavior when punishment was delayed by 2 or 30 seconds. While poor suppression was due in part to the animals not linking the behavior to the consequence, Camp also surmised that the animals continued performing the punished behavior because with the delayed timing, they were unsure whether the punishment absolutely would occur. To understand, consider this. When people are dieting, they know to avoid copious amounts of high-calorie foods. However, because the foods taste so good, they eat them anyway to reap the immediate taste rewards. The reasoning is that it's not absolutely a given that these calories will make it to their thighs. Maybe the calories will get exercised off or the items are less fattening than they thought. However, if every time they ate desserts their thighs immediately ballooned before their eyes, they would no longer eat high-calorie desserts when on a diet. (Figure 2.6-F)

2.6.6 Punishment can strengthen the undesired behavior.

Another point that's more crucial with punishment than with other categories of learning (covered in later chapters) is that punishment must occur every time the animal performs the undesirable behavior. If the pet is only punished sometimes (on a variable schedule of punishment), she will also be receiving rewards sometimes (variable schedule of reinforcement). Rewards that occur on a variable schedule have the greatest strength. For instance, using the trash can example again, if your dog raids the garbage can, you could set up a booby trap by placing several mousetraps in the can and covering them with a light veil of trash. The next time she investigates the trash, the sudden loud snapping sounds scare her away. This punishment keeps the trashcans safe for a while, but several days later, she tries again. For the second time, the booby trap goes off just as planned. This time, she stays away for several days more. But because rubbish raiding has been so successful and fun in the past, she tries once more. This time the trash is unguarded by mousetraps, so her gamble pays off with a jackpot. While this one reinforcement for pilfering the trash might not seem like such a big deal, now the dog is suddenly on a variable schedule of reinforcement. The raiding has now turned into a more exciting game because, like the slot machines at a casino, the outcome or prize is less predictable.

2.6.7 Punishment can suppress some behaviors, thus masking the underlying emotional state.

Some people use punishment to decrease aggression, and it can work. However, it frequently only suppresses a pet's external warning signs, such as a growl or a raised lip, without addressing the underlying association or emotional state. The consequence later might be that instead of giving a warning, the dog suddenly bites.

2.6.8 Punishment can lead to a poor association and a poor bond.

When punished, the pet associates the punisher with unpleasant events and the bond between human and animal companion might weaken. Furthermore when punishment is a primary means for fixing behaviors, it can make the owner resentful of the pet and can cause owners to punish for prolonged periods. In fact in humans it's been reported that 70% of child abuse cases were attempts to discipline through the use of physical punishment that escalated out of control (Kadushin and Martin 1981). The proper way to use an aversive is to dole it out with no emotion and preferably use some form of remote-controlled aversive so it can be independent of any associations with the punisher.

2.6.9 Punishment fails to show the animal appropriate behavior.

Even when punishment is executed appropriately, it fails to show the animal what the desired behavior is. Without a replacement behavior, the animal could choose to perform the undesirable behavior in spite of the punishment. Additionally, punishment has been shown to be more effective when subjects are reinforced for an alternate appropriate behavior (Perry and Parke 1975).

2.7 Establishing Leadership and Modifying Behavior Without Force

If dominance theory is not a good model for understanding and modifying most behaviors in our pets, what is? Generally, what humans seek is the ability to influence their pets to willingly perform desirable behaviors (e.g., positive leadership), not dominance or merely control over resources. Maybe we want our pets to consistently come when called, or remain lying down across the room or pay attention to us on a walk rather than barking at a squirrel. Humans can choose to try to influence behavior through force, like a dictator or a bully. Or we can choose to gain leadership by rewarding desirable behavior.

According to foremost management theorist and professor Peter Drucker, consistency and predictability are key factors in leadership (Benowitz 2001). Influencing others through force is generally not recommended by management theorists for managing humans. It generates passive resistance, requires continual pressure by the manager and causes subordinates to disobey (Benowitz 2001). Similar effects are expected when force is used with pets. Instead, humans can gain influence, higher rank and priority access to resources without force by controlling all resources and using them as motivators for rewarding good behavior.

DEFINITIONS OF LEADERSHIP

In the fields of business management and sociology, leadership is a hot topic but a trait that is often ill-defined (Barker 1997, Kaiser et al. 2008). As a result, there are many different definitions.

Accepted definitions state that leadership is "the process of influencing activities of an individual or group to achieve a certain objective in a given situation" (Dubrin 1990 in Barker 1997) or "establishing direction and influencing others to follow that direction" (Benowitz 2001) or "exercising influence in a group of strangers or obtaining high status in a social system" (Kaiser et al. 2008). By these definitions, the influence or rank may be gained through coercion or through rewards. Other management theorists more specifically state that with leadership, followers must follow willingly (Knowles and Saxberg 1971, Kaiser et al. 2008).

When defined in the broader manner, different leadership styles such as "autocratic" and "participative" and "laissez-faire" may be described. The autocratic style in which the manager makes the decisions without allowing others to participate is most similar to a dominance-subordinate relationship in animals. This style of leadership is generally not recommended by management consultants and professors because it generates passive resistance, tends to require continual pressure and direction from the leader and is usually not a good tactic for getting the best performance from a team (Benowitz 2001). Additionally, those managers who rule through coercive power (the ability to punish) "most often generate resistance which may lead workers to deliberately avoid carrying out instructions or to disobey orders" (Benowitz 2001).

The method of withholding all resources from the pet and using them only to reward appropriate behaviors has been called Nothing in Life Is Free, No Free Lunch or the Learn to Earn Program, and there are various versions. All of them stress rewarding desirable behavior and removing the reward for bad behaviors. In one version (Yin 2004), the dog can first be taught to automatically sit and look at the owner for treats (kibble from her regular daily meals). That is, when the dog is hungry, the owner stands completely still with food hidden in his hand and just waits for the dog to sit—no verbal cue, no hand signal, no touching the dog—he just waits. Once the dog sits, the owner immediately gives her the treat. When the dog understands that she must choose on her own to sit in order to receive the treat that she wanted, she should be required to automatically sit and remain seated when she wants to be petted, go out the door or have her toy tossed, and for each kibble. By requiring this behavior, the dog is learning self control and to look to the owner for permission for access to a resource she wants. There

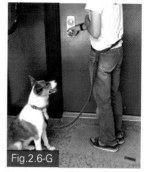

Fig.2.6-G

Fig.2.6-G: This dog has learned to automatically say please by sitting in order to earn the privilege of going out the door. This is part of the Learn to Earn Program for building leadership skills in the human member of the animal-human team.

is no battle of wills between dog and owner; the dog is just taught a new way to receive all of the resources that she used to get for free, and she's taught that inappropriate behaviors are not rewarded *(Video 3)*. Once the owner has decided on the rules, he must communicate the rules to the pet by reinforcing the correct behaviors immediately as they occur; i.e., within 1 second. He must also prevent the pet from receiving rewards for undesirable behaviors. For instance, when dogs want to be petted, they frequently jump on their owners instead of sitting calmly. If this happens, owners must clearly remove their attention by holding completely still, turning their head away or turning their back to the dog and then standing still. These behaviors make it clear to the dog that she is not receiving attention. But once the dog sits, the owner must immediately reward her and then continue intermittently rewarding as she is sitting so that the dog learns to remain seated.

Leadership is established when humans

1. set clear rules for behavior;

2. communicate the rules by rewarding correct behaviors as they are occurring or within one second;

3. consistently reward these desirable behaviors and remove rewards for undesirable behaviors until the pet develops good habits.

The rules must be reinforced consistently until they become a habit for the dog in all instances where sitting is required. If the owner pets the sitting dog and the dog starts to get up, the owner must immediately remove attention or he will unintentionally reward the dog for excited, uncontrolled behavior. If the owner later sits on the floor and allows the dog to climb into his lap without first automatically sitting and waiting for a cue, he is also rewarding uncontrolled behavior. The dog must earn attention by sitting calmly every time she wants it.

Leadership is established when the human sets clear rules for behavior and effectively communicates the rules by always rewarding the correct behaviors as they occur and preventing or immediately removing rewards for undesirable behaviors. The owner must reward the desired behaviors frequently enough that they become a habit. When owners can meet these three criteria, they will be seen as predictable, dependable and trustworthy in the eyes of their pet. Now, rather than complying out of fear, pets can choose to follow human direction because doing so leads to rewards. Such a model fosters a better understanding of the underlying cause of improper behavior and leads to a strong bond between animals and humans, rather than an antagonistic approach to living with animals.

References

American Veterinary Society of Animal Behavior. 2007. AVSAB Position Statement–Punishment Guidelines: *The use of punishment for dealing with animal behavior problems.* http://www.avsabonline.org/avsabonline/index.php?option=content&task=view&id=119 (accessed June 27, 2008).

American Veterinary Society of Animal Behavior. In press. AVSAB position statement: *The use of dominance theory for dealing with animal behavior problems.*

Azrin, N.H. 1960. Effects of punishment intensity during variable-interval reinforcement. *Journal of the Experimental Analysis of Behavior* 3:123-42.

Azrin, N.H., W.C. Holz, and D.F. Hake. 1963. Fixed-ratio punishment. *Journal of the Experimental Analysis of Behavior* 6:141-48.

Azrin, N.H., H.B. Rubin, and R.R. Hutchinson. 1968. Biting attack by rats in response to aversive shock. *Journal of the Experimental Analysis of Behavior* 11(5):633-39.

Barker, R. 1997. How can we train leaders if we don't know what leaderhip is? *Human Relations* 50(4): 343-62.

Barnett, J.L., G.M. Cronin, T.H. McCallum, and E.A. Newman. 1993. Effects of "chemical intervention" techniques on aggression and injuries when grouping unfamiliar adult pigs. *Applied Animal Behaviour Science* 36:135-48.

Benowitz, E.A. 2001. *CliffsQuickReview: Principles of Management.* New York: Hungry Minds.

Bernstein, I.S. 1981. Dominance: The baby and the bathwater. *Journal of Behavioral and Brain Sciences* 4:419-57.

Boitani, L., F. Francisci, P. Ciucci, and G. Andreoli. 1995. Population biology and ecology of feral dogs in central Italy. In *The domestic dog: Its evolution, behaviour and interactions with people,* ed. J. Serpell, 217-44. Cambridge: Cambridge University Press.

Bouissou, M.F. 1972. Influence of body weight and presence of horns on social rank in domestic cattle. *Animal Behavior* 20:474-77.

Camp, D.S., G.A. Raymond, and R.M. Church. 1967. Temporal relationship between response and punishment. *Journal of Experimental Psychology* 74(1):114-23.

Capitanio, J.P. 1985. Early experience and social processes in Rhesus macaques (Macaca mulatta): II. Complex social interaction. *Journal of Comparative Psychology* 99(2):133-42.

Capitanio, J.P. 1999. Personality dimensions in adult male Rhesus macaques: Prediction of behaviors across time and situation. *American Journal of Primatology* 47:299-320.

Capitanio, J.P. Written communication with author, May 21, 2008.

Coppinger, R., and L. Coppinger. 2002. *Dogs: A New Understanding of Canine Origin, Behavior, and Evolution*. New York: Scribner.

Domjan, M. 2003. *The Principles of Learning and Behavior*. 5th ed. Belmont, Calif.: Wadsworth/Thomson Learning.

Drews, C. 1993. The concept and definition of dominance behavior. *Behaviour* 125:284-313.

Drobatz, K.J., H. Saunders, C. Pugh, and J. Hendricks. 1995. Noncardiogenic pulmonary edema in dogs and cats: 26 cases (1987-1993). *Journal of the American Veterinary Medical Association* 206: 1732-36.

Goodman P. Written communication with author, June 19, 2008.

Goodwin, D., J.W.S. Bradshaw, and S.M. Wickens. 1997. Paedomorphosis affects agonistic visual signals of domestic dogs. *Animal Behavior* 53:297-302.

Herron, M, F.S. Shofer and I.R. Reisner. 2008. Safety and efficacy of behavior modification techniques used by dog owners. In 2008 ACVB/AVSAB *Scientific Paper and Poster Session. New Orleans, La.*, July 18, 2008.

Kadushin, A., and J.A. Martin. 1981. *Child Abuse: An Interactional Event*. New York: Columbia University Press.

Kaiser, R.B., R. Hogan, and C.S. Bartholomew. 2008. Leadership and the fate of organizations. *American Psychologist* 63(2):96-110.

Klinghammer E. Personal communication with author, June 22 1999.

Knowles, H.P., and B.O. Saxberg. 1971. *Personality and Leadership Behavior*. Reading, Mass.: Addison-Wesley.

MacDonald, D.W., and G.M. Carr. 1995. Variation in dog society: Between resource dispersion and social flux. In *The Domestic Dog: Its Evolution, Behaviour and Interactions with People*, ed. J. Serpell, 199-216. Cambridge: Cambridge University Press.

Martinez, M., A. Calvo-Torrent, and M.A. Pico-Alfonso. 1998. Social defeat and subordination as models of social stress in laboratory rodents: A review. *Aggressive Behavior* 24:241-56.

Mech, L.D. 1999. Alpha status, dominance, and division of labor in wolf packs. *Canadian Journal of Zoology* 77:1196-1203.

Mech, L.D. 2008. What ever happened to the term alpha wolf? *International Wolf* 18(4):4-8.

Pauli, A.M., E. Bentley, A.K. Diehl, and P.E. Miller. 2006. Effects of the application of neck pressure by a collar or harness on intraocular pressure in dogs. *Journal of the American Animal Hospital Association* 42(3):207-11.

Perry, D.G., and R. Parke. 1975. Punishment and alternative response training as determinants of response inhibition in children. *Genetic Psychology Monographs* 91:257-79.

Price, E.O. 2002. *Animal Domestication and Behavior*. New York: CABI Publishing.

Rushen, J. 1988. Assessment of fighting ability or simple habituation: What causes young pigs to stop fighting? *Aggressive Behavior* 14:155-167.

Wagnon K.A., R.G. Loy, W.C. Rollins, and F.D. Carroll. 1966. Social dominance in a herd of Angus, Hereford and Shorthorn cows. *Animal Behavior* 14:474-79.

Yin, S. 2004. *How to Behave So Your Dog Behaves*. Neptune City, N.J.: TFH Publications.

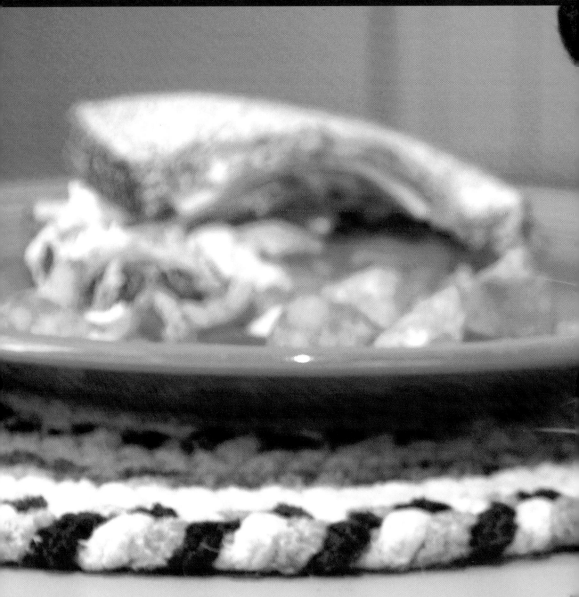

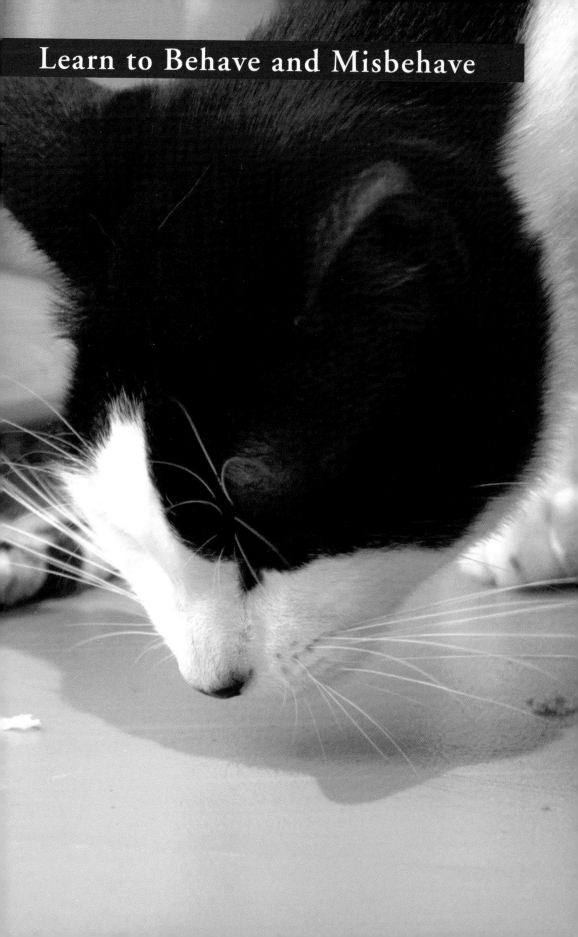

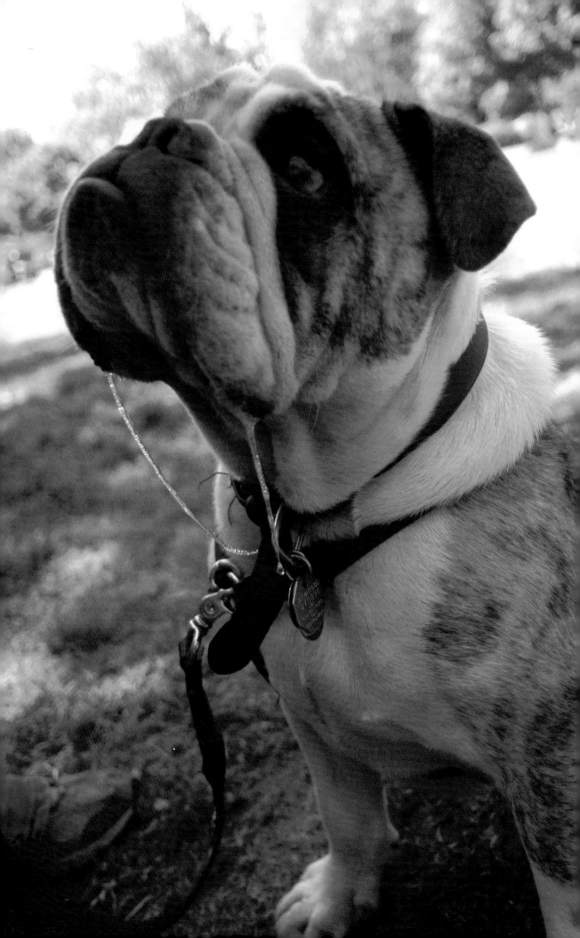

CHAPTER 3.
CLASSICAL
CONDITIONING
a.k.a Associative Learning

The young calico cat eyes the bowl as if savoring the sight. A scent from the warmed food wafts up. It's the same food she ate ravenously one meal ago, but she won't touch it now and it's the fourth type of food she's been through. Each one she devours encouragingly, but then she refuses the next meal.

What's happened? This kitty with a liver shunt eats the meal and then feels sick afterwards. She associates the illness with the food and consequently learns to avoid that food in the future. She has learned through **classical conditioning** to avoid the new foods. (Figure 3-A) Classical conditioning is one of the two major mechanisms of learning in animals, and animals learn through classical conditioning every day. To understand the concept, it's important to first know the history.

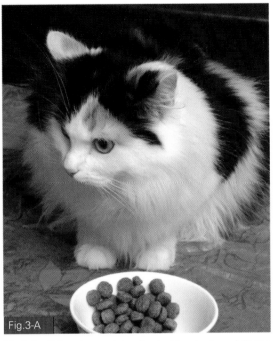

Fig.3-A

Fig.3-A: This cat associates food with a feeling of illness due to a liver shunt.

3.1 Pavlov's Dog

In the early 1900s, a Russian physician and researcher named Ivan Pavlov was studying digestion in dogs (Hunt 1993). He fed meat powder to dogs and then measured their salivation. After several repetitions, he noticed that dogs frequently began salivating before food entered their mouths. The salivation was triggered by the sight of food and the sound of people approaching with their meal. Upon this discovery, he changed the focus of his research and began investigating these "psychic secretions." Pavlov paired feedings with the sound of a stimulus that previously had no meaning to the dogs. He chose a bell because animals don't normally have any innate response to bells. He rang the bell and then immediately presented the food. After doing this many times, he found that when he tested the dogs by ringing the bell in the absence of food, the dogs salivated.

These results can be explained by the following: The food on its own elicits an involuntary physiological (and emotional) response—one that occurs without conditioning or training. Consequently, this stimulus is called an **unconditioned stimulus** and the salivation response is an **unconditioned response**. After pairing the neutral stimulus bell with the food enough times, the bell elicits the salivation even in the absence of food. Thus, the bell starts off as a neutral stimulus, but when paired enough times with food, it essentially takes on the same meaning as the food. It becomes a **conditioned stimulus**—one that was learned—and it elicits the salivation, which is now called a **conditioned response** because it was trained.

3.2 Classical Conditioning and the Gastrointestinal System

Since Pavlov's findings, the process of classical conditioning (a.k.a. associative learning) has been found to work across many different stimulus-response systems. In the 1950s, John Garcia and his colleagues at the Radiologic Defense Laboratory at Hunter's Point in San Francisco found that rats developed a taste aversion to solutions they were drinking as they were irradiated (Garcia and Koelling 1966). This aversion was presumably due to the association of the food with the nausea developed upon irradiation. Similarly, most humans have had an experience in which they have eaten a particular food while or immediately prior to becoming ill and subsequently have developed an aversion to that food.

3.3 Classical Conditioning and the Immune System

Classical conditioning can affect the immune system, too. There have been anecdotal reports of classical conditioning and learned allergic reactions. A 19th century medical journal reported that a patient with a known allergy to roses experienced an asthma attack when exposed to an artificial rose (MacKinzie 1886, cited in Russell 1984). More recently, researchers have found that guinea pigs can be trained to exhibit a histamine release in response to a novel odor (Russell et al. 1984). (Figure 3.3-A) The guinea pigs were immunologically sensitized to bovine serum albumin (BSA) by injecting BSA into the foot pad, leading to a histamine release. Then, during classical conditioning training, each guinea pig was injected with saline as a control on 5 separate occasions and BSA on 5 separate occasions. Injections were spaced one week apart to allow the animal to recover from any allergic reaction, and the order of injections was randomized. The injections were paired with 1 of 2 odors. One odor was paired with BSA and the other was paired with saline. The odors used were sulfur-smelling dimethyl-sulfide and fishy-smelling triethylamine. Half the animals received dimethylsulfide paired with BSA and triethylamine paired with saline. The other half received triethylamine paired with BSA and dimethylsulfide paired with saline. After the 10 training trials, each animal underwent test trials. In the first trial the researchers presented the odor that had been paired with BSA—dimethylsulfide in half the guinea pigs and triethylamine in the other half—but in the absence of a BSA injection. In the second trial the odor that had been paired with saline was presented in the absence of saline injection. The third trial was a repeat of trial one. All 8 guinea pigs showed marked histamine response on presentation of the odor that had been paired with BSA. Thus, the odor paired with BSA had become a conditioned stimulus. The histamine response level was comparable to the response that would have been elicited by an allergen. Conversely, when exposed to the odor that had been paired with the control saline injection, the histamine release was minimal.

Group 1 guinea pigs: 5 training trials and 3 test trials with each odor

TRAINING PHASE			TESTING PHASE	
PAIRING OF ODOR WITH INJECTION				
Odor	+ Injection	= Result	Odor ⟶	Result
DMSO (sulfur smell)	+ BSA (allergen)	= Histamine response	DMSO in the absence of any injection ⟶	Histamine response
Triethylamine (fishy smell)	+ Saline (control)	= No histamine response	Triethylamine in the absence of any injection ⟶	No histamine response

Group 2 guinea pigs: 5 training trials and 3 test trials with each odor

TRAINING PHASE			TESTING PHASE	
PAIRING OF ODOR WITH INJECTION				
Odor	+ Injection	= Result	Odor ⟶	Result
DMSO (sulfur smell)	+ Saline (control)	= No histamine response	DMSO in the absence of any injection ⟶	No histamine response
Triethylamine (fishy smell)	+ BSA (allergen)	= Histamine response	Triethylamine in the absence of any injection ⟶	Histamine response

Fig.3.3-A

Fig.3.3-A: Response to odors that had previously been paired with BSA (allergen) or saline injection (control).

3.4 Applications to Daily Interactions With Pets *(Video 1)*

Given that the types of classically conditioned responses and stimuli can vary so greatly, one would expect that classical conditioning is a common phenomenon that takes place every day. And this is true; animals are constantly making associations both in our presence and our absence. Unfortunately, they are often making detrimental associations with respect to humans and other animals, objects or environments. (Figure 3.4-A) One such association occurs in training situations. Many trainers use methods that focus on the use of strong corrections, including shock collars. A study by Schilder and van der Borg (2004) on working dogs in the Netherlands revealed that dogs who had been trained using shock collars showed signs of fear, stress and pain when shocked. They yelped, lowered their tail, crouched, flicked their tongue and lowered their ears in response to the shock. These dogs also showed subtle but consistent signs of fear and stress during obedience training, protection training and while free-walking with their handler both on the training ground and in the park during sessions when they were not shocked. The signs included lip-licking, raising a paw and a lowered ear position. The results indicate that the dogs learned to associate the situations, environments and handlers with the pain and fear induced by the shock collar. In some instances, the dog also associated the command with a shock. In these cases, when a dog had been shocked following a command and the command was given later, the dog immediately yelped upon hearing the command in the absence of the shock.

In addition to developing a learned fear response to their handlers, animals can develop aggression when techniques involving fear and pain are applied (Azrin et al. 1968). This finding has been demonstrated in many species, ranging from rats to humans (Berkowitz 1983; Overall 1997). The aggression can be directed toward the object causing

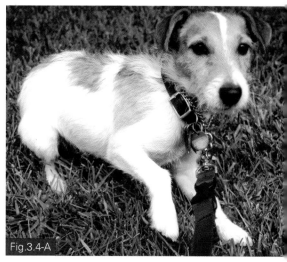

Fig.3.4-A: A study on working dogs revealed that those who had been trained using shock collars showed signs of fear, stress and pain when shocked. They yelped, lowered their tail, crouched, flicked their tongue and lowered their ears in response to the shock.

the fear and pain, or it can be redirected toward humans, other animals or inanimate objects. Consequently, when aversive methods such as shock collars or choke chain corrections are used to correct behaviors such as barking or lunging at dogs or people, they could have the unintended effect of creating a more negative association of pain or fear with the object, person or animal that the dog was reacting to. In turn, the inappropriate behavior might escalate to overtly aggressive behavior.

This type of negative association does not occur solely during owner-supervised interactions or interactions on the owner's property. It occurs within the context of the veterinary hospital, too, and starts even before the client has made it to the hospital. For example, when a client brings a new kitten to your veterinary hospital for the first time, she puts the kitten into a travel carrier—a new experience for the cat—and drives to the hospital in a car. Along the way, the kitten might salivate or vomit due to nausea induced by the ride. When he arrives at the hospital, the kitten smells and hears foreign scents and sounds, causing an additional fear response. Then in the exam room, he receives a painful vaccination.

While the exam may have seemed to go well because the kitten did not hiss or struggle, a visit 3 weeks later might reveal something different. This time when the owner brings the crate out, the kitten hides. He has been classically conditioned to associate the crate with the pain, fear and nausea of his last trip to the hospital, and he's having an involuntary physiological response. Once he arrives at the hospital for his second visit, rather than stiffly lying sternal with his ears back and head low—a posture indicating fear—he hisses and yowls. He has been trained to associate the hospital and the veterinarian with

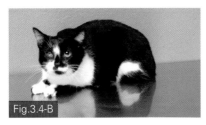

Fig.3.4-B

Fig.3.4-B: Due, in part, to the frightening events associated with the veterinary visit—the car ride, foreign sights, sounds and smells in the waiting room, and the pain of the vaccination, this kitty has been classically conditioned to fear both the veterinary hospital and the crate that it arrives in. These fears are not likely to decrease on their own.

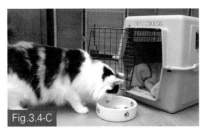

Fig.3.4-C

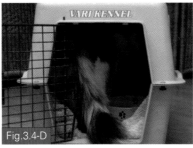

Fig.3.4-D

Fig. 3.4-C, D: Fears can be reversed through desensitization and classical counterconditioning. To carry out this process with the crate, the owner could feed the cat his meals right outside the crate. Then gradually move the food farther into the crate until the cat readily goes into the crate to eat. (For more details on this and car rides, refer to Chapter 6.)

aversive conditions and now, when he can't escape the situation, he responds aggressively. At this point, if the kitten is restrained and vaccinated, his anxiety, fear and aggression might remain at the same level or it could increase both within the visit and on future visits. (Figure 3.4-B)

While we might unintentionally classically condition undesired associations in our clients' pets, these problems can be alleviated by classically conditioning a different association (Yin 2004; Wright et al. 2005). For instance, we can train the fearful kitten to associate the crate, car ride and veterinary hospital with food, thus eliciting all of the pleasurable physiological changes that come with food. (Figures 3.4-C and 3.4-D) This is called classical counterconditioning because it involves countering the association that was previously classically conditioned with a new association.

Usually with counterconditioning, we start with the stimulus at low intensity because the animal will be too fearful of the regular-intensity stimulus to eat the food. Then we gradually increase the intensity in small increments. This process is termed systematic desensitization. Thus, to countercondition to the crate, start by feeding the cat his meal outside the crate at whatever distance he will approach and eat the food without hesitation. When he eats comfortably in one location for at least one meal, move the food closer and closer for the next meals and finally into the crate. Doing this slowly enough should result in the kitten comfortably eating the food while he's in the crate. When the kitten will walk into the crate and lie down in anticipation of food or in the absence of food, he has been successfully counterconditioned. This training usually takes less than 1 week in both dogs and cats and requires little extra time. Training will progress quickest if we make the association clear by presenting the food immediately when the aversive situation or stimulus is present (the crate) and remove the food when we remove the aversive stimulus. Furthermore, the desensitization steps should be incremental such that the animal shows little or no fear response during the sessions.

The pattern of desensitization and counterconditioning is the same regardless of the situation. With the car ride aversion, feed the kitten his daily meal in his crate within the stationary car. When he comfortably eats his food at this level of stimulus several days in a row, turn the car on for a short period. The next step would be to take him on a short car ride around the block. (If the ride triggers a salivation or vomiting response from earlier classical conditioning, an antiemetic might be needed for the first several sessions or food can be kept to a minimum for the first short rides.) Next, the kitten should be counterconditioned to the aspects of a veterinary hospital that cause fear, such as unfamiliar people, injections and nail trims. (Figure 3.4-E) This can be performed by the owner at home.

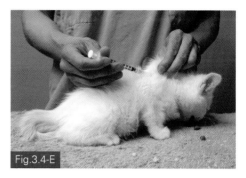

Fig.3.4-E

Fig.3.4-E: For vaccinations, one could start by giving a treat and simultaneously rubbing the kitten in the injection site. Contact should cease immediately when the kitten finishes the treat. Additional steps include grasping the fur for a second, grasping for longer periods of time, pinching the skin softly and shaking it, poking the tented skin with a capped needle and finally, injecting. The kitten should be eating the entire time while you are rubbing, grasping and pinching the skin.

References

Azrin, N.H., H.B. Rubin, and R.R. Hutchinson. 1968. Biting attack by rats in response to aversive shock. *Journal of the Experimental Analysis of Behavior* 11(5):633-39.

Berkowitz, L. 1983. The experience of anger as a parallel process in the display of impulsive, "angry" aggression. In *Aggression: Theoretical and Empirical Reviews, Vol. II, Theoretical and Methodological Issues*, ed. R.G. Geen and E.I. Donnerstein, 103-33. New York: Academic Press.

Garcia, J., and R.A. Koelling. 1966. Relation of cue to consequence in avoidance learning. *Psychonomic Science* 4:123-24.

Hunt, M. 1993. *The Story of Psychology*. New York: Anchor Books.

Overall, K.L. 1997. *Clinical Behavioral Medicine for Small Animals*. St. Louis, Mo. :Mosby.

Russell, M., K.A. Dark, R.W. Cummins, G. Ellman, E. Callaway, H.V.S. Peeke. 1984. Learned histamine release. *Science* 225(4663): 733-34.

Schilder, M.B.H., and J.A.M. van der Borg. 2004. Training dogs with help of the shock collar: Short and long term behavioural effects. *Applied Animal Behaviour Science* 85:319-34.

Wright J.C., P.J. Reid, and Z. Rozier. 2005. Treatment of emotional distress and disorders—Non-pharmacologic methods. In *Mental Health and Well-being in Animals*, ed. F.D. McMillan, 145-58. Ames, Iowa, :Blackwell Publishing.

Yin, S., 2004. *How to Behave So Your Dog Behaves*. Neptune City, N.J.: TFH Publications.

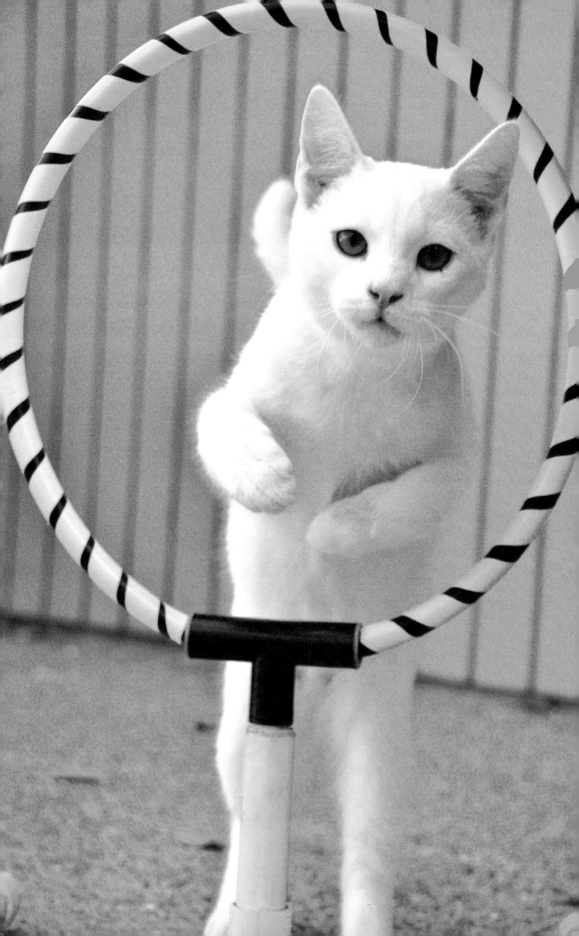

CHAPTER 4.
OPERANT CONDITIONING BASICS
Learning by Trial and Error

It's 7 a.m. on a spring day overlooking the heavily treed yards of a suburban neighborhood. A strange sound breaks the early morning silence. Clank. Clank clank…then it's quiet for several seconds. Then clank clank clank…more silence. A curious scrub jay flies down from a distant branch and sits on the fence to observe. She's heard this noise before, but this is the first time she's gone for a closer look. It's a blue cube, being pushed around by a dog. The jay cocks her head one way and then the other to get a better view. Then she sees it. Something falls out of the cube. "Come on, just a little bit more." She cautiously waits until the dog rolls the cube a few feet farther before sneaking down to the grass. Inconspicuously, the bird looks right, then left, then grabs it. Score! It's dog kibble. She eats it, grabs another piece to cache and flies away.

The scrub jay has just learned that whenever she hears the clanking sound of the dog's Buster Cube—a plastic toy that dispenses kibble when the dog rolls it around—she should fly down to the yard. If the dog misses some of the kibble, it's an easy meal for the jay. She learned this through operant conditioning, also known as trial and error learning.

With operant conditioning, the animal repeats behaviors that have desired consequences and avoids behaviors that lead to undesirable consequences. *(Video 1)* For instance, bears, raccoons, dogs and rats raid garbage cans because they've learned through trial and error that doing so leads to finding food. (Figures 4-A and 4-B) Similarly, songbirds visit bird feeders regularly in order to find food. When the bird feeders are consistently left empty, the birds no longer visit.

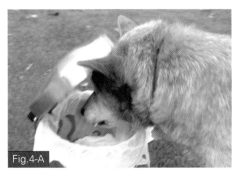
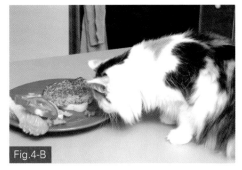

Fig. 4-A, B: This dog is examining the garbage can contents and this cat has jumped on the counter because they frequently find food when they do so. Since dogs evolved as scavengers, it should be no surprise that they are as good as bears, raccoons and rats at learning to raid food sites. Similarly, cats in the wild need to find food for a living so jumping on the counters for the occasional accidental food rewards, as well as the fun of exploring, should be expected.

4.1 The 4 Categories of Operant Conditioning

There are several important terms to know regarding operant conditioning. A good understanding of these terms (Figure 4.1-A) will enable you to evaluate the knowledge of trainers and behavior consultants with whom you'll be dealing, as well as that of companies designing products for behavior modification. The terms are the crux of learning theory, which is a major area of psychology. Those who state that their methods are based on psychology or science might not be qualified to make this statement if they do not know these definitions and their applications fluently.

Figure 4.1-A: 4 categories of operant conditioning

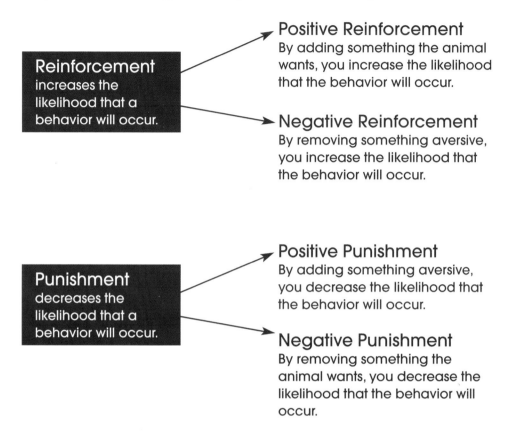

Reinforcement increases the likelihood that a behavior will occur.

Positive Reinforcement
By adding something the animal wants, you increase the likelihood that the behavior will occur.

Negative Reinforcement
By removing something aversive, you increase the likelihood that the behavior will occur.

Punishment decreases the likelihood that a behavior will occur.

Positive Punishment
By adding something aversive, you decrease the likelihood that the behavior will occur.

Negative Punishment
By removing something the animal wants, you decrease the likelihood that the behavior will occur.

4.1.1 Reinforcement vs. punishment.

The first two terms to learn are **reinforcement** and **punishment**. Reinforcement is anything that increases the likelihood that a behavior will occur again (Lindsay 2001; Yin 2004). For example, if you call your dog and give her a treat when she comes to you, she is more likely to come the next time you call her. Punishment is anything that decreases the likelihood that a behavior will occur again (Lindsay 2001; Yin 2004). If you call your dog and then yell at her and give her a leash correction because she took too long to come, she is less likely to come the next time you call her.

4.1.2 Positive vs. negative.

The second set of terms is **positive** and **negative**. Positive and negative do not mean good or bad; rather, think of them as a plus sign or a minus sign. Positive means adding something and negative means subtracting something.

4.1.3 The 4 categories of operant conditioning.

These terms can be combined, leading to 4 categories of operant conditioning: positive reinforcement, negative reinforcement, positive punishment and negative punishment.

4.1.3a With positive reinforcement, adding something the animal desires increases the likelihood that the behavior will occur again. For instance, cats can be trained to come to you by rewarding them with a treat when they walk over and sit in front of you. (Figures 4.1-B and 4.1-C)

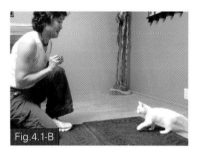 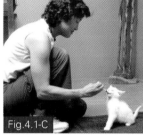

Fig.4.1-B

Fig.4.1-C

Fig.4.1-B, C: Positive reinforcement: By rewarding this kitty with treats or food she likes for walking over and sitting, we increase the likelihood that she will repeat this behavior.

4.1.3b With negative reinforcement, removing something aversive increases the likelihood the behavior will occur again. For example, if we teach a dog to come when called by hooking him to a leash, pulling with constant pressure and then releasing the pressure when the dog takes a step toward us, we are using negative reinforcement. The dog will eventually learn to come to you to avoid being pulled. (Figures 4.1-D and 4.1-E) If using this technique, it is imperative that the pressure stops as soon as the animal starts performing the correct behavior; otherwise, she will not know which behavior turns off the pressure.

Fig.4.1-D, E: Negative reinforcement: The behavior of moving forward when the handler walks or pulls on the leash will increase if the handler immediately releases pressure on the leash (removes an aversive) as soon as the dog begins to step forward.

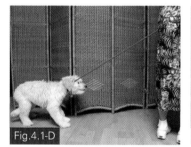 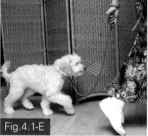

Fig.4.1-D

Fig.4.1-E

Negative reinforcement can be thought of like nagging. Often kids dislike cleaning their bedrooms, but if their parents tell them over and over to clean it, they will usually do so to avoid more nagging. Of course, it's important that the nagging stop as soon as the child starts to clean the room. When given a choice between learning new behaviors and forming new habits through positive or negative reinforcement, most people prefer positive reinforcement.

4.1.3c Punishment can also be positive or negative. The concept people are most familiar with is positive punishment, although they might not know that term. With **positive punishment**, adding something aversive decreases the likelihood that the behavior will occur again. For instance, if your dog raids the garbage and you whack her with a newspaper while she's performing the act, she will be less likely to raid the garbage again—at least when she knows you can see her or are close enough to whack her with a newspaper. (Note: I am not advocating this technique; it is just an example.) (Figures 4.1-F,G,H)

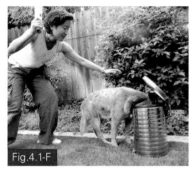 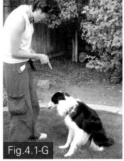 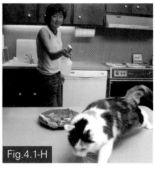

Fig.1-F, G, H: Positive punishment means adding anything that decreases the likelihood of a behavior occurring again. It could be physical punishment such as whacking the dog with a newspaper (which I don't recommend); verbal punishment if it causes the animal to cower, run away or otherwise look fearful; or a squirt of water if it causes the animal to run away. If it's aversive to the animal and decreases the behavior, it is a punishment. If it seems aversive to you but not to the animal, then it is not a punishment.

4.1.3d With negative punishment, removing something the animal desires decreases the likelihood that the behavior will occur. For instance, kittens often climb on or claw you when you are feeding them in an attempt to grab the treat more quickly. If you remove the treat as soon as the kitten starts to raise her paw, you will decrease the pawing, climbing behavior. (Figures 4.1-I and 4.1-J)

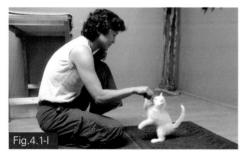 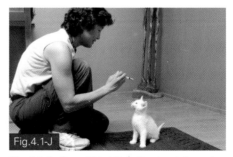

Fig.4.1-I: Negative punishment: This kitten is pawing to get to the treat more quickly.

Fig.4.1-J: By withholding the treat from her when she paws, she will be less likely to paw for it again.

4.2 Systematic Classification of Training Techniques

The operant conditioning categories seem straightforward at first, but often when one starts classifying training techniques, it starts to become confusing. Some techniques fall into more than one category, depending on how you describe the behavior and the technique. To avoid confusion, approach classification in a methodical way. One such way is as follows:

1. First, define the behavior you're talking about and decide whether you want to increase or decrease that behavior. If the goal is to increase the behavior, you will, by definition, use reinforcement. If the goal is to decrease the behavior, you will, by definition, use punishment. For example, say your dog greets you by jumping all over you. You want to change this behavior. You can define two goal behaviors: Either train him to stop jumping on you or train him to greet you by, for example, sitting calmly. If your goal is to train him to stop jumping, then by definition you'll be using punishment. If your goal is to train the more appropriate behavior of sitting for attention, then you'll be using reinforcement.

2. Next, decide whether you're adding something or subtracting something to determine if the operant category will be negative or positive. If you yank the dog's collar to make him stop jumping, you are adding something the dog finds aversive to decrease the behavior. Consequently, you are using **positive punishment**. (Note: I'm not advocating that you yank the dog's collar; I'm just using this as an example.) Alternatively, you might opt to remove the attention your dog wants by standing motionless and completely ignoring her. By doing so you will decrease the jumping behavior, so you are still using punishment. In this case, though, you are using **negative punishment**, because you're removing something she wants.

If your goal is to train the dog to greet by sitting, you will be using positive reinforcement or negative reinforcement. If you wait until the dog sits and then give her a treat for sitting, you are using **positive reinforcement**. If you hook the dog up to a leash and choke chain and step on it so that it tightens causing pressure and then release the pressure immediately when she sits, you're using **negative reinforcement**.

4.3 Distinguishing Between Positive Punishment and Negative Reinforcement

Techniques for negative reinforcement and positive punishment can be similar. Many commercial companies use the term "negative reinforcement" because it sounds friendlier, when really what they're describing is positive punishment. The primary difference is the emphasis on the goal behavior. In the majority of cases where we use aversives in training, our goal is to stop a behavior rather than to focus on strengthening an appropriate desirable behavior. (Figure 4.3-A)

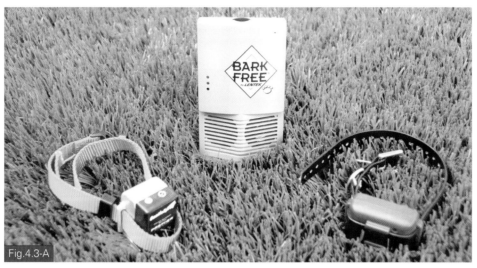

Fig.4.3-A: Positive punishment or negative reinforcement? Anti-bark collars and ultrasonic devices are not designed to reward dogs for quiet behavior; instead, they are designed to inhibit barking. Thus, these products are positive punishment products. Such products are often only effective short term because they fail to remove the underlying motivation for the undesirable behavior and fail to train a desired behavior which the dog can perform instead. Punishment techniques are more likely to be effective when used in combination with positive reinforcement (Perry and Park 1975).

4.4 A General Approach to Solving Behavior Problems

Although animals in the wild learn through all 4 categories of operant conditioning, at home and in specific training sessions, the category that generally works best for humans interacting with animals is positive reinforcement. Consequently, while we tend to solve behavior problems by asking how we can stop or punish an undesirable behavior, we should focus instead on how to reinforce an alternate appropriate behavior and how to avoid reinforcing the undesirable behavior. Thus, step 1 in solving common behavior problems is to first identify possible reinforcers for the undesirable behavior so that we can avoid reinforcing it. Step 2 is to decide on a behavior you would rather have the animal perform. Note that in many cases, you don't actually have to identify the reinforcer for the undesirable behavior.

> To fix a behavior problem, ask what behavior you would rather have and reinforce that behavior instead. Also remove reinforcements for undesirable behavior.

Example 1: Your friend complains that his dog is too excited when they play ball. She jumps up and down and tries to grab the ball. He thinks the dog can't be trained using toys because she is "over-motivated" or "overexcited." In operant conditioning terms, why does she jump for the ball and how can you fix this problem? (Figures 4.4-A to 4.4-F)

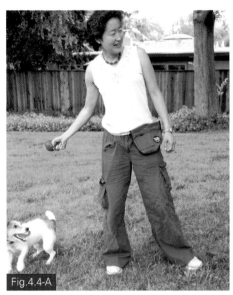 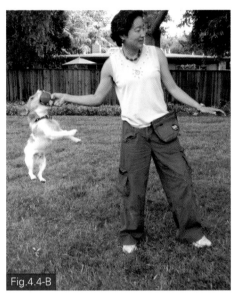

Fig.4.4-A, B: Step 1a: Identify the reinforcer for the undesirable behavior; i.e., what is reinforcing the dog's jumping at the ball? Jonesy grabs toys out of people's hands because he can get them faster that way. He's frequently rewarded by getting the toy when he jumps. In other words, he has received positive reinforcement for jumping and grabbing the toy out of the thrower's hands.

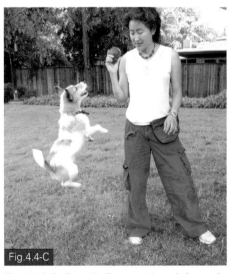 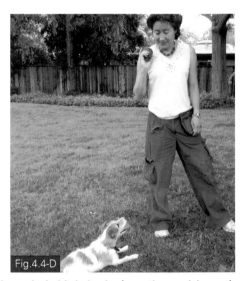

Fig.4.4-C, D: Step 1b: Remove the reinforcer for the undesirable behavior (negative punishment). If the thrower removes the toy whenever Jonesy starts to jump—thus removing what he wants— Jonesy will quickly learn that jumping will not work, so he will stop jumping.

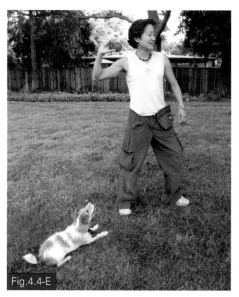
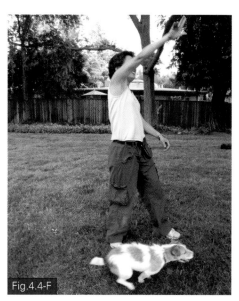

Fig.4.4-E, F: Step 2: Reinforce an appropriate behavior instead (positive reinforcement). Now the thrower only tosses the ball if Jonesy is lying down calmly. Note that you can preemptively set the situation up so that the dog automatically performs the appropriate behavior and doesn't have the opportunity to perform the undesirable behavior. For instance, you can hold the ball close to you and up high while standing stationary and preparing to toss it, rather than dangling the toy around as you walk or are getting ready to throw it. Or you can have the dog sit and give him treats while you get ready to toss the ball. Repeat this exercise until it becomes a habit for the dog to sit until you toss the ball.

Example 2: Every morning your cat wakes you up at 5 a.m. She cries and cries and even climbs all over you when you're lying in bed. Sometimes you push her off the bed, but she continues anyway until you feed her. Why does the cat wake you up every morning? Because you're reinforcing her behavior by getting up to feed her, and you're interacting with her when she jumps on the bed. Ignore her completely and feed her only after she's quiet, preferably at a time that's convenient for you. Note: If you can't stand the noise, lock her in a separate room with toys and a bed or in a cat carrier or dog crate at night (refer to Chapter 6 to learn how to carrier train a cat).

Example 3: This scheme for solving problem behaviors can also be used immediately in the veterinary clinic. For the excitable but hungry dog who jumps on people and will not hold still for examination, first quickly teach her to sit for rewards (treats). Give her the first treat for free to make sure she likes them and realizes that you have them. Hold the next treat in your closed hand close to you but well above her nose level so she has to look up to see it. Wait until she offers a sit—you can be taking a history simultaneously—and immediately reward once she sits and before she gets up. You can lure her into a sit with the treat if needed the first few times. Then, continue giving treats for the calm sit behavior. Avoid commanding the dog. You wouldn't want to hear someone commanding you or your child sharply to sit or hold still during a doctor's exam. The sit exercise should look like a game to the dog. If you're worried about what the clients think, just tell them that you're waiting to see how long it takes their dog to figure out that she should sit in this situation to earn the treats.

The treats should be small enough that the dog finishes them with one bite or within 1-2 seconds. When you examine an energetic dog or a fearful or nervous dog, have the owner or your technician give rewards for calm sits or for standing still. At first, make the dog's task easy by quickly examining only one area, such as an eye. The goal is to be quick enough that the dog has a good chance of remaining stationary and calm, thereby earning a reward. As the dog learns to remain calm for short procedures, increase the length and difficulty of the task. The entire process can take just a few extra seconds or minutes, yet it can save you an exponential amount of time and manpower in future visits. It also teaches the dog that you are consistent, predictable and trustworthy. Owners can practice with their pets at home, too. As an added benefit, both the pet and the owner will start to associate you and the hospital with pleasant experiences.

4.5 Shaping Complex Behaviors

Usually when we're training a behavior, we can't reach the goal behavior in one step. We have to start with a behavior that we can train, and gradually train behaviors that are closer to our goal behavior. In other words, we shape the behavior through incremental steps called successive approximations.

Example 1: *(Video 2)* To train a dog to perform a somersault, you could first teach her to touch a target (a ball on the end of a stick) with her nose when you put the target right in front of her nose. Reward the dog with a treat when she performs this. When she's good at that step, teach her to touch the target held when it is down lower, until she can consistently perform this step. Next, hold the target down even lower so she has to reach closer to the ground. Then, in incremental steps, hold the target between her legs so she starts bending her head under and between her legs. If she offers some forward motion while doing this, or if you have her stand on something so her rear end is higher than her front end, you can eventually get a somersault. (Figures 4.5-A to 4.5-D)

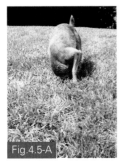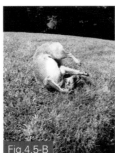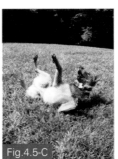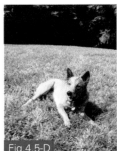

Fig.4.5-A to D: A shaped behavior: Zoe performs a somersault, which she learned through several shaping steps.

Example 2: Say you want to take a photo of your dog with your two chickens. The chickens can be kept in the shot by tossing food in the area, but you want the dog to lie down and remain there for the 30 seconds you need to take the photo. If you've already trained the dog to lie down for 30 seconds without distractions, should she also be able to lie down while you take a photo with two chickens present? No. You must train her to lie down with the distractions of the chickens and you

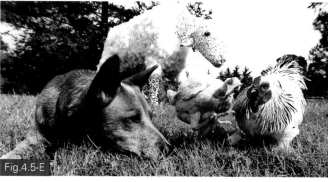

Fig.4.5-E: A shaped behavior: Several training steps were required to get Zoe to lie down next to the chickens for this photo.

handling the camera. Start with her farther away from the chickens and give frequent treats. Then gradually move the chickens closer. Next, give treats less often. (Figure 4.5-E)

4.6. When the Shaping Plan Stalls

Frequently, a rough shaping plan is devised but things don't go as expected. When a shaping plan doesn't work, it's due to one of three problems:

1. **Going on to step 2 before the animal knows step 1**. Just because an animal can perform a behavior correctly a few times does not mean that she knows the behavior well. This is clear when you consider how humans learn. In chemistry class, for instance, even if you can do several problems, it doesn't mean you know the concept well. You have to do many more problems over and over. With animals, strive for 80-100% correct responses before moving on to the next step. To make things simpler, choose a number—say, 5 or 10 correct responses in a row—and see if this criteria results in the pet performing well on new steps. In cases where you are going for 10 correct responses in a row, if the behaviors are complex or your pet gets bored repeating them, you can intersperse other exercises in between or spread out the training over several sessions.

2. **Skipping steps**. The trainer might expect too much from the animal by accidentally skipping steps. For instance, just because a dog can touch a target in front of her nose does not mean she will touch the target when it is placed between her legs. Similarly, just because you perform multiplication problems well doesn't mean that you can do calculus problems correctly. If the animal is doing well at one step and poorly at the next step (60% or fewer correct responses), go back and add additional steps in between.

3. **Staying on the same step for too long**. Trainers can also err by staying on the same step too long. For instance, food rewards should be used temporarily and only in the early learning and habit-forming stages of a specific behavior or exercise; then they should be faded away. Many owners use food to reward heeling or walking

next to them on a loose leash. The problem arises when they fail to systematically increase the criteria for earning the food so that less food is needed. That is, they continue giving frequent treats for heeling on walks when really they should be requiring that the dog go longer distances to earn a treat, until eventually treats are no longer required, at least in low-distraction situations, and can be replaced by other reinforcers. Once this stage of heeling on walks is reached, trainers could then reserve treats for heeling primarily in the higher distraction situations such as when going from the car to the dog park or when passing a cat. If they practice in these high-distraction situations enough and systematically increase the number of steps or amount of time the dog must heel and focus on them prior to rewarding with the treat, they can also fade away treats in these situations.

4.7 Timing, Criteria and Rate of Reinforcement

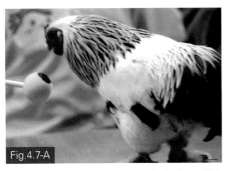

Fig.4.7-A

Fig.4.7-A: The importance of timing: This chicken is learning to peck the black dot on the target. To learn the task, he must be rewarded immediately after he pecks the black dot.

Timing: The reinforcement or punishment must occur as the behavior is occurring, within 1 second or before the next behavior occurs. Animals learn to perform the behaviors that are reinforced, not the behavior you think you reinforced or meant to reinforce.

Now you know the principles of operant conditioning. But implementing them effectively requires practice, because, like playing tennis or a musical instrument, training is a technical skill. In this particular "sport," the keys to success are good timing, well-defined criteria and the correct rate of reinforcement.

4.7.1 Timing.

With animal training, timing is critical. The reinforcement or punishment must occur as the behavior is occurring, within 1 second or at least well before the next significant behavior occurs. For instance, if you're teaching a chicken to peck a black dot, what happens if she pecks the dot and you start to deliver the food reward, but she's moving so quickly that she also pecks outside the dot before grabbing the food? The chicken will learn that pecking outside the dot leads to food rewards, so she thinks that's what she's supposed to do. (Figure 4.7-A) The take-home message here is that animals learn to perform the behaviors that are reinforced, not the behaviors that you think you reinforced or meant to reinforce.

4.7.2 Well-defined criteria.

To train successfully, you must firmly establish the criteria for the behavior you want, so that you can be clear and consistent. That means the picture of what you want should be so clear in your mind that if you describe the criteria to someone else, he or she will reward the exact behavior that you pictured. With the chicken example, the chicken might sometimes hit the center of the dot, sometimes hit right at the border and sometimes grab at the dot and rip at it. You must decide exactly which behavior to reinforce. If you only want the chicken to peck at the center, then you must only reward when she pecks the center of the dot. Otherwise you will get all of the above pecking behaviors. (Figure 4.7-B)

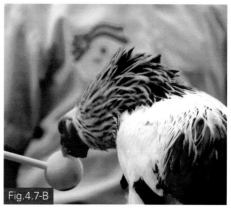

Fig.4.7-B: The importance of criteria: This chicken pecked just outside the black dot. If the criterion is to peck in the center of the dot, then the trainer must be careful to only reward pecking the center.

Criteria: To train successfully, you must firmly establish the criteria for the behavior you want, so that you can be clear and consistent. That means the picture of what you want should be so clear in your mind that if you describe the criteria to someone else, he or she will reward the exact behavior that you pictured.

The Bridging Stimulus: Sometimes it's difficult to convey to the animal exactly when she has performed a correct behavior because the animal is moving quickly and it's hard to get the treat to her at the moment she is performing the correct behavior or within 1 second. It can also be difficult if the animal is far away or is looking away from you when performing the correct behavior. In these cases, we can use a bridging stimulus to tell the animal when she has done something right. First, teach the animal that a novel, conspicuous sound—such as a clicker—means food is coming. Do this by pairing the click with food. That is, every time you make the clicker sound, deliver food to the animal within 1 second. Once you've classically conditioned the association between clicker and food, use the clicker to mark when the animal has done something right. Now, instead of getting the food to the animal immediately so that she knows when she has done something right, you can just use the clicker sound, which will cause her to stop what she's doing, orient in your direction and look for the treat reward. As a bridging stimulus, the clicker bridges the gap between the correct behavior and the food reinforcement. Follow the click immediately with a reward every time to avoid diminishing the association.

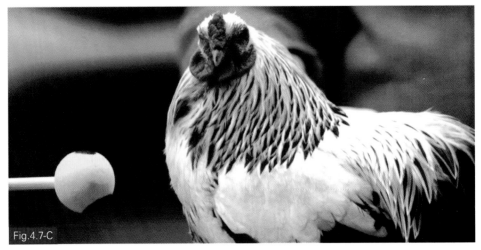

Fig.4.7-C: Reinforcement rate must be high enough: Animals need a high rate of reinforcement to keep them interested in training. This chicken looks bored because the task is too hard; consequently, he is not receiving rewards frequently enough to keep him interested.

4.7.3 Rate of reinforcement.

When working with chickens, exotics, cats, piglets and other animals off leash, you have to reinforce their behaviors enough to keep them interested in the game; otherwise, they'll just wander away. (Figure 4.7-C) With dogs and horses, we often force them to stay near us by using a leash or lead rope; however, they also need a high enough reinforcement rate to stay focused on us and do what we ask. The leash or lead rope is just a safety device to keep the dog or horse out of trouble. We should really rely on our good timing, well-defined criteria and correct rate of reinforcement to keep the animal interested in sticking with us during training.

4.7.3a Continuous rate of reinforcement. When animals (and people) are first learning a behavior, reinforce the behavior on a **continuous ratio**. That is, every time they perform the behavior correctly, reinforce the behavior until they know it well. Be sure to choose a behavior that's easy enough for the animal to perform repeatedly in rapid succession. If the animal has a hard time figuring out what she's supposed to do, she will get bored or frustrated and give up. To us, it seems like the pet has a short attention span. However, if we choose behaviors that the pet can perform correctly in rapid succession, we build what's called **behavioral momentum**, which makes the behavior less resistant to change.

This phenomenon is gaining attention in human psychology research. A study by Dube et al. (2003) looked at developmentally disabled children performing computer game tasks. When on a high rate of reinforcement, their behavior was more resistant to disruption by an alternate source of reinforcement, compared with when they were on a low rate of reinforcement. Similarly, a correlation study looking at behavioral momentum in college basketball games found that when teams were playing well and thus on a high rate of reinforcement within the last three minutes, they responded better to adversity than when the behavioral momentum was low (Mace et al. 1992).

4.7.3b Variable ratio of reinforcement. Once the pet performs the behavior correctly at least 80% of the time and you can bet money that she'll perform it on cue the next time, either switch to a **variable ratio** of reinforcement (VR) or raise the criteria. With a variable ratio of reinforcement, the animal doesn't know which time the correct behavior will earn the reward. You reinforce the behavior on average every 2, 3, 4, 5 or more times (VR 2, VR 3, VR, 4, VR 5, VR 5+) depending on your goals and the animal's training level. This is how slot machines work. As a gambler, if the odds of winning are 1/1000, you know you'll win, on average, every thousandth time, but you don't know exactly which time that is. It could be the next time, 100 pulls later, or after 1,500 pulls. Because you don't know, you try harder. Variable ratio reinforcement is the most effective schedule of reinforcement, which is why so many people are hooked on gambling.

When implementing a variable ratio of reinforcement, remember that VR refers to an average ratio. Using VR 5, for example, you would offer treats on average for every fifth behavior, but sometimes surprise the animal by rewarding on, say, the third, fourth or seventh correct behavior. Rewarding exactly every fifth behavior (called a **fixed ratio**) might result in some animals becoming lazy for the first three times and then performing better on the fourth and fifth time. When using variable ratio reinforcements, start with a low ratio. If your pet consistently performs well (80-90% of the time or 5-10 times in a row for easy behaviors), then move onto a higher VR.

4.8 Motivation *(Video 3)*

All animal species are motivated by 3 innate reinforcers: food, the need to avoid pain and danger, and the need to reproduce. For general training purposes, opportunities to engage in reproductive acts are not a practical reinforcer, and using aversives that generate fear is fraught with side-effects (refer to Chapter 2). That leaves food as a common motivator. All animals have to eat to survive. So if we alter the manner in which they are fed, we can use food to our advantage for training purposes.

In addition to these 3 innate reinforcers, different species and individuals are motivated by different things. Predator species such as dogs tend to enjoy chasing objects and fetching toys, especially ones that squeak like wounded prey. For animals who live in groups, especially those for whom being in a herd or flock provides safety, social reinforcement is a strong motivator. As every animal is an individual, when choosing a reinforcer it's essential that you use the reward that motivates the animal in that context or at that point in time.

Reinforcer strength changes dynamically based on the animal's state or the environmental context. We can control the strength and type of reinforcer that's appropriate by controlling the animal's environment. For instance, to use food as the reward, make sure the cat or dog is hungry by measuring her daily food allowance and subtracting her reward allotment from this. Also, train her before she has received her meal, or use all of her regular food allotment for training purposes until she's well behaved.

4.8.1 Use the appropriate motivator for the context.

Be sure to use what's motivating to the pet in the given context. To do this, observe the pet's body language carefully and interpret her behavior correctly. (Figures 4.8-A to 4.8-D)

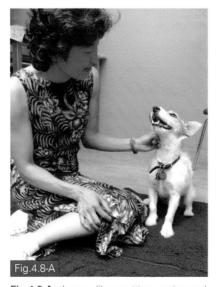

Fig.4.8-A: Jonesy likes petting, praise and attention in the house.

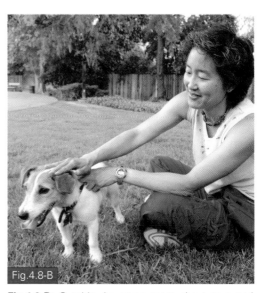

Fig.4.8-B: Outside, he cares more about toys and food. He's ignoring me when I pet him. If I use petting and praise as a reward in this context, I am wasting my effort and training ineffectively.

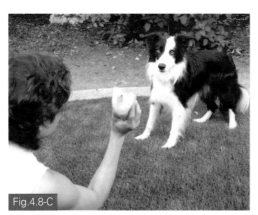

Fig.4.8-C: This dog loves toys. He's focused on this toy and is waiting for me to throw it for him.

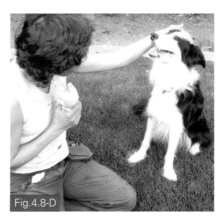

Fig.4.8-D: Unlike Jonesy, he's also motivated by praise and petting, even when there are toys in sight. Here, he looks at me and leans against the hand that is petting him.

4.8.2 Use all of the pet's motivators to your advantage for the most efficient training. (Figures 4.8-E,F,G)

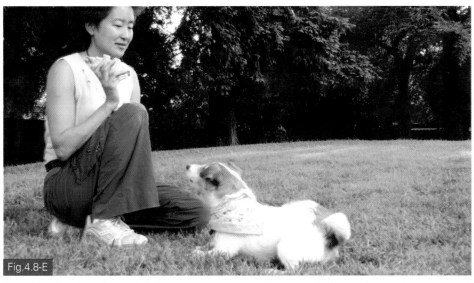

Fig.4.8-E

Fig.4.8-E: Use all motivators (reinforcers) to train. Jonesy learned to lie down using food as the reward. But here, I practice using toys as the reward instead, since I am planning to toss the toy in a game of fetch.

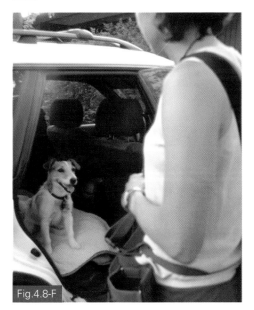

Fig.4.8-F

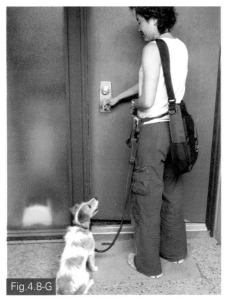

Fig.4.8-G

Fig.4.8-F: Here, the reward for sitting and waiting politely is that I will let him out of the car.

Fig.4.8-G: Here, the reward for sitting is that Jonesy gets to go into the house, where he will immediately run to the water bowl or to see whether the other dogs have been fed.

4.9 Communication *(Video 4)*

Many factors determine whether our pets perceive the message we intend to give. One is timing. If we fail to reward the animal as the desirable behavior is occurring or shortly thereafter, it will be difficult for her to understand which behavior we want. Another factor is our body language and verbal cues. Often when a pet fails to respond to our commands, we think of her as stubborn or stupid, especially if the pet is in a nondistracting environment and she has been rewarded frequently. One major cause of poor performance is the animal's inability to decipher our signals.

4.9.1 Visual cues take precedence over verbal cues.

While we humans are used to communicating by talking, this might not be the best mode of communication with animals. Research by Mills (2005) looked at which signal type takes precedence in dogs. Mills trained dogs to respond to verbal "right" and "left" cues, as well as a visual pointing cue for the same behaviors. To guard against bias that could be created by the order of teaching, half the dogs were initially trained using verbal cues and the other half using visual cues.

The researchers tested the dogs by placing a container of treats on either side of the dog—one box on the right and one on the left. When they gave the "left" cue, the dog got the food reward if she ran to the box on the left. If she ran to the wrong box, she got no reward. Once dogs consistently responded correctly to verbal or visual cues alone, the cues were given together, with a twist. The researchers gave a verbal signal for one direction and a visual signal for the other at the same time to see which one the dogs would follow. For anyone whose dog competes seriously in agility, the results were predictable: The dogs consistently followed the visual pointing cue and ignored the verbal cue. This dynamic plays out on every agility course—a dog will usually go where her handler's body is pointing rather than where the handler might be verbally trying to send her.

This bias toward the visual makes it imperative for us to realize that when working with dogs, they might be reading signals we're not aware of. So when your voice tells the dog to do one thing but your body tells her to do another, she's not being stubborn—she could just be reading a different message than the one you think you're sending. It's also important to realize that when training an animal, if you are teaching a verbal cue and a visual cue simultaneously, the animal will most likely learn only the most salient cue, the one that is most relevant and stands out from the rest of the environment. In most cases this is the visual cue. This phenomenon is called **overshadowing** (Yin 2004; Domjan 2003). A more effective way to teach two different cues is to train the visual cue

> When simultaneously given a verbal and a visual cue signaling different behaviors, the dog will most likely follow the visual cue.

first and then train the verbal cue by uttering the verbal cue immediately followed by the visual cue. Thus the verbal cue predicts that the visual cue will appear.

4.9.2 Dogs interpret all of our visual signals at once.

Even when we're purposefully sending visual commands to our dogs, such as in the obedience trial ring or during long-distance work, there's more to the signal than we might think. Fukuzawa and his colleagues (2005a) found that dogs look at the entire body, not just one part, to determine what we want. In this study, the researchers looked at the dog's response to different visual "right" and "left" cues. They compared eye movement and head movement to the right or left with pointing right or left but keeping the eyes and head looking forward. The 6 dogs in the study found the hidden food source faster when both signals were presented together. This suggests that dogs are taking in the whole picture of what's going on. That is, they don't look at our hands or our head; they look at our entire body. As a result, if all signals are not consistent, the dog can become confused.

In the same study, researchers (Fukuzawa et al. 2005a) also found that subtle visual cues are involved in giving a verbal cue when they looked at the response to tape recordings and found that dogs didn't respond as though these recordings were a real-time human voice. In this experiment, a "come" or "sit" command was given in one of 4 conditions: from a person sitting in a chair; from the same person wearing sunglasses to prevent his giving visual eye cues; and from each of these conditions again, but with the command being issued from a tape recorder behind the person. Dogs made many more errors when the tape recorder was used. Such errors could be attributed to the dogs distinguishing a difference between the tape-recorded and live-voice commands, but another hypothesis is that dogs also rely on lip movement or some other indication that the human is speaking to them. In fact, in a fifth variation, the handler uttered the "come" or "sit" cue while looking away from the dogs, and the dogs again made many errors, indicating that the orientation of the handler is important.

4.9.3 Subtle differences in verbal cues can affect how well an animal responds.

Variations in verbal commands can also confuse dogs. Fukuzawa et al. (2005b) performed a series of studies to test this. First, they tested slight variations in the commands to see if dogs recognized them as the same words. They taught dogs to stand and stay, and then from 5 feet away, the trainer gave either a "come" command or a "sit" command. Once the dogs reliably responded correctly, the researchers changed the command words slightly. In place of "sit," they used "chit," "sat" and "sik," and in place of "come" they used "tum," "keem" and "kufe." The researchers found that dogs did not respond as well to the similar-sounding words. That is, they were able to recognize that the similar-sounding words were not the same as the commands they had learned. This indicates that due to slight differences in how people pronounce words, obedient response to one person's commands won't necessarily transfer to another person unless the phonemic characteristics are mimicked.

4.9.4 Emotional content of the verbal cue is important.

Yet another significant aspect of verbal cues is the emotional content. Mills and his colleagues (Mills 2005; Mills et al. 2005) trained dogs to reliably come or sit when a handler was standing 5 feet away behind a screen. He and his colleagues then tested the dogs to see how they responded to different emotional contents. The commands were uttered in a neutral tone; a happy tone, with the inflection ascending; an angry version, with the tone descending; and a gloomy version, in which the handler sighed first. Dogs responded more predictably when the tone was positive, but when the command was said in an angry or gloomy manner, there was more variation in their responses.

> Dogs respond more predictably when your tone of voice is positive than when a command is stated in an angry or gloomy manner.

4.9.5 Take-home messages on communication.

1. Be aware of visual signals, as they might override verbal commands.

2. Make sure all of your signals (visual and verbal) mean the same thing and are coordinated, or your message could look more like a dubbed version of Godzilla than a clear-cut cue.

3. When you do use verbal cues, make sure everyone says them exactly the same way, or train your dog that the slight variations mean the same thing.

4. If you want your dog to respond correctly to your verbal commands when you're out of sight or facing away, you'll have to specifically train her to do so.

5. Remember that dogs respond more predictably when the tone is positive than when the tone is gloomy or angry.

Remember that when communicating with our pets, it's not just what we say, it's also how we say it and whether our visual and verbal cues are sending the same message. Once we're more aware of the signals we send to our pets and how they perceive them (based on their responses), we can reduce the everyday frustrations and open a clearer line of communication between us and them.

References

Domjan, M. 2003. *The Principles of Learning and Behavior.* 5th ed. Belmont, Ky.: Wadsworth/Thomson Learning.

Dube, W.V., W.J. Mcilvane, and K. Mazzitelli. 2003. Reinforcer rate effects and behavioral momentum in individuals with developmental disabilities. *American Journal on Mental Retardation* 108(2):134-43.

Mills, D.S., Fukuzawa, M., and J.J. Cooper. 2005. The effect of emotional content of verbal commands on the response of dogs (*Canis familiaris*). In *Current Issues and Research in Veterinary Behavioral Medicine-Papers Presented at the 5th International Veterinary Behaviour Meeting,* ed. D Mills, E.

Leving, G. Landsberg, D. Horwitz, M Duxbury, P. Mertens, K. Meyer, L. Radosta Huntley, M. Reich and J. Willard, 217-20. West Lafayette, Ind.: Purdue University Press.

Fukuzawa, M., D.S. Mills, and J.J. Cooper. 2005a. More than just a word: Non-semantic command variables affect obedience in the domestic dog. *Applied Animal Behaviour* 91:129-41.

Fukuzawa, M., D.S. Mills, and J.J. Cooper. 2005b. The effect of human command phonetic characteristics on auditory cognition in dogs. *Journal of Comparative Psychology* 119(1):117-20.

Lindsay, S.R. 2001. *Handbook of Applied Dog Behavior and Training.* Vol. 2: Etiology and assessment of behavior problems. Ames, Iowa: Iowa State University Press.

Mace, F.C., M. Shea, and J. Nevin. 1992. Behavioral momentum in college basketball. *Journal of Applied Behavior Analysis* 25:657-63.

Mills, D.S. 2005. What's in a word? Recent findings on the attributes of a command on the performance of pet dogs. *Anthrozoos* 18:208-21.

Perry, D.G., and R. Parke. 1975. Punishment and alternative response training as determinants of response inhibition in children. *Genetic Psychology Monographs* 91:257-79.

Yin, S., 2004. *How to Behave So Your Dog Behaves.* Neptune City, N.J.: TFH Publications.

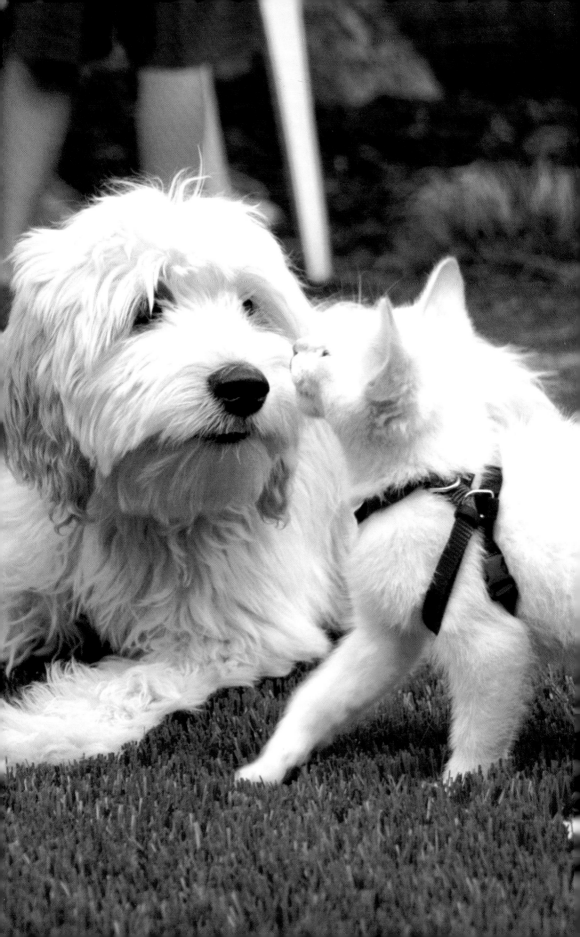

CHAPTER 5.
METHODS OF
Behavior Modification

*"Desensitizing a Very Dog-Aggressive Beagle—3 Weeks Into Training,"
reads the title on the YouTube video. The words partially obscure the
Beagle who is lying tensely in the middle of the floor, his leash attached
to a pinch collar sitting snuggly around his neck. A leashed puppy
springs in and out of the video, approaching randomly from different
directions like a Superball bouncing off an uneven floor. The puppy
clearly just wants to play. The Beagle clearly does not. He remains
lying down, but his panting, lip-licking and furtive glances toward
the puppy whenever the pup comes into striking range betrays his fear.
Finally, as the puppy approaches his face, he flashes his teeth in a
warning, not once but 3 times. The trainer pets him in hopes that
he will stop, but by the third time it's clear that due to the puppy's
continued advances, the Beagle's fear is escalating. A sharp jerk with
the leash and pinch collar quickly curbs the warning behaviors. The
Beagle now tries to avoid looking at the puppy. He cowers several times
as the trainer's hands wave above him in the air. "The dog is doing
much better. I can do this to your dog, too," states the ending
text on the video.*

109

While the trainer in the video was using a method of modification called **habituation**, the type of habituation he was using was clearly not **desensitization** (described in detail later in this chapter). Rather, he was doing the exact opposite by **flooding** the Beagle (exposing the animal to the full-force stimulus) when he presented the puppy at a distance at which the Beagle was clearly nervous. Furthermore, the trainer combined the flooding with positive punishment by giving a pinch collar correction when the Beagle tried to protect himself.

The use of flooding and punishment in this type of situation is akin to taking someone who is intensely fearful of spiders and making her sit near spiders that are crawling around. Any moves to scream, shoo the spiders away or protect herself would be met with physical corrections. The idea is that her actions of screaming or trying to kill spiders could be stopped in this manner, and with no detrimental emotional effects on the person being treated. In other words, the trainer was addressing the outward signs of fear (raised lip, growling, snapping) while failing to address the underlying motivational state driving the aggressive behavior.

Veterinary behaviorists and Certified Applied Animal Behaviorists typically recommend desensitization and counterconditioning (DS/CC) as the crux of behavior modification in animals. When trainers and dog owners misunderstand the terminology being used, they incorrectly perform techniques with the idea that they are doing exactly what such behaviorists recommend. So it's imperative to understand what the common methods of behavior modification actually are. This chapter explains the 4 methods of modification and provides examples of when and how to use them.

The 2 major classes of behavior modification are habituation and counterconditioning. Habituation can be further divided into flooding and desensitization, and counterconditioning can be broken down into classical counterconditioning and operant counterconditioning.

5.1 Habituation (Figure 5.1-A)

In nature, animals are constantly bombarded with stimuli. A myriad of sounds, smells, sights and tactile sensations stimulate their nervous system. If they attended to each one, they would quickly develop sensory overload. So how do they know which stimuli should incite a startle response and which to ignore? One way is through the process of habituation. Habituation is when a response to a novel stimulus, such as the sound of a train or the sight of a car, diminishes over time due to repeated exposure to the stimulus in the absence of any aversive or pleasurable experience (Leussis and Bolivar, 2006). In other words, habituation means that the animal "gets used to it."

We're all familiar with habituation because it happens to us all the time. If you live in a peaceful neighborhood and then move into one with train tracks nearby, initially the sound of the trains keeps you up all night. Over time, though, you notice the trains less and less until you often don't even realize that one went by. Animals such as dogs and cats commonly have to habituate to loud sounds, too. *(Video 1)*

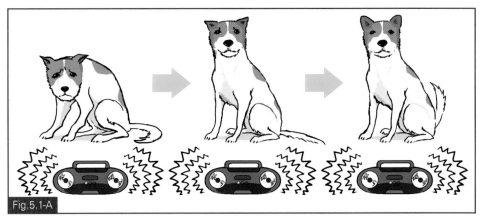

Fig.5.1-A

Fig.5.1-A: With **habituation**, the animal's response to the stimulus gradually decreases due to repeat exposure with no positive or negative consequences. So initially he may be fearful of the sound from a radio, but over time, since there are no negative consequences, the fear response diminishes.

Habituation is one of the simplest and most common forms of learning. One of the major functions of habituation is to teach animals what not to fear. As discussed in Chapter 1, the default setting for animals in nature is to be fearful of all objects and other animals that they have not specifically identified as being safe. This is why wild animals don't come walking out of the woods to congregate with humans around the campfire like characters in an animated cartoon. Fear has an important survival value. Those who aren't naturally afraid of new things are most likely to end up on some predator's dinner plate. (Figures 5.1-B,C,D)

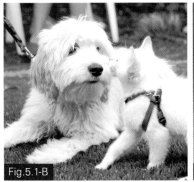
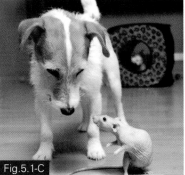
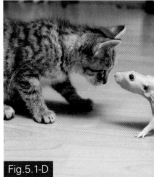

Fig.5.1-B   Fig.5.1-C   Fig.5.1-D

Fig.5.1-B, C, D: The white kitten and naked rat have been socialized to many animals, people and environments during their sensitive period for socialization. As a result, they have generalized their habituation. The kitten expects dogs to be friendly and the rat expects the same from dogs and cats. This generalized habituation or socialization to many different species, individuals and environments is important for animals living as companions to humans. The same degree of habituation in an animal living in the wild would greatly shorten the animal's lifespan, though. In fact, because the Jack Russell Terrier greeting the rat has a history of killing wild rats in his yard, it's likely that if this pet naked rat encountered him for the first time outside in an unsupervised situation, she would also be dead.

Habituation accounts for why the local squirrel seems to be teasing your dog by standing in a tree just out of reach, and it explains why deer can graze near a road with many passing cars. Initially, the squirrel is afraid of your dog and the deer is afraid of cars, but because both the tree and the road regions contain resources such as food, they watch warily and stick around. When nothing bad happens to them, they learn that from their safe spots in the tree and on the side of the road, the barking dog on the ground and the moving cars passing by are not dangerous. Consequently, they do not flee.

Habituation is context specific. When our pets habituate to certain stimuli, like loud noises and new objects, we're surprised that they still react to the same stimuli in different surroundings or contexts. That is, they don't generalize. It's important for habituation to be specific at first. If the squirrel learns that he's safe from the dogs when he's in a tree and then also holds his position when the dog rushes over to him when he's on the ground, habituation will have led to his early demise. Similarly, if the deer that learns that moving cars on the road are safe remains stationary the first time a car pulls to the side of the road, he could possibly end up mounted on a wall. Habituation can generalize, but usually only after the animal has habituated to the specific stimuli under many different contextual variations. (Figures 5.1-E and 5.1-F)

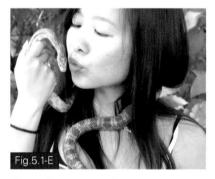

Fig.5.1-E: Iris is comfortable holding the corn snake. However, just because she has habituated to one type of snake doesn't mean she will generalize this to all snakes.

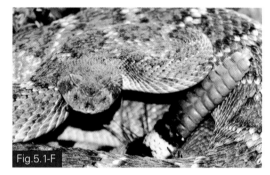

Fig.5.1-F: If Iris did generalize to all snakes and tried to pick up this venomous one, she would be injured and possibly die.

Habituation can be divided into two subcategories: flooding and desensitization.

5.1.1 Flooding.

With flooding, the animal is exposed to the full-force stimulus (Yin 2004; Wright et al. 2005). Inexperienced pet owners commonly try this with their animals. They introduce their cat to a dog by holding the cat in place while the dog comes up to greet him, or they get their dog used to having his toenails trimmed just by holding him down while trimming his nails. Ideally, the dog would gradually get used to the stimulus. But more often, if the animal is extremely fearful, several problems can occur.

Problem 1: Animals can become sensitized to the frightening stimulus. (Figure 5.1-G) That is, they become more fearful and reactive. For instance, at first it may take a fairly loud sound or a large spider to elicit a fear response. But once sensitized, even a soft sound or a picture of a spider may cause a fearful reaction. (Figures 5.1-H, I, J)

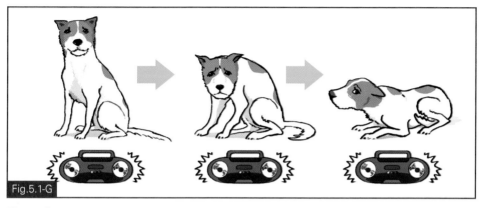

Fig.5.1-G: With **sensitization**, the animal becomes more fearful of the frightening stimulus. Here the dog initially has a moderate fear response to the radio. Over time, his response to even low-level sound becomes severe.

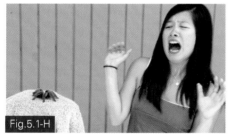

Fig.5.1-H: While Iris likes snakes, she is afraid of spiders. Some people suggest that animals (and humans) should just face their fears by being placed into the situation that causes them to be fearful. If you were afraid of spiders, would having spiders placed on or near you for extended periods of time teach you to face your fear?

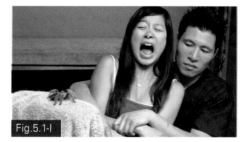

Fig.5.1-I: Holding Iris stationary so that she has to "face her fears" while the spider is placed near her does not make Iris feel more comfortable. She remains afraid. In fact, doing this can sensitize her to spiders such that she starts having nightmares. She could even generalize her fear to pictures of spiders and fake spiders.

Fig.5.1-J: In fact, even flooding her with toy spiders makes her anxious. Her internal emotional state is not changing.

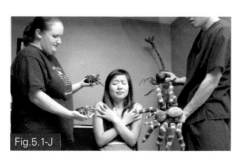

Problem 2: The animal exposed to flooding might never improve. A second problem with flooding is that, even if the animal does not become sensitized to the stimulus, he might simply never improve. (Figures 5.1-K and 5.1-L) Similarly, you may have a spider in your house that you see every day, but you may never get used to or feel comfortable around it.

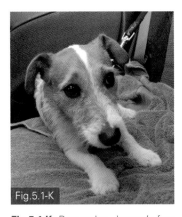

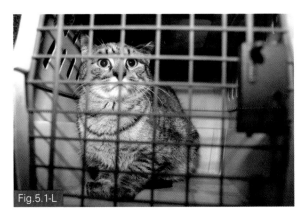

Fig.5.1-K: Remember Jonesy's fear of car rides? (see Chapter 1) He remained afraid even after riding in the car 5 times a week for up to 4 hours at a time over the course of a year.

Fig.5.1-L: Patients in veterinary hospitals are commonly flooded. Other dogs and cats, loud sounds and unfamiliar people are all presented at high intensities or too close. On repeated visits, fearful cats usually do not improve. If kept under these conditions long enough (hours, days or weeks), some might improve while others would remain fearful.

5.1.2 Desensitization.

A more useful form of habituation is desensitization. With desensitization, the stimulus is initially situated far away from the animal or somehow made weaker or less intense. (Figures 5.1-M,N,O) When the pet gets used to the low-level stimulus, the strength of it is gradually increased or it's moved closer (Yin 2004; Wright et al. 2005). Ideally, the level would increase slowly enough so that the animal never reacts fearfully, or barely reacts to the stimulus; otherwise, he could become sensitized. Stimulus intensity should only be increased when the animal has no reaction at the current level.

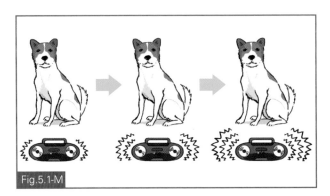

Fig.5.1-M: With **desensitization**, the animal is exposed to the stimulus at increasing intensity levels. Ideally, the animal should never react strongly to the stimulus and the intensity should only increase once the animal reliably has no fear response at the current level. That is, the stimulus should always be presented below the animal's fear threshold.

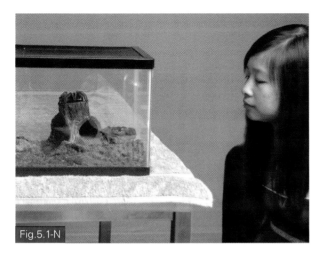

Fig.5.1-N

Fig.5.1-N: This is the correct first step in the desensitization process for Iris. Here, she can get used to the spider at her own rate. It's in a terrarium from which she knows it can't escape and get to her. She can choose the distance at which she's comfortable. If you're attempting to desensitize an animal and he displays a fear posture or tries to get away, then the animal is above his fear threshold and you are desensitizing incorrectly, or not at all.

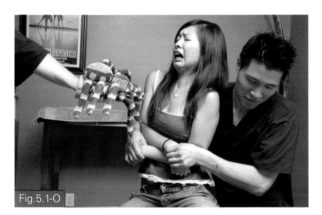

Fig.5.1-O

Fig.5.1-O: Often we start with a stimulus level that seems low to us, but if the animal shows a strong response then we are actually flooding, not desensitizing. For instance, here we attempt to desensitize using a puppet spider. The fact that Iris has a strong fear response tells us that she is not being desensitized. Our goal with desensitization is to get little or no fear response at each step.

While desensitization usually works better than flooding, if used alone it is still a fairly weak form of behavior modification. It works best with objects or stimuli that only induce a weak fear response. If you were extremely fearful of spiders, imagine how long it would take for you to get used to having them around just through desensitization. You might get used to having a spider around in a terrarium and not think twice about it. But even if you sat next to the terrarium for an hour a day, the next step of having the spider outside of its enclosure might be difficult. And working up to the step where you're never startled by the spider no matter where it suddenly appears could take a very long time.

But there is a solution. Desensitization can be combined with two more powerful methods of modification: operant and classical counterconditioning (Wright et al. 2005). When performed appropriately, both of these methods can change the underlying emotional state that drives the behavior.

5.2 Counterconditioning

(Videos 2 and 3)

The goal of counterconditioning is to change the emotional/physiological response to a stimulus or to train an alternate incompatible behavior. It goes a step further than habituation when applied appropriately, because when addressing fear, it emphasizes an actual positive response as its goal, whereas desensitization strives to achieve only a neutral response to the stimulus.

5.2.1 Classical counterconditioning. (Figures 5.2-A and 5.2-B)

With classical counterconditioning, a new association is classically conditioned. In other words, we train a different emotional and physiological response to the situation. For instance, if a cat is fearful of carriers, he's taught that good things happen when he's near the carrier (e.g., he gets food when he goes near or into the carrier). If a dog is fearful of loud noises, we teach him to associate tasty dog treats or play with the loud sounds. Initially, the carrier or loud noise elicits a fear response that includes a spike in corticosteroids (stress hormones) and triggers a behavioral response—either flight, fight or freeze—as a manifestation of the internal emotional state. Our goal is to teach the cat or dog an incompatible emotional response, so we give treats regardless of the animal's behavior. The idea is that by changing the emotional state, the behavior will then change, too. Usually, counterconditioning is combined with desensitization (DS/CC). *(Videos 4-7)*

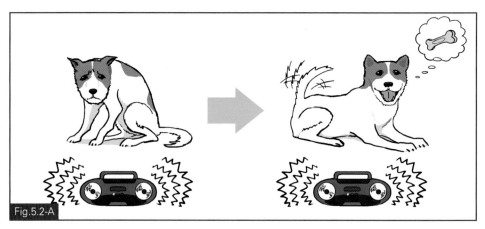

Fig.5.2-A

Fig.5.2-A: Classical counterconditioning focuses on changing the animal's emotional response to a stimulus. For instance, if a dog is fearful of sound from a radio, we can pair food or play with the stimulus so that we classically condition a positive emotional response.

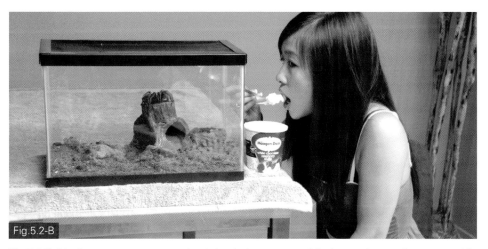

Fig.5.2-B

Fig.5.2-B: Iris demonstrates an example of classical counterconditioning as she eats ice cream while looking at the spider. If she only gets to eat ice cream when she's around the spider, she can quickly learn to associate the spider in the terrarium with positive experiences. This is different from desensitization or habituation, through which she would just learn to tune out the spider or get used to its presence but not actually learn to associate it with something positive.

5.2.2 Operant counterconditioning. (Figure 5.2-C)

Operant counterconditioning is when an animal is trained to perform an alternate, incompatible behavior (Wright et al. 2005). For instance, if a dog lunges and barks every time he sees another dog, train him to watch you and perform tricks so that he focuses on you whenever he sees a dog. The routine changes from "see other dogs and bark like a maniac" to "see other dogs and pay attention to my owner," because doing so will earn treats for good behavior.

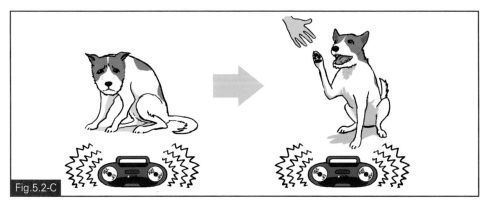

Fig.5.2-C

Fig.5.2-C: With operant counterconditioning, the animal is rewarded for performing an alternate, incompatible behavior. So if the dog growls and barks at the radio he fears, you can train him to instead focus on you and perform tricks. For operant counterconditioning to be effective, the alternate behavior must be one the animal enjoys so that the underlying emotional state can be changed too.

As with classical counterconditioning, pair this with desensitization. Start at a distance where the stimulus is weak and gradually work your way closer. For operant counterconditioning to work in this type of case, it's imperative to get the animal to focus on you instead of on the object causing the reaction. Many trainers mistakenly make their dog sit or lie down and continue to focus on the stimulus in this high-arousal situation. Consequently, the dog may not be barking or lunging at the object, but his mind and attention are still on the object.

Additionally, in cases where the animal is aggressive to or fearful of another animal or object, be sure to use positive reinforcement and make sure the animal is performing behaviors he enjoys. This is essential because it is still important to change the underlying emotional state that's driving the behavior. Every time operant conditioning is used, classical conditioning is also occurring. So the animal is learning not only an alternate behavior, but also an association. If an aversive is used, the animal might learn to associate the other dog or person with pain or a bad experience, which could make him act more aggressively. That is, if the underlying emotional state is not addressed, then the outward emotional response is not likely to change permanently. *(Video 8)*

> When you are using operant counterconditioning to modify behavior in aggressive or fearful animals, be sure to use positive reinforcement and make sure the animal is performing behaviors he enjoys. Every time operant conditioning is used, classical conditioning is also occurring. So the animal is learning not only an alternate behavior, but also an association. If an aversive is used, the animal might learn to associate the initial stimulus with pain or a bad experience, which could make him act more aggressively. That is, if the underlying emotional state is not addressed, then the outward emotional response is not likely to change permanently.

5.3 Use and Misuse of the Behavior Modification Methods

While the general population tends to jump right to flooding, the most effective behavior modification method is actually the combination of desensitization and counterconditioning. A study by Poppen (1970) compared the effects of flooding, desensitization, classical counterconditioning and classical counterconditioning paired with desensitization (DS/CC) for eliminating rats' fearful responses to a tone that had previously been paired with shock. Rats who received DS/CC improved significantly faster and more effectively than those who received the other modification techniques. *(Video 9)*

Casual observers watching someone tossing treats to a fearful, barking dog in hopes of modifying the behavior through DS/CC might ask, "But aren't you rewarding the barking behavior?" *(Video 10)* It turns out that the underlying change in emotional state induced by the classical counterconditioning outweighs the operant conditioning that might occur (Wright et al. 2004). In laboratory counterconditioning studies performed on rats who have been trained to associate a tone with an aversive such as a shock, the rats typically freeze due to fear when they hear the tone, even in the absence of the shock. If the tone is then paired with food many times, such that the rat receives food when he's performing the freezing behavior, the freezing does not increase. Rather, it decreases and instead the rats tend to orient to the feeder and salivate.

So why might owners imagine that their dog seems to bark more with classical counterconditioning? One explanation is that they are classically counterconditioning in an ineffective manner. This is most likely to occur if the owner uses classical counterconditioning without combining it with desensitization. Doing so makes it difficult to keep the dog in the desired alternate emotional state (below his reactivity threshold). A similar situation occurs when food is not tossed frequently enough or play isn't intense or interactive enough to keep the dog in the desired emotional state. Occasionally, behaviors such as the barking that accompanies fear can be reinforced; however, because the emotional state changes, the characteristic of the barks as well as the attitude and behavior of the dog changes.

One case that illustrates this point is the Treat and Train Professional Dog Training System clinical trial (Yin 2008). During the trial, dogs were taught to run to a rug and lie calmly in the face of door-related distractions. Several of the participating owners did accidentally reward barking behavior temporarily. When they were counterconditioning dogs to the knocking of the door, they unknowingly presented the knocking stimulus too loudly at first, causing the dogs to bark, and then they intermittently rewarded the dogs after they barked. The tone of the barks changed from the low-pitched, harsh, unmodulated barks characteristic of dogs in a disturbance situation (Yin and McCowan 2004) to a higher-pitched, more pitch-modulated and more tonal bark that was consistent with play. The dogs also adopted different postures. Whereas before they had been tense and highly aroused, now their tails wagged and they showed less tension. Also, when they barked, their attention was not always directed at the door; they would bark and then look at the Treat and Train as if expecting treats. And, in spite of rewarding the barking behavior, the dogs barked less than they had before starting the protocol. In each case, when the owners later paired desensitization with classical counterconditioning correctly, the barking decreased drastically.

Definitions

Habituation can be divided into flooding and desensitization.

- Flooding: Present the stimulus full force until the animal stops reacting to it. The animal no longer notices or responds to the stimulus because the stimulus has no aversive or pleasurable consequences.

- Desensitization: Present the stimulus at a low level so that the animal does not respond to it, and gradually increase the strength of the stimulus until the animal no longer responds even to the full-force stimulus. For desensitization to work well, be sure the animal has no response at the given level of stimulus before moving on to the next level.

Counterconditioning can be divided into classical counterconditioning and operant counterconditioning.

- Classical counterconditioning: Train an association that's opposite to a previous, classically conditioned association. Remember that with classical counterconditioning, the animal's emotional state and physiological response is changing, which should result in a behavioral change.

- Operant counterconditioning: Train an alternate behavior that's incompatible with the problem behavior. Usually, for operant counterconditioning to work, the animal must associate the alternate behavior with pleasurable consequences so that the underlying emotional state that drives the behavior also changes.

References

Leussis, M.P., and V.J. Bolivar. 2006. Habituation in rodents: A review of behavior, neurobiology, and genetics. *Neuroscience and Biobehavioral Reviews* 30:1045-64.

Poppen, R. 1970. Counterconditioning of conditioned suppression in rats. *Psychological Reports* 27:659-71.

Wright, J.C., P.J. Reid, and Z. Rozier. 2005. Treatment of emotional distress and disorders—Non-pharmacologic methods. In *Mental Health and Well-being in Animals*, ed. F.D. McMillan, 145-58. Ames, Iowa: Blackwell Publishing.

Yin, S. 2004. *How to Behave So Your Dog Behaves*. Neptune City, N.J.: TFH Publications.

Yin, S., E. Fernandez, E. Richardson, S. Pagan, and D. Snyder. 2008. Efficacy of a remote-controlled positive reinforcement protocol for training dogs to behave at the door. *Applied Animal Behaviour Science* 113:123-38.

Yin, S., and B. McCowan. 2004. Barking in domestic dogs: Context specificity and individual identification. *Animal Behaviour* 68:343-55.

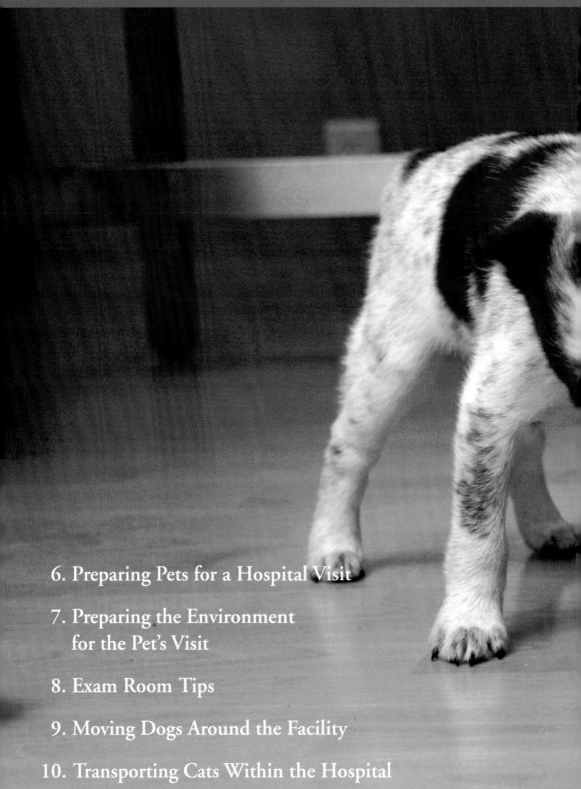

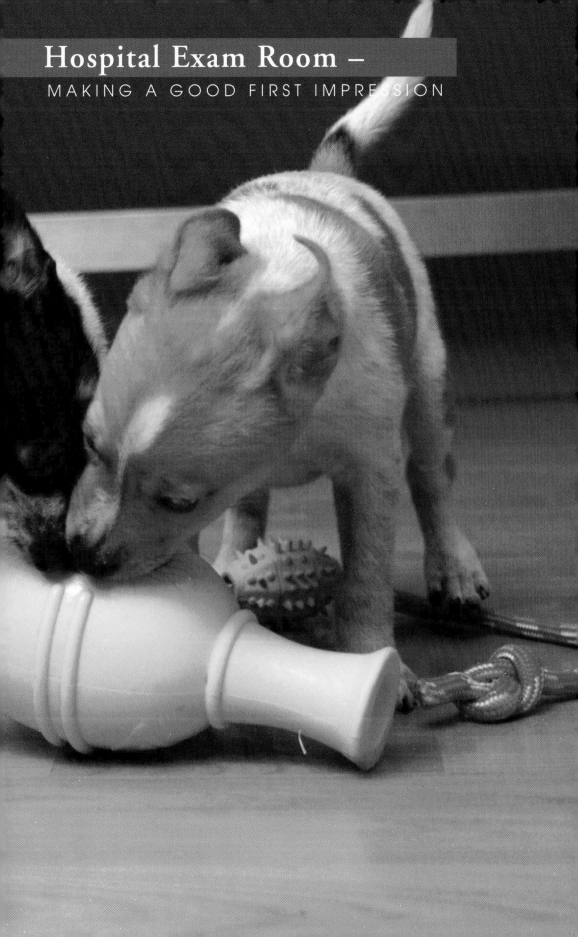

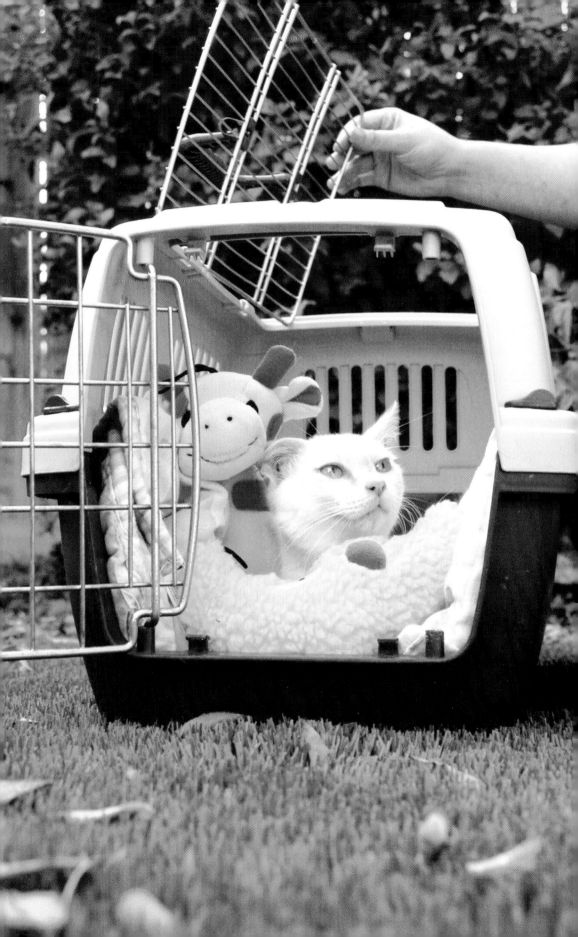

CHAPTER 6.
PREPARING PETS
For A Hospital Visit

It's a scene right out of a movie. The victim's kidnapped, stuffed in a little box, taken on a bumpy ride and then left in a strange room where she waits anxiously. Her fear pulses erratically with each glimpse of the strangers holding her captive.

Check list to help owners prepare their pets for a great veterinary visit.

Owners should first train their pet to:

- enjoy being in the travel crate (be sure to make it comfortable; include a towel for cats);

- love car rides.

They should bring:

- a hungry pet;

- a meal that you withheld that day;

- treats;

- a favorite toy;

- a towel or bandana sprayed with Feliway for cats or Dog Appeasing Pheromone (DAP) for dogs, if these have been shown to decrease anxiety in their pet. Catnip (for cats) and lavender oil (for dogs) can also decrease anxiety in some patients.

Sounds like fiction, but it's a regular event for most of our feline patients and many of our canine patients, too. To them, being tossed in a crate or carrier and forced to ride in a car are about as enjoyable as being abducted by aliens. With such a harrowing preview of the plot to come, it's no wonder they arrive in a state of yellow alert. If they've also never learned to enjoy, or at least accept, new people and other pets, then sitting in a waiting room filled with these potential predators places them in the role of a prisoner waiting to become the main course in a tribal feast.

While we can't thoroughly address possible issues of fear until we actually see them for the first time, we can at least ensure that they arrive at the hospital in a happy state. Provide clients with simple instructions for teaching their pets to enjoy their crates and car rides. Then make sure the pet enters the hospital hungry, and tell the client to bring their pet's withheld meal along with treats and even a favorite toy. These steps will improve the likelihood that we can make the visit enjoyable and even win the dog's or cat's trust.

6.1 Crate Training Is a Good Thing!

To those who are new to the concept of crate training, confinement in such a small space might seem like some sort of medieval torture. But free-roaming dogs seek shelter in small, enclosed spaces and feral cats hide in small, dark spaces to avoid being eaten by coyotes and other predators. In fact, anyone who's visited a person with cats knows that when unfamiliar people enter their home, many cats immediately run for

Crate or carrier training usually takes less than a week, even with the most cranky cat or an adult dog.

cover in places much smaller than a comfy travel carrier. Based on this natural history, one can see how pet dogs and cats can easily be trained to perceive a travel carrier or crate as a cozy cave or a home away from home (and one that can be taken with them wherever they go). In fact, all dogs and cats should be trained to enjoy being in a travel carrier or crate so they feel comfortable traveling. For dogs, in particular, learning to enjoy staying in their crates for extended periods of time can be important for teaching them that it's okay to be alone in their "bedroom." Then they'll be less likely to develop anxiety when separated from their owners down the road. Both dogs and cats can even be trained to sleep quietly in their crates at night.

Training pets to see their crate or carrier as their personal bedroom is simple even for cranky cats and adult dogs, and usually takes less than a week. It's all about teaching them that great things happen when they're in their crate (classical conditioning). The great thing we will use is food. Throughout the process, other motivators can be used, as well.

6.2 Crate Training Dogs

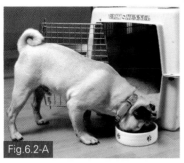

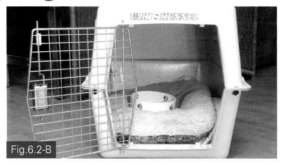

Fig.6.2-A: If the dog really dislikes being confined, start by feeding his daily meals just outside the crate.

Fig.6.2-B: When he's comfortably eating his meals in this new location, move the food just inside the crate so he has to stick his head in to eat. If he's the type of dog who will get scared if he hits the door when going in or out, start with the door removed from the crate.

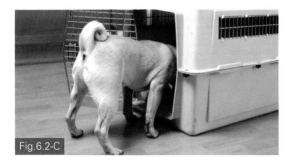

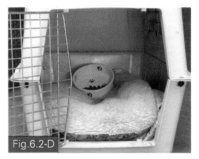

Fig.6.2-C: The dog should readily stick his head inside the crate. If he's comfortable, he'll eat his entire meal without backing out to look around.

Fig.6.2-D: Gradually move the food dish farther inside the crate until the dog easily goes all the way into the crate.

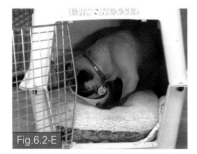

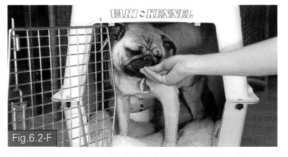

Fig.6.2-E: For most dogs, reaching this point takes less than 3 days of twice-daily feedings.

Fig.6.2-F: Once he's finished with his meal, give him several treats (or kibble) in a row to encourage him to wait in his crate rather than dart out. If the dog is the type to dart out, shove the treat right into his face so that your hand and the treat act like a stop sign blocking his exit.

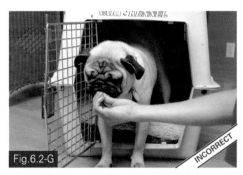

Fig.6.2-G, Incorrect: If the dog is coming out of the crate, either you aren't reaching in far enough or you're delivering the treat too slowly, which makes him think you want him to grab it.

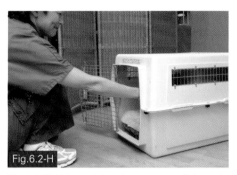

Fig.6.2-H: When giving the treat, reach into the crate and put the treat all the way up to the dog's face, so that you don't accidentally make him come forward out of the crate to get it.

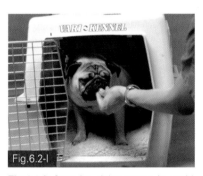

Fig.6.2-I: Start by giving treats in rapid succession, quickly enough to keep him inside. Then slow the rate of giving so that he learns to wait in the crate for 3-5 seconds between treats.

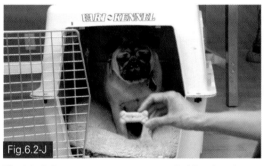

Fig.6.2-J: Between treats, your treat-holding hand must be far enough from the dog that you're not luring him out. Try tossing the treats or kibble in to him. If he reaches for the treat when you're holding them outside the crate, pull the treat away quickly so that it's clear to him that he doesn't get it.

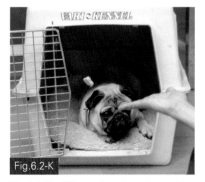

Fig.6.2-K: When the dog is waiting calmly in his crate, toss the treat inside or hand it to him. Repeat this process for 5-10 treats.

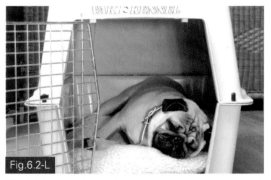

Fig.6.2-L: How do you know when he loves his crate? He will randomly go in it and lie down to rest on his own.

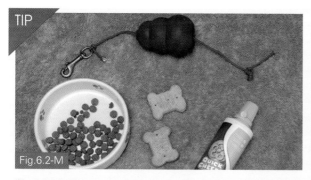

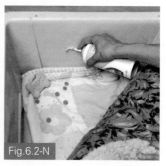

Fig.6.2-M, Tip: Hide tasty treats in the crate for him to find throughout the day. The goal is to have him learn to explore the crate for treats. Consider rigging a Kong toy with treats in it to remain in the crate. To do this, place a rope through the Kong and add a clasp so that you can clip it to the bars of the crate. Fill the Kong with part of his meal or treats, perhaps mixing in some canned food and freezing it to make it last longer.

Fig.6.2-N, Tip: Hide treats under bedding and in the back of the crate so that he has to go all the way inside.

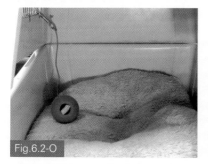

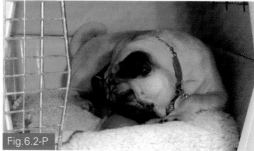

Fig.6.2-O, Tip: Tether a filled Kong toy in the crate so the dog has to eat it there and can't drag it out.

Fig.6.2-P, Tip: The Kong toy makes the meal into a puzzle for the dog—like eating a bone. It allows for a longer period of practice with the door closed. The dog is learning that being in the crate is a pleasant experience.

6.2.1 Teaching dogs to stay in their crate for extended time periods.

Dogs should learn to rest quietly in their crates for extended periods of time; this will help them learn to remain calm when separated from their owners. Many puppies whine and bark when you leave them alone because they want to be where the action is. When this behavior is rewarded at an early age, it can progress to severe separation anxiety such that you can never keep the dog confined in the house or even in a room because he will bark persistently and destroy everything.

Proper crate training helps prevent the development of anxiety and barking when dogs are separated from their owners by a barrier or left alone in the house. For some dogs, the pleasant association already established with the crate is enough to teach them to remain quiet and calm when left in it. For others, as soon as they finish their meal or Kong toy, they start to whine or bark to be let out. These dogs must be specifically trained to be quiet in the closed crate. It's not enough to just have treats in the crate and hope their pleasant experience allows them to rest quietly in the closed crate at all times.

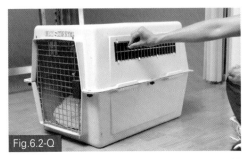
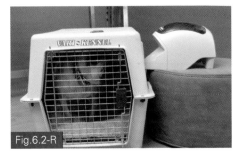

Fig.6.2-Q: Dogs who vocalize in the crate should be rewarded intermittently for being calm and quiet instead. Hang out near the crate and periodically toss treats inside (perhaps do this while you are watching television). Then systematically increase the interval between treats so that you can use fewer and fewer treats. Also, gradually increase your distance from the crate. The dog should eat the treats immediately; failure to do so indicates that the dog is anxious or not hungry and the food is no longer a reward.

Fig.6.2-R: Alternatively, use the MannersMinder remote-controlled, automated dog training system (formerly known as the Treat 'n Train). The food-dispensing portion of the machine can be set to release kibble or round treats at rates of every 3, 5, 7, 10, 15, 20, 25, 30, 45, 60, 120 and 300 seconds. Start with the treats dispensing frequently enough so that the dog does not become anxious and bark. Then systematically teach the dog to remain quiet for longer time periods by increasing the interval between treats. If he does bark, stop giving treats until he's quiet again so that he's not accidentally rewarded for barking. The dog should be let out before he becomes satiated. Eventually, the dog will no longer need treats to remain quiet. Either his meal or treats can be used for the training session.

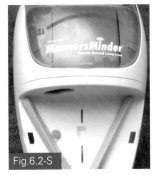
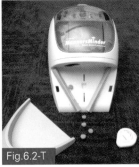
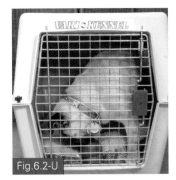

Fig.6.2-S, T: To adapt the MannersMinder for dispensing into crates, remove the food bowl and fold two 3 x 5 index cards and attach them with tape to form a chute. Treats can be dispensed using a remote control or the MannersMinder can be switched to automatic so that it dispenses at a rate that you set.

Fig.6.2-U: To extend the meal when not using a MannersMinder, give the dog a bone or provide a filled Kong.

6.2.2 Teaching the cue word, "kennel" or "crate."

If you want the dog to go into the crate upon hearing a verbal cue, follow the steps below.

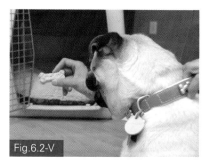

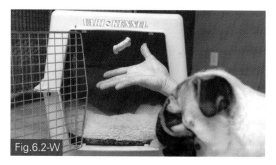

Fig.6.2-V: Once the dog anticipates crating by running in as soon as he sees you bring food, teach him the cue word "kennel" by keeping him outside the crate until you put his meal in it. Hold his collar so he can't get into the kennel. Next, say "crate" or "kennel" right before you release your hold on his collar and let him run into the crate.

Fig.6.2-W: Practice training this cue word randomly throughout the day by walking with the dog toward his crate and saying "kennel" or "crate" right before tossing a treat inside. Say the cue word before you toss the treat so he learns that the word predicts his chance to earn a treat by running into the crate. Alternatively, you can hold his collar so he doesn't have a chance to run into the crate until after you say the cue word, followed by releasing his collar.

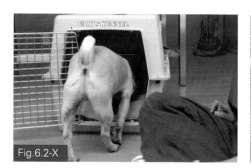

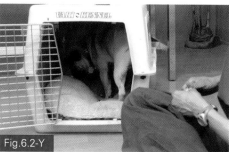

Fig.6.2-X, Y: Once the dog goes inside, toss more treats to the back. You're trying to teach him to stay in there and wait for you to toss more treats.

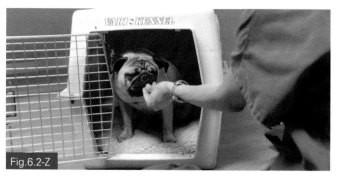

Fig.6.2-Z: Once he turns around to face the crate door, give him treats for sitting or lying patiently inside. Increase the interval between treats so he learns to wait longer to get his treat.

6.2.3 Switching from lure to reinforcement to train entering on cue.

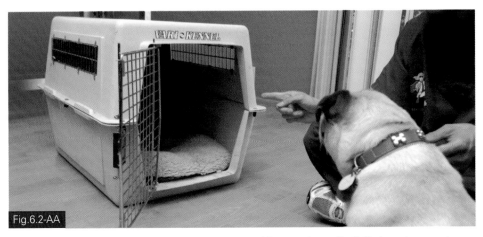

Fig.6.2-AA: When you toss the treat into the crate and he runs in readily 5-10 times in a row in one session, try it without a food lure. To switch from lure to reinforcement, first hold the dog's collar while he's facing the crate. Because he's gotten lots of rewards when in the crate, he'll want to go in. Hide a treat behind your back or in your hand, or even have one already in his kennel (one that he didn't see you put in there). Say "kennel" and then release his collar.

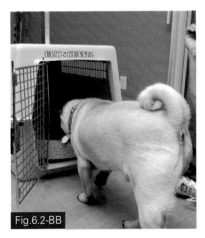

Fig.6.2-BB: Because he's reliably gone into the crate 5-10 times immediately prior to this, he should do so easily now.

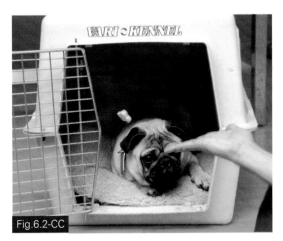

Fig.6.2-CC: After the dog is in, toss him the treat. Again, throw in additional treats to reward him for staying put.

6.2.4 Using other reinforcers.

If you think the dog will be difficult, add other reinforcers to speed the training. Use the things that most motivate the dog. If he loves to play fetch, then try a tennis ball. If he craves attention, maybe even whining and barking for it, then train him that the best way to get your attention is to go lie quietly in his crate.

Toys *(Video 1)*

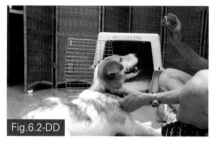

Fig.6.2-DD: Start by using the toy as a lure; show it to him.

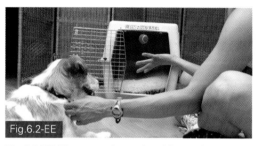

Fig.6.2-EE: Then toss the toy in while you hold the dog's collar.

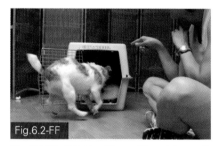

Fig.6.2-FF: Tell him "kennel" and immediately release his collar so he has the opportunity to run into the crate.

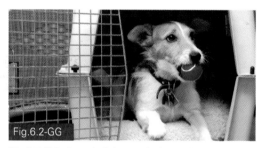

Fig.6.2-GG: Once he's in, try playing with him while he remains in his crate. Have him give you the toy or trade the toy for treats. Then toss the toy back in again.

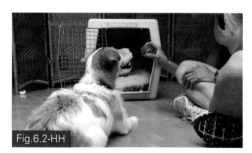

Fig.6.2-HH: Once the dog can perform the above exercises with a toy 5-10 times in a row, start the next step where you switch to using the toy as a reinforcer rather than using it to lure him in. Begin by either showing him the ball or hiding it behind your back.

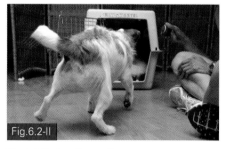

Fig.6.2-II: Say "kennel' but don't toss the toy in. Because he's performed the previous step so many times, he should automatically run in. If he doesn't, then continue to work on the previous step.

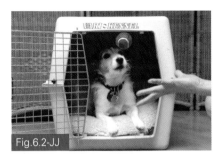

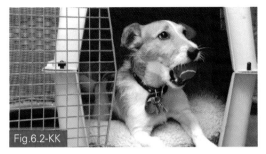

Fig.6.2-JJ: Once he's in, toss the toy before he runs out.

Fig.6.2-KK: Repeat this until he consistently runs in right after you say "kennel" and stays there, expecting you to toss the ball in. Some dogs may prefer that you toss the ball away from the kennel so they can play fetch.

Petting and attention

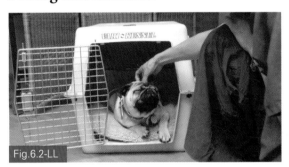

Fig.6.2-LL: Some dogs love petting and even demand it by whining or barking. For these dogs, crate training should focus on petting the dog when he goes into the crate. Once he's in, pet him in 5- to 10- second intervals. Stop for 5-10 seconds, then repeat the petting to reward for remaining quiet and in the crate.

6.3 Carrier Training Cats

Carrier training cats is identical to training dogs, but fewer steps are required.

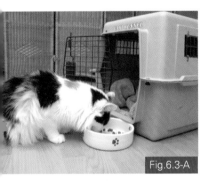

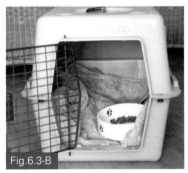

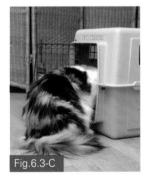

Fig.6.3-A: If the cat really dislikes being confined, start by feeding her daily meals just outside the carrier.

Fig.6.3-B: When she's comfortably eating her meals in this new location, move the food just inside the carrier so she has to stick her head in to eat.

Fig.6.3-C: She should readily stick her head in. When she's comfortable, she'll eat the meal without backing out to look around.

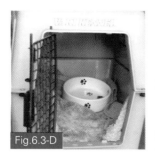

Fig.6.3-D

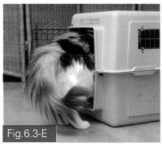

Fig.6.3-E

Fig.6.3-D: In this manner, gradually move the food dish farther in until the cat easily goes all the way into the carrier.

Fig.6.3-E: For most cats, getting to this point takes less than 3-4 days.

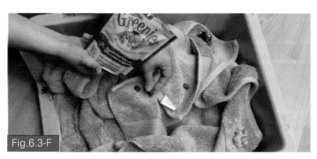

Fig.6.3-F

Fig.6.3-F: Hide tasty treats or toys (whichever she's most motivated by) in the carrier for her to find throughout the day. The goal is for her to learn to explore the carrier for treats or toys.

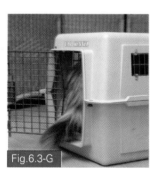

Fig.6.3-G

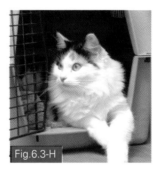

Fig.6.3-H

Fig.6.3-G: The cat should always readily enter the carrier and walk out in a relaxed manner. If she looks vigilant or rushes out, then work in more gradual steps.

Fig.6.3-H: How do you know when the cat loves her carrier? When she randomly enters and lies down to rest on her own. Some cats even choose to sleep in their carriers.

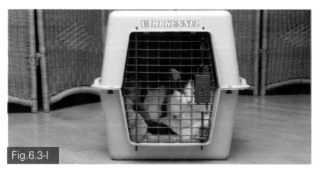

Fig.6.3-I

Fig.6.3-I: Once the cat comfortably enters her carrier to rest, the carrier door can be closed during her meal, and she can be kept in the carrier for short periods of time. Gradually work up to enclosing her for longer sessions. This step is optional for cats, whereas for dogs it's required. Cats often adapt better than dogs to being in travel carriers.

Completing all of these simple steps will leave you with a hound or housecat that thinks his crate or carrier is a heavenly haven.

6.4 Training for Car Rides

Dogs and cats should be kept safe in vehicles either by confining them in travel crates or seat-belting them in place. Without restraint, some dogs won't wait until arriving at the park to start playing; to them, the car is their moving playground. Other pets are just a nuisance in the car and can distract the owners enough to cause a car accident. Additionally, when the driver is forced to suddenly swerve or stop, unrestrained pets are easily injured.

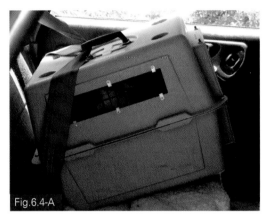
Fig.6.4-A

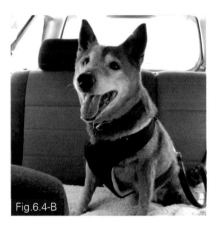
Fig.6.4-B

Fig.6.4-A: Cats and small dogs can travel in their safe-haven carrier, which should be belted to prevent the pet from being jostled about. A rough ride can cause the pet to become fearful.

Fig.6.4-B: A dog who won't be in a travel carrier should be on leash with someone holding the other end or seat-belted so that she remains somewhat stationary.

The First Car Ride

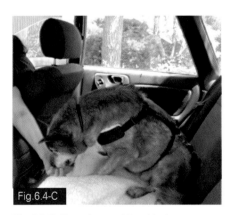
Fig.6.4-C

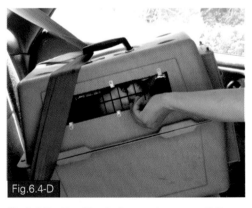
Fig.6.4-D

Fig.6.4-C: Start the car ride with the pet on an empty stomach. Give treats during the ride so that the pet associates it with good things. If she's hungry, she'll eat the treats once she's somewhat relaxed.

Fig.6.4-D: Hand-feed the treats sequentially or just toss a bunch into the crate or onto the seat. Note that if you're driving to a veterinary visit, limit the number of treats given in the car so the pet does not get satiated, since food may be used for counterconditioning at the hospital.

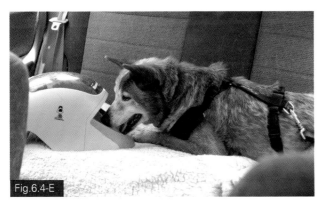

Fig.6.4-E: If traveling alone, consider using the MannersMinder to dispense treats for both dogs and cats. This works best if they have already gone through part of the protocol for traveling and the animal has been previously trained using the MannersMinder. For dogs who learned to down-stay using the MannersMinder, require the dog to lie down first before having the machine automatically release treats.

Be sure that the first ride is short so that the pet doesn't have time to get nauseous. And consider the driver's driving skills—don't make the pet sick with fast turns and sudden stops. End in a location that your dog or cat likes. For most cats, this means returning home. Practice these short car rides until your pet acts relaxed all the time, then increase the driving distance. Usually, after only a few rides, dogs will be comfortable in the car; cats might require a few more trips.

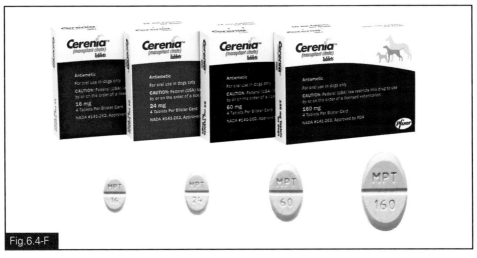

Fig.6.4-F: If the dog gets car sick, consider trying Cerenia (Pfizer Animal Health, New York), an antimetic (maropitant citrate) for motion sickness. Cerenia should be given at least 2 hours before travel but after food has been withheld for 1 hour, for fastest absorption. Because each treatment lasts 24 hours, it can be given 1 hour after the dog's dinner the night before the dog will travel in the car. To prevent gastric upset, it should be wrapped loosely in a small amount of food such as peanut butter, spreadable cheese or deli meat slices. Wrapping tightly in food such as placement in Pill Pockets, hot dogs or sausage will delay the absorption of the medication.

6.5 Using Food as a Motivator

Owners should bring their pets to the hospital hungry. Ask them to withhold the previous meal and instead bring it along on the visit, in addition to some of the pet's favorite treats. We want to use food to give the pet a good experience, and this way the animal can get a meal's worth of food in the hospital. Encourage owners to start offering treats in the waiting room. That means that by this point the pet should not need many treats during their car ride to the hospital, or she will no longer be motivated to eat treats during the hospital visit.

In general, cats are less likely than dogs to eat—initially, at least—during a hospital visit. But unless the cat is wasting away and looks like a skin-covered skeleton, she's most likely eating enough to maintain her weight, which means she is food-motivated. She just might not eat when you want her to. One way to get a cat motivated to eat is to have the owner switch from free-feeding to a twice-a-day meal plan. Start by putting down the cat's food and taking it away as soon as she turns away from the food dish. The food can be offered again in 15 minutes or stored until the next mealtime. In general, if food is offered 3-4 times per day, then by the third day she should be

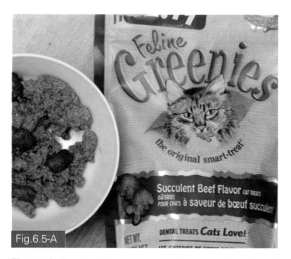

Fig.6.5-A

Fig.6.5-A: To get older cats interested in new foods and treats, mix the new product into their regular meals. At first they might eat around the treats, but eventually if the treats come with their food on a regular basis, they'll try them and get used to them.

on a regular feeding pattern of 2 daily meals. Just as a free-roaming cat quickly learns that she has to eat when she has the chance, a thin, picky housecat will, too.

While dogs, who evolved as scavengers for at least 15,000 years, quickly learn to eat everything in sight, cats can be pickier about what they put in their mouths. It's helpful to have cats accept a variety of foods. We can ensure that cats don't grow up finicky by providing them with many different foods when they're young. To get older cats interested in new foods and treats, mix the new product into their regular meals. (Figure 6.5-A) At first they might eat around the treats, but eventually if the treats come with their food on a regular basis, they'll try them and get used to them. If the treat is tasty, they might even prefer it to their kibble or canned food, at which point it can be reserved for special occasions. Once the cat is regularly eating her treats, use the treats as well as her regular food to reward good behavior throughout the day.

Remind clients that treats should make up no more than 10% of a pet's daily diet and that they should decrease the amount of regular food being fed. Ideally, the pet would work for her regular kibble or canned food and treats would be reserved for more distracting situations.

To download these protocols in pdf form so that they can be posted on your hospital web site and provided to clients, go to www.nerdbook.com/ lowstresshandling

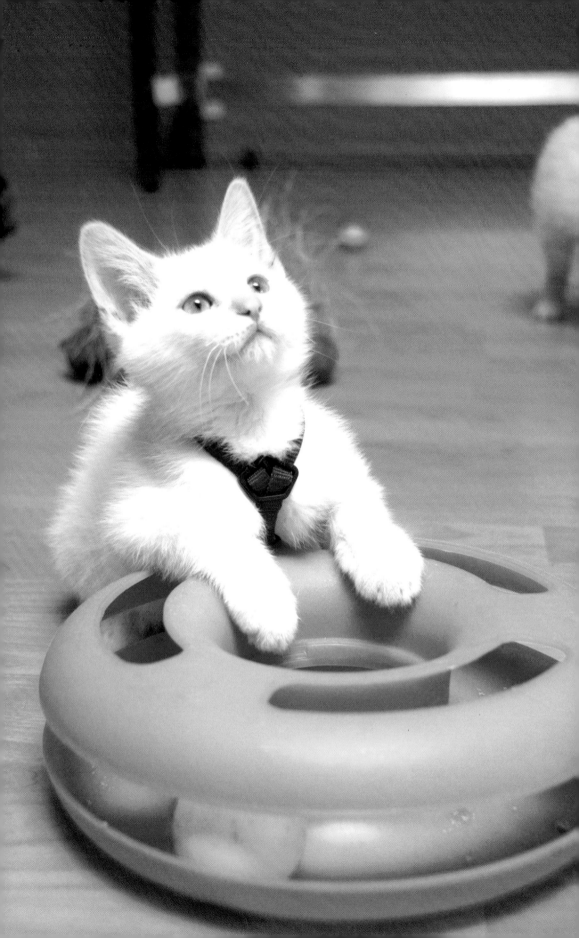

CHAPTER 7
PREPARING THE ENVIRONMENT
For the Pet's Visit

The record from the referring vet gave the reason for the visit: "Caution" stamped in red. "Extremely aggressive to technicians and veterinarians when they approach," stated the description in the file. "Doesn't like anyone and no one can get close." Then the patient, a middle-aged blonde Cocker Spaniel, walked into the behavior consult room, tail wagging, and immediately sat for treats. "Wow! She usually doesn't do that at the vet hospital," said her owner incredulously. "Usually by this point they're asking me to muzzle her."

So what's the difference? This hospital doesn't look like a hospital. The waiting room is quiet, rather than filled with barking dogs. The upstairs lobby is carpeted and the behavior room has both throw rugs and plush chairs. For the little blonde Cocker, visiting this hospital is more like visiting the home of a friend. Additionally, in the reception area she got a yummy treat while her owner checked her in. Normally she'd be too nervous in the hectic hospital environment to take treats, but in this comfortable environment she was more relaxed. She also didn't have to sit on a cold, uninviting metal scale. This hospital's scale was covered with a comfortable towel or rug. In the exam room, where she might start becoming scared, the first things she experienced were a happy voice and her favorite treats.

> The environment the pet enters sets the tone for the appointment. It's imperative to start with a pet-friendly environment that will put even the less-socialized pets at ease. Doing so will cut down the amount of counterconditioning necessary, the number of technicians required and the chemical restraint needed to deal with patients.

The environment the pet enters sets the tone for the appointment. It's imperative to start with a pet-friendly environment that will put even the less-socialized pets at ease. Doing so will cut down the amount of counterconditioning necessary, the number of technicians required and the chemical restraint needed to deal with patients. The following are examples of ways to improve the hospital setting.

7.1 The Entry

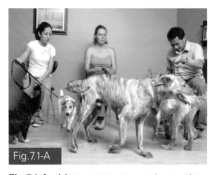

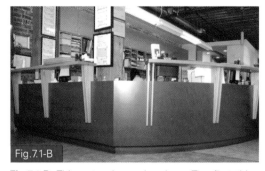

Fig.7.1-A: Many pets are anxious when they go to the hospital. They are often fearful of other animals or people. If they step into the hospital and this is the first thing they see, they could immediately become fearful.

Fig.7.1-B: This setup is much calmer. The first thing dogs and cats see is a reception desk. People waiting at the desk will most likely be looking away from them rather than staring at them. Few dogs and cats will be directly in the line of sight. In this hospital, the waiting areas are recessed to the right and left.

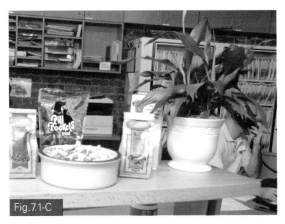

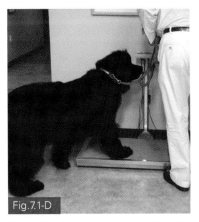

Fig.7.1-C: Treats should be placed in strategic locations such as the reception desk, so that the receptionists can give treats to the dogs and cats. This immediately builds a positive relationship with the patients and clients.

Fig.7.1-D: Another ideal location for treats is near the scale. This dog refused to get on the scale until treats were offered. For weighing cats, each exam room should have its own cat scale.

7.2 The Waiting Room *(Video 1)*

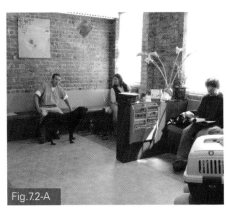

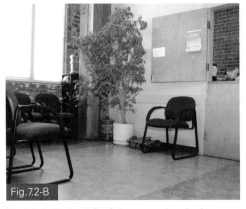

Fig.7.2-A: Provide species-specific waiting areas. In this hospital, to the right of the entry door is a large, recessed waiting room. This dog-only waiting area is further subdivided by a short visual barrier so that animals can still be somewhat separated. The room has a television set and coffee for the comfort of the clients. Keeping clients comfortable helps keep the patients comfortable.

Fig.7.2-B: To the left of the entry door in the same hospital is a small, recessed cat-only waiting room. Consider using a Feliway pheromone diffuser (Ceva Animal Health, Lenexa, Kansas) as it can have a marked calming effect on some cats.

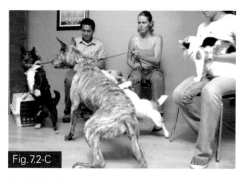

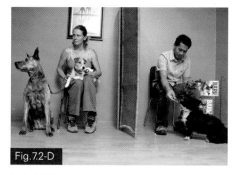

Fig.7.2-C: Crowded multi-species waiting rooms that lack dividers can lead to anxiety for both feline and canine patients. Once aroused, these patients often are fearful or aggressive for the rest of their visit.

Fig.7.2-D: Even small rooms can be subdivided easily by using inexpensive privacy screens.

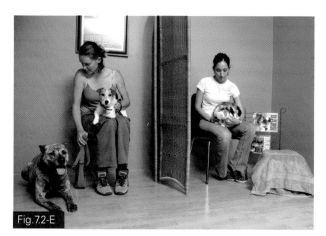

Fig.7.2-E: Hospitals should have separate cat and dog areas. Providing towels to drape over cat carriers can help cats feel more secure and alleviate some fear, since this will prevent them from seeing other cats. Whenever possible, place both cats and dogs who are nervous in the waiting room into a quiet exam room as quickly as possible.

7.3 The Scale

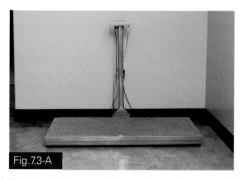

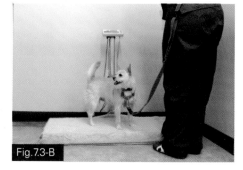

Fig.7.3-A: For many dogs and cats, the second fearful event in the hospital is being forced onto a metal foreign object—the scale.

Fig.7.3-B: Scales can be made appealing by placing a towel or rug on them. Non-slip drawer liners can be placed under the towel, if needed.

7.4 The Exam Room

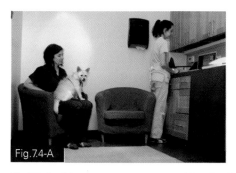
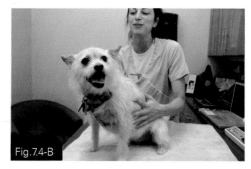

Fig.7.4-A: Many exam rooms are cold and uninviting. This behavior consult room is comfortable. A majority of dogs who are fearful in veterinary hospitals become comfortable in this particular room. Just adding a washable bath rug or throw rug makes the room cozier for the pet. The exam table folds out from the counter, allowing for more space in the room.

Fig.7.4-B: The dog pictured here has a history of fear aggression, especially at the veterinary hospital. But in this comfortable, quiet room, the technician is easily able to get the pet into a happy play mode. She relaxes and enjoys being petted. Notice the towel on the table for comfort. This particular hospital uses many towels. Due to the volume of towels used, they invest in a laundry service. This allows technicians to spend time treating patients rather than doing laundry or calling for repair service for the washer and dryer.

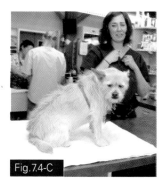
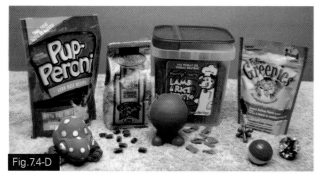

Fig.7.4-C: Here is the same dog in the busy treatment room. She is quiet, occasionally cowers and looks as if she is falling asleep. She did not respond to petting from her owner, who is standing next to her. It might be better to perform her treatments or procedures in a private exam room to encourage a good experience and allow her to become more comfortable with each visit.

Fig.7.4-D: Be sure the exam room has a variety of treats and a few rubber or vinyl toys that can easily be cleaned, or inexpensive toys that can be sent home as a gift to the owner. Generally, soft treats such as Lean Treats (Butler Animal Health Supply, Dublin, Ohio) are preferable, but some dogs like hard treats such as Liver Biscotti (Premier Pet, Richmond, Virginia). Many cats won't eat treats at the hospital, however in hospitals where the environment is comfortable, the cats are not first exposed to seeing other animals, and patients are given time to habituate to the exam room, 50% of the cats may eat treats. Cats tend to like tuna, baby food, Feline Greenies, canned food and even canned cheese. Treats and toys used in the exam rooms can also be sold through the hospital.

7.5 Treatment Areas and Kennels

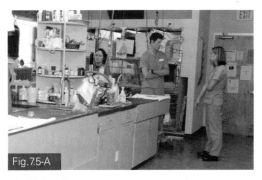

Fig.7.5-A

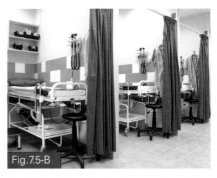

Fig.7.5-B

Fig.7.5-A: The treatment area is frequently the noisiest, most high traffic area of the hospital. This is unfortunate, because sick or fearful pets need a comfortable, quiet environment. Often the sickest animals – including those who are fearful of unfamiliar people, animals and places – are kept in this high stress situation because they must be monitored carefully.

Fig.7.5-B: Note that in human hospitals, patients get private or semi-private rooms with curtains surrounding their bed. We should do our best to provide a similarly restful environment for pets.

Decrease visual contact

Both cats and dogs should be kept in rooms or kennels in which they are unable to see other animals. This usually means the cages are facing a wall rather than another cage. Additionally the hospital should be kept as quiet as possible. Provide cats with hiding spots.

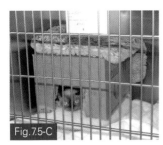

Fig.7.5-C

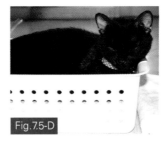

Fig.7.5-D

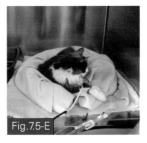

Fig.7.5-E

Fig.7.5-C: Kennels for cats should include hiding places, like this inexpensive cardboard box. Towels can also be draped over a portion of the cage door. A pad on top of the box provides an elevated spot for cats who feel more secure when they can survey their surroundings.

Fig.7.5-D: Baskets or boxes can also be placed so that cats will sleep in them rather than hiding in their litter box.

Fig.7.5-E: For those situations where a catheter is used and it must be visible, make a pet bed from twisted towels.

Reduce noise

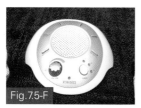

Fig. 7.5-F

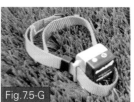

Fig. 7.5-G

Fig.7.5-F: Reducing noise: A white noise machine such as SoundSpa (HoMedic, Commerce Township, Michigan) can be played to help dampen sudden noises.

Fig.7.5-G: In situations where one dog is barking incessantly, the citronella antibark collar (Premier Pet, Midlothian, Virginia), which squirts a short burst of citronella spray when the dog barks, may be used. It has been shown to decrease barking in dogs in a veterinary hospital setting without negative effects on the barking dog (Moffat et al. 2003). But because it's a punishment, it has the potential to increase stress or fear and dogs wearing it should be monitored for such signs. Also because jingling tags and the sound of nearby dogs barking can trigger the spray, dog tags should be removed and the collar only used when the problem involves just one barker.

Pheromones and aromatherapy

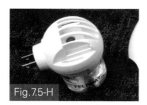

Fig. 7.5-H

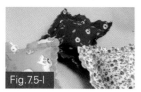

Fig. 7.5-I

Fig.7.5-H, I: Pheromones and aromatherapy: For cats, Feliway diffusers can be used in waiting rooms, exams rooms and treatments rooms to decrease anxiety. It can also be sprayed on towels or bedding. It has a marked effect in some cats. Catnip pillows can be made and given to cats who become calm rather than aroused in its presence. For dogs, Dog Appeasing Pheromone (Ceva Animal Health, Lenexa, Kansas) spray as well as lavender or chamomile oil can be placed on their bedding (Graham et al. 2005).

7.6 The Take-Home Message

These environmental changes are simple but will have a huge impact on the wellbeing of your patients. The lower their stress level, the faster they will recover and the easier they will be to treat. Always remember that noise, as well as the sight and sound of animals and people they fear, will cause pets to become anxious. If you were recovering in a noisy hospital filled with spiders and snakes, it would be difficult to relax enough to recover quickly. Keep this in mind when thinking of ways to devise better healing environments.

References

Graham, L., D.L. Wells, and P.G. Hepper. 2005. The influence of olfactory stimulation on the behaviour or dogs housed in a rescue shelter. *Applied Animal Behaviour Science* 91: 143-153.

Moffat, K.S., G.M. Landsberg, and R. Beaudet. 2003. Effectiveness and comparison of citronella and scentless spray bark collars for the control of barking in a veterinary hospital setting. *Journal of the American Animal Hospital Association* 39:343-348.

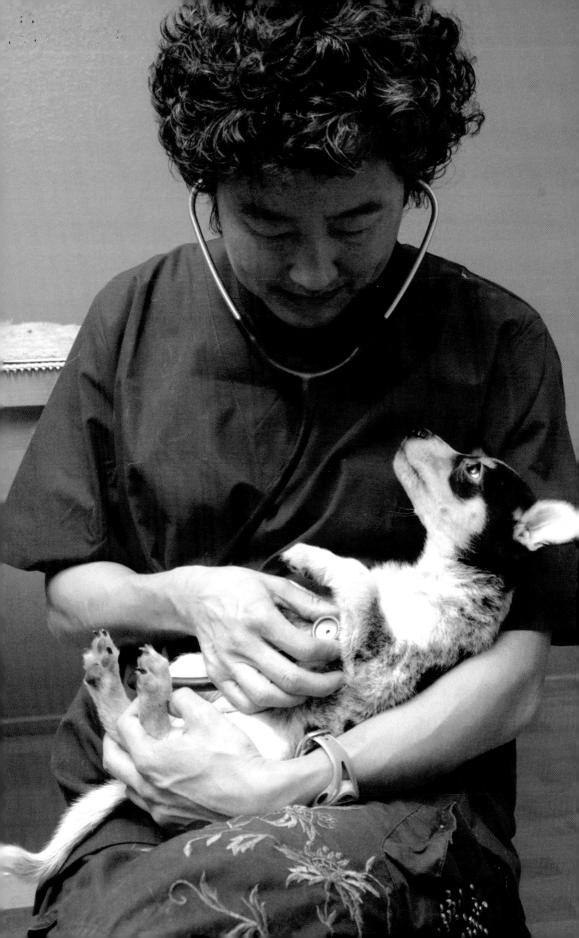

CHAPTER 8.
EXAM ROOM
Tips

My daughter's dentist is great. The first time I took Delaney there, the whole time we were in the waiting room she kept telling me, "There's no way I'm getting in that chair." I thought, "Oh, this is going to be interesting." When it was her turn, the dental hygienist greeted her by saying, "What a pretty dress you're wearing." And immediately Delaney was putty in their hands. She climbed up into the chair and sat through everything just fine. She's been good there ever since. They really know how to deal with kids.

Kelly Moffat, DVM, diplomate ACVB

Delaney's dentist office specializes in dealing with children. The staff is trained to know how to handle kids, and they understand the importance of saying the right thing and greeting in the right manner. This chapter focuses on what veterinarians and staff can do in the exam room: what to "say," how to greet and what to do to make pets see employees as friends rather than foes.

8.1 Toys and Treats

Have toys and treats available so that clients will be encouraged to try playing with their pets prior to the exam.

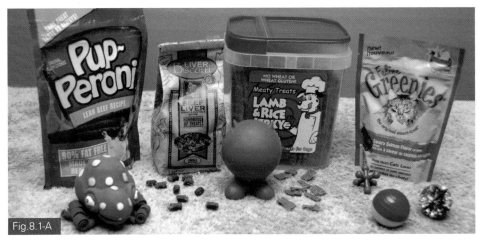

Fig.8.1-A

Fig.8.1-A: Treats should be broken into bite-sized pieces that the dog or cat can finish in 1-2 seconds. Giving 5-10 small treats is better than giving one large treat. Owners of healthy (non-anorexic) pets, as well as puppies or kittens, should be told to withhold food and bring the meal to the exam, so it can be used for training. Most kittens and up to 50% of adult cats in a comfortable hospital environment will eat tuna, baby food, Feline Greenies or the canned food they usually get. The majority of dogs will also eat during the exam if the set-up instructions mentioned in Chapter 7 are followed. For dogs, semi-moist treats such as Lean Treats (Butler Animal Health Supply, Dublin, Ohio) generally work better than dry treats; however, many dogs like Liver Biscotti (Premier Pet, Midlothian, Virginia) better than some semi-moist treats. Treats and some toys can also be sold through the hospital.

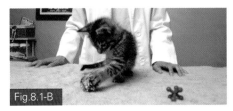

Fig.8.1-B

Fig.8.1-B: For cats and kittens, use inexpensive toys that can be given away. Or provide plastic, rubber or vinyl toys that can be sprayed with disinfectant and rinsed.

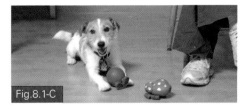

Fig.8.1-C

Fig.8.1-C: For dogs and puppies, vinyl and rubber toys are also a good choice, since they can be sprayed with disinfectant and then rinsed.

8.2 Greeting Cats Correctly

(Also review Chapter 1)

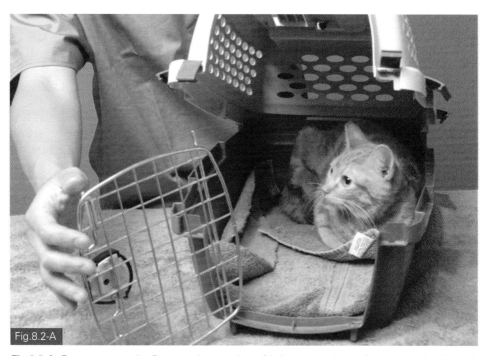

Fig.8.2-A: For many cats, the first greeting consists of being dumped out of a carrier or having their carrier shaken so that they will fall out like a loose apple from a tree. This immediately confirms their fear that you will handle them roughly, and it can cause them to become agitated or aggressive. For cats who are fearful and want to stay in their carrier, take the time to disassemble the carrier. This one act of patience can prevent you from being bitten or scratched during the exam.

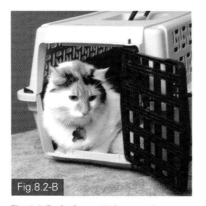

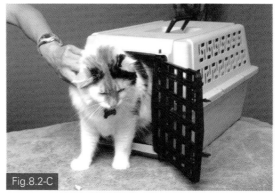

Fig.8.2-B, C: Cats will frequently come out of their carriers willingly if the owner opens the carrier door while waiting in the exam room or if the door is kept open during the initial history-taking. Some shy cats are more likely to come out of their carrier if the opening faces the wall. Often, elevating the back of the carrier slightly will encourage the cat to step out.

8.3 Greetings Dogs Correctly

(Also review Chapter 1)

Some dogs are immediately comfortable at the veterinary hospital. Others are clearly nervous. Still others appear friendly at first until you get close to them and lean over them the wrong way.

Why the difference? Imagine someone walked into the room carrying a big, hairy spider. If you're not particularly fearful you might smile, say hi and then quickly walk away. But if they then placed the spider too close for your fear level, your attitude might suddenly change. The same thing goes for our pets.

Watch the dog's body language

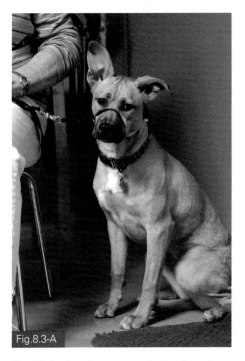
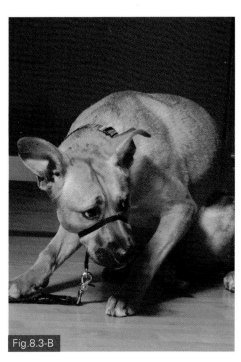

Fig.8.3-A

Fig.8.3-B

Fig.8.3-A: If a dog appears aloof or just sits or stands looking at you, be aware that she might be fearful or anxious. Many dogs whom people consider as having aloof temperaments or describe as "one-man" dogs focus only on their owners because they are afraid or unsure of other people.

Fig.8.3-B: When a stranger approaches this particular dog, she cowers, making her fear much more obvious. The dog should not have to cower for you to recognize that she is fearful.

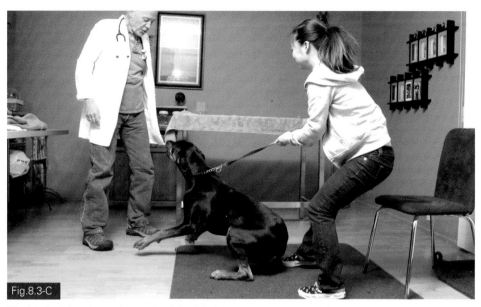

Fig.8.3-C: Other dogs who are fearful might lunge and bite instead of cowering, especially if they are approached incorrectly. A correct greeting is essential for everyone's safety, including the receptionists. Muzzling all dogs is not an option because many dogs become more fearful and aggressive when they have a muzzle on. Additionally, once they have it on, they might never let you or the owner muzzle them again.

Avoid direct eye contact

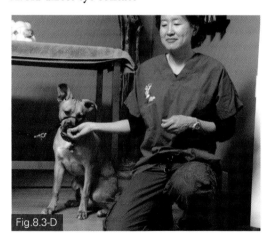
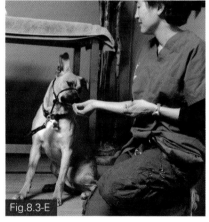

Fig.8.3-D: With this extremely fearful dog, I approach her backwards and then squat down to her level while approaching. I previously tossed a few treats on the floor, and she took them. Now I hold one out for her while avoiding eye contact.

Fig.8.3-E: Once she's comfortable taking the treats with my back turned, I turn toward her slightly to see how she feels with this level of face contact. She readily takes a steady stream of treats. If a dog you're working with is still uncomfortable at this point, refer to Chapter 14, Handling Difficult Dogs.

Avoid leaning over or reaching for the dog: Example 1

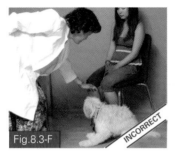
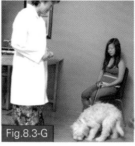
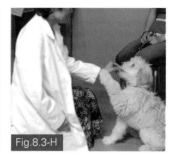

Fig.8.3-F   Fig.8.3-G   Fig.8.3-H

Fig.8.3-F, Incorrect: Bad greeting: Avoid walking into the dog's personal space and leaning over her. Instead, spend an extra 10 seconds to greet her appropriately. By doing so, you'll save time because you (1) won't need to muzzle her; (2) can examine her by yourself so you don't need to find a technician to help; (3) don't have to deal with her trying to struggle and get away. The owner will also be happier with your skill level and the rapport you now have with her pet.

Fig.8.3-G, H, Correct: Good greeting: Toss treats to the dog so that she's moving around in a relaxed state, then hand treats to her without bending over her. She is much more relaxed now and shows no signs of fear. To understand personal space, try this exercise: Start with 2 people standing 10 feet apart facing each other. They can then walk toward each other and stop when they still feel comfortable. Then they should take 2 steps closer; ask them, "How does this feel?" (exercise contributed by Amanda Eick-Miller).

Avoid leaning over or reaching for the dog: Example 2

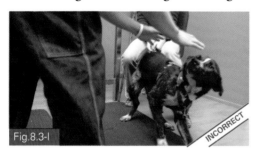
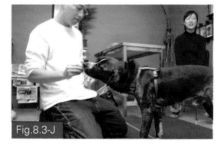

Fig.8.3-I   Fig.8.3-J

Fig.8.3-I, Incorrect: Bad greeting: The greeter in this photo is leaning forward to pet the dog, who cowers. The dog could have easily chosen to lunge and bite rather than cowering. In fact, although he usually cowers in this situation, if one day he lunges instead, then this—defensive aggression—is likely to become his default fear behavior. The switch to defensive aggression is more likely to happen if the dog is highly aroused or has had other fearful experiences (such as waiting in a lobby filled with dogs he's afraid of) just prior to this event. If this occurs in the vet hospital, then the hospital is the stimulus that has triggered his switch from a fearful dog who flees to one who becomes aggressive. Once this occurs, the dog is possibly on a path to euthanasia.

Fig.8.3-J, Correct: Good greeting: Now the greeter is giving treats. Notice that he is not reaching out toward the dog. Rather, he's holding the treat and letting the dog come to him. If the dog didn't approach, the greeter would toss treats first instead. The fact that this dog is coming into the man's personal space to take the treat—and doing so with an upright posture—indicates that he is more comfortable now. If he were leaning backward while taking the treat, then he would be showing he's still not comfortable in the situation.

Avoid leaning over or reaching for the dog: Example 3

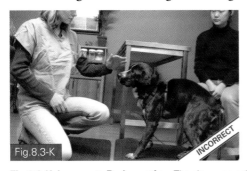

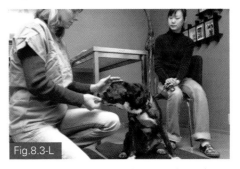

Fig.8.3-K, Incorrect: Bad greeting: The dog was calm when the technician stood next to him and even when she squatted down, but when she suddenly reached for him, he cowered. She didn't even have to lean over him the way the previous greeter did to get this reaction. Avoid suddenly reaching for any part of the dog.

Fig.8.3-L, Correct: Good greeting: Here the technician has already given him 5-10 treats and he is comfortably leaning his head into her personal space to get them. She is counterconditioning him to her outstretched hand by reaching out slightly just after he starts taking treats. She will remove her hand as he finishes the treat. The goal is to have the dog never look at her hand or act anxious or fearful that her hand is reaching toward him. (see Chapter 14) This counterconditioning process can take just seconds.

Avoid leaning over or reaching for the dog: Example 4

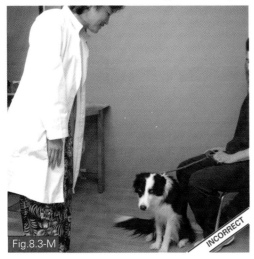

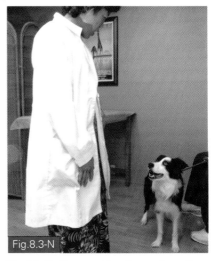

Fig.8.3-M, Incorrect: Bad greeting: This dog is looking down and away from me because I just walked into the room and tried to soothe him by saying "It's okay" in a quiet voice. If you went to the dentist's office and the hygienist kept telling you soothingly "It's going to be okay," you would probably become more apprehensive about what was about to happen. A calm tone of voice is not likely to change the dog from a fearful emotional state to a happy one.

Fig.8.3-N, Correct: Good greeting: Here, as I entered the room I talked to the dog in a happy voice ("jollying")—not a baby voice, but the voice you'd use if you were giving a pep talk or cheering your kids on at a soccer game. This switched his emotional state from one of fear to one of happiness and playfulness.

8.4 Examine the Pet Where She's Comfortable

In the carrier

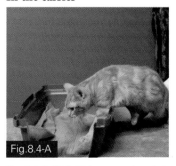
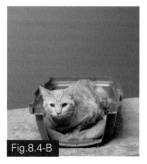
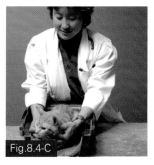

Fig.8.4-A, B, C: This cat prefers being in her carrier. Cats can be examined in their carrier if they are more comfortable there. *(Video 1)*

Under towels

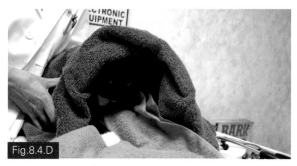
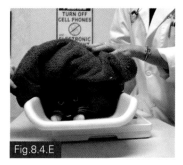

Fig.8.4-D, E: Other cats feel more comfortable if they are hidden under a towel during the examination. This one is even being weighed in the towel. Many cats prefer being examined on the scale because the raised sides make them feel more secure. Refer to Chapter 17 for details on examining cats using a towel.

On your lap

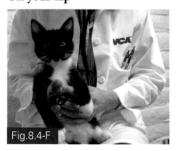
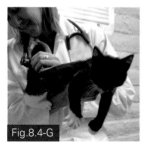
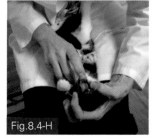

Fig.8.4-F, G, H: Kittens and some cats will hold still better if they are in your lap. A full exam can often be performed in this position. Often the cat may be more comfortable if she is facing her owner. It can be helpful to place a towel in your lap before placing the kitten on your lap.

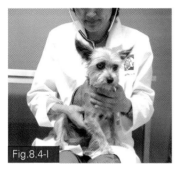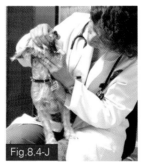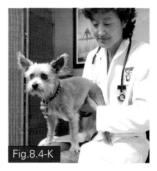

Fig.8.4-I, J, K: Like kittens, little dogs who are used to sitting in people's laps might also be more comfortable being examined in your lap rather than on the table.

On the floor

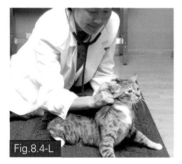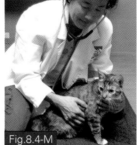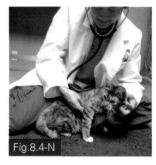

Fig.8.4-L, M, N: This cat is comfortable being examined on the floor but does not need to be scruffed. Only scruff cats when scruffing is needed and causes the cat to become calmer (not just immobilized). *(Video 2)* This cat can be restrained simply by placing a hand in front of her chest. Scratching her behind the ear also works to keep her in position.

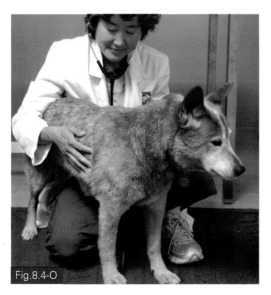

Fig.8.4-O: Dogs don't need to be examined on the exam table. This particular dog, Zoe, is comfortable being examined on the floor. Don't put the dog on the table just to make her fearful enough to hold still. It's better to learn how to restrain appropriately so that you can examine the dog where she's comfortable. Placing a dog on the table so that she has less room to move around is appropriate only if the dog is comfortable there.

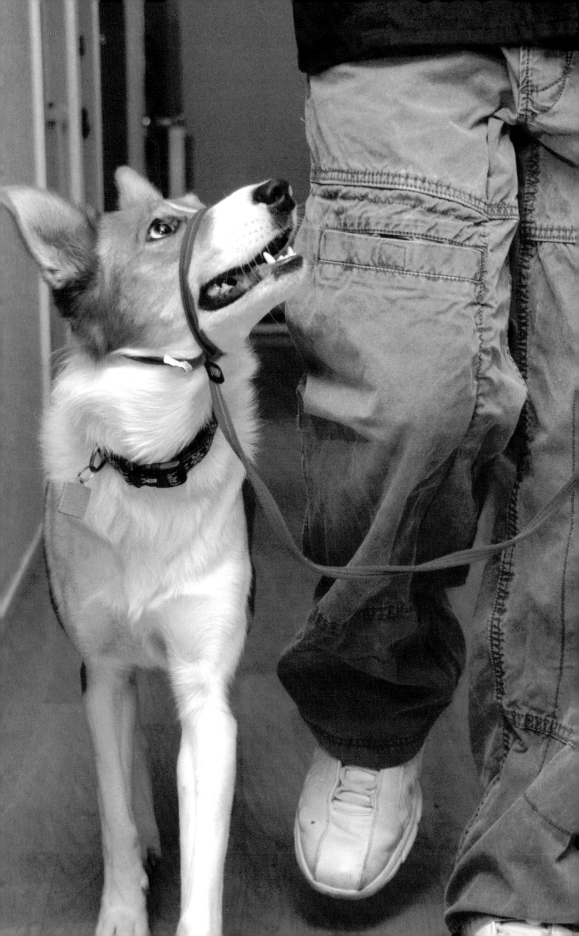

CHAPTER 9.
MOVING DOGS
Around The Facility

"Ruff! Ruff! Bark! Ruff! Bark!" The sound of an 80-pound angry German Shepherd echoes off the concrete kennel walls. Two technicians stand tentatively in front of the kennel, contemplating how they will get the Shepherd out. One technician starts to open the gate, a slip lead extending from the end of her arm. The dog backs away a few steps before lunging a step forward. The technician slams the gate shut. "Should we get the rabies pole?" she asks. Just then, a third technician walks up. The others back away from the kennel, all eyes on her rather than the dog. She stands with her side facing the dog, opens the gate, calmly reaches in with the loop of the slip lead and places it over the barking dog's head. Once the leash is on, the dog immediately quiets down and follows the technician out.

Everything you do—from the way you greet the dog to how you get it in and out of a kennel or cage—tells the dog something about you. Subtle differences in how you get dogs into and out of cages, walk them from one location to another and lift them make the difference between whether they view you as someone who can guide them or someone who might lead them astray. This chapter provides simple tips for performing all of these maneuvers safely and efficiently, and in a way that enables the dog to trust and be confident in you.

9.1 Removing Dogs From Their Kennels

9.1.1 Method 1: Remaining outside the kennel.

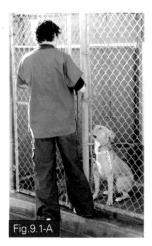

Fig.9.1-A

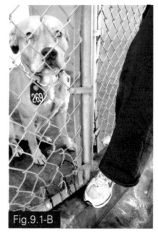

Fig.9.1-B

Fig.9.1-A,B: Stand at the gate opening with your side to the door. Face the door hinges if you're opening the gate outward. Place your foot in front of the gate so that the dog cannot push the gate open. When you open the gate, place your knee between the gate and the fence if needed to help prevent the dog from pushing by you.

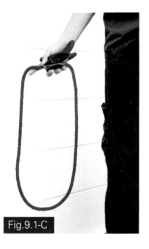

Fig.9.1-C

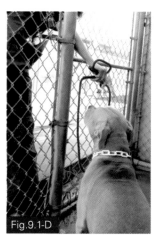

Fig.9.1-D

Fig.9.1-C,D: Make a big loop with the leash, and then open the gate just wide enough to reach your arm through. Using the arm closest to the kennel, reach in with the leash. Place the loop over the dog's neck with just one hand.

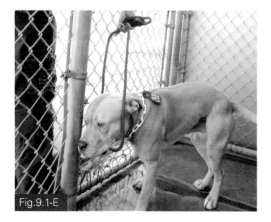

Fig.9.1-E

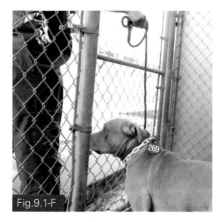

Fig.9.1-F

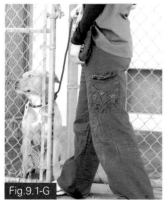

Fig.9.1-G

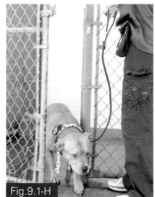

Fig.9.1-H

Fig.9.1-E to H: Drop the loop and tighten it around the dog's neck by pulling up on the leash. Once the dog is secured with the leash, open the door and let him walk through. The leash should be loose to allow him to walk out on his own. If you need to use the leash to keep him from bolting, shorten it.

WHAT'S WRONG WITH THESE PICTURES?

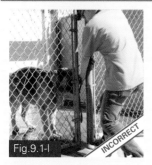

Fig.9.1-I

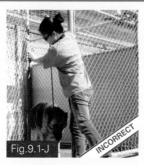

Fig.9.1-J

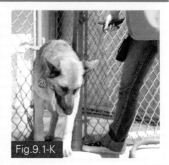

Fig.9.1-K

Fig.9.1-I, Example 1, Incorrect: The handler is reaching in with the wrong arm. She should reach in with the arm that's closer to the fence.

Fig.9.1-J, Example 2a, Incorrect: Here she tries to tighten the leash by extending her arm. When handling a leash, keep it at a length that allows your hands at stay at waist level.

Fig.9.1-K, Example 2b, Correct: Because the handler shortened the leash, she can keep her hands at waist level.

9.1.2 Method 2: Letting dogs come to the front of the kennel on their own.

Some dogs will not come to the front of the kennel if you are blocking the exit. But many of them will come out if you open the gate slightly and stand aside. This method works well for dogs who are moving or jumping around too much to get the leash on them via Method 1, or for those who are focused on just getting out of the kennel. It's also effective for dogs who are territorial or fearful and are barking and jumping at the gate.

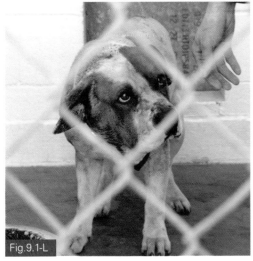

Fig.9.1-L: For dogs who stay in the back of the kennel, reaching in with the leash or even just a hand can appear threatening. This dog cowers when a hand reaches toward him.

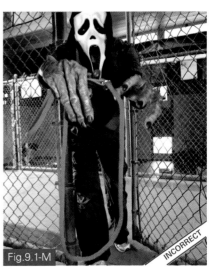

Fig.9.1-M, Incorrect (dog's view): If dogs are fearful, no matter how friendly you are, you could still look scary to them, especially if you reach into their personal space.

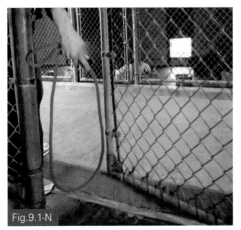

Fig.9.1-N, Correct: Instead of reaching in while facing the dog, place the leash loop in front of the door opening.

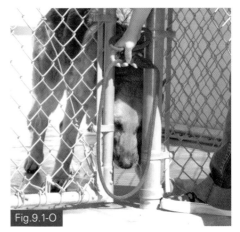

Fig.9.1-O: The loop should be large enough and low enough that the dog's head goes through but his front legs do not.

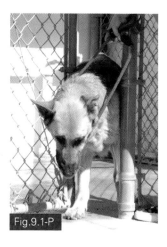

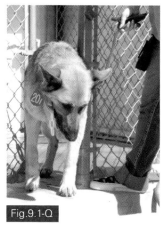

Fig.9.1-P: Be sure the loop is around his neck.

Fig.9.1-Q: Let the loop tighten as the dog walks out.

9.1.3 Method 3: Going inside—for dogs who won't come to the front of the kennel. *(Videos 1-4)*

Many dogs are so fearful that they just cower at the back of the run. Some might bark in the safety of the kennel, but as soon as they see you approach or it's clear that you're about to enter, they run to the back. Often handlers are afraid of these dogs and use rabies poles on them. Doing so makes the dogs even more fearful and can elicit defensive aggression. This primes them to be more aggressive in future interactions and causes tranquilizers to be less effective. In general, dogs who cower and back away when they realize that you're going to enter can be taken out of the kennel safely and with little stress to the dog or handler if you approach correctly and have good leash-handling skills. This requires practice on your part. To build your own confidence, start with dogs who are small enough that they don't scare you. If you're fearful, dogs will know it from your body language, making them feel more threatened or at least less comfortable.

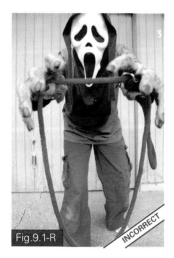

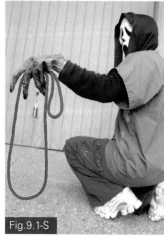

Fig.9.1-R, Incorrect (dog's view): Entering with a leash while facing the dog can be menacing to the dog. This can cause the dog to defend himself aggressively.

Fig.9.1-S, Correct (dog's view): Approaching backwards or sideways is less threatening.

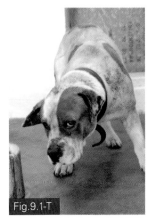
Fig.9.1-T

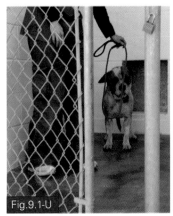
Fig.9.1-U

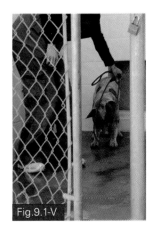
Fig.9.1-V

Fig.9.1-T, Example 1: This fearful junkyard dog was confiscated by animal control using a rabies pole. He was considered a "caution" animal. With proper techniques he could have been walked safely using a slip lead, with less stress to both the dog and the handler.

Fig.9.1-U: Avoid approaching head-on. Here, I back up steadily at a 45-degree angle to the dog; when I get close, I hold out the loop of the leash. *Note: Do not walk away from a fearful dog with your back fully turned. He could attack as you're walking away because as the distance increases and the dog sees that you're not watching, he builds up enough confidence to attack defensively.*

Fig.9.1-V: Dogs tend to lower their head when they see the leash coming, so you'll have to lean or bend down a little to get the leash over the head. Minimize leaning so that you can give the dog as much personal space as possible. Note that I am positioned along the wall so that the dog has a visible escape route in the direction of the leash loop. If I stood in front of the dog instead, he would feel trapped and possibly be more likely to react defensively.

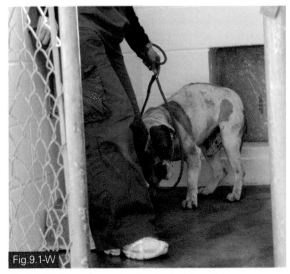
Fig.9.1-W

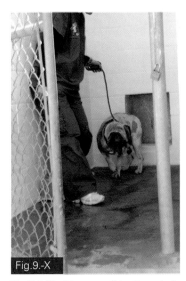
Fig.9.-X

Fig.9.1-W: Sometimes the dog backs himself into a corner. In this position, he's more likely to attack defensively if you pressure him too much by moving toward him too quickly or in a threatening manner.

Fig.9.1-X: Move confidently, calmly and slowly to avoid triggering defensive aggression. Good leash-handling skills are imperative.

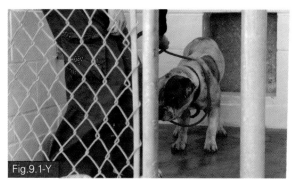

Fig.9.1-Y

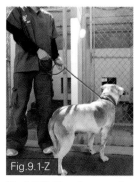

Fig.9.1-Z

Fig.9.1-Y: Move slowly enough that the dog never has to move faster than a slow walk but quickly enough to get the loop around him. **Avoid a sudden grab, as this can cause him to go into emergency escape mode**. Once in this mode, he's more likely to make a reactive decision to bite defensively. To help prevent a chase, block off escape routes such as the door behind the dog. If dogs notice access to an escape route, they might dart away from you (again, going into emergency escape mode).

Fig.9.1-Z: Usually, once the dog has a leash on, he no longer tries to escape. This dog walked readily out of his kennel and is now standing more relaxed outside of it.

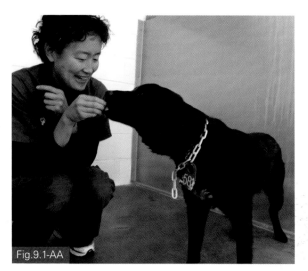

Fig.9.1-AA

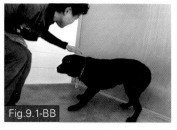

Fig.9.1-BB

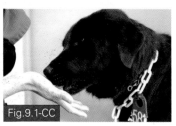

Fig.9.1-CC

Fig.9.1-AA: Jollying the dog by talking to him in a happy tone can cause many fearful dogs to immediately change their demeanor to one of happiness or even playfulness. Using soothing, repetitive words most likely will have no effect on the dog since it won't switch him to an alternate emotional state. You can tell by the dog's response whether talking is helpful or not. Use only the methods that work for that particular dog. Adjust your techniques based on the dog's response. When I offer treats and talk to this dog in a happy voice, she walks up to me and takes the treats. Notice that I don't reach out to give the treat; I let her come to me.

Fig.9.1-BB, CC: Tossing treats can also effect an immediate change in many dogs. At first, they're fearful and unsure about you, but when you toss treats they learn that you're a source of good things. This dog is fearful and cowers when I improperly reach for her, even though she took a few treats from me earlier. But after tossing additional treats and letting her approach at her own pace again, she soon walks right up and takes the treats again.

WHAT'S WRONG WITH THIS PICTURE?

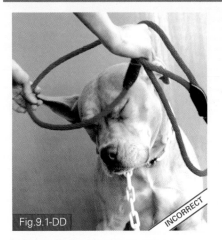

Fig.9.1-DD

INCORRECT

Fig.9.1-DD, Incorrect: This handler needs two hands to get the loop over the dog, which can be threatening to fearful dogs. For the safety and comfort of both you and the dog, become proficient at using the one-handed technique.

9.1.4 Avoid using a rabies pole, if possible.

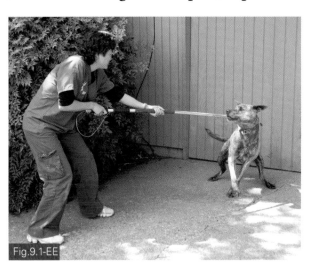

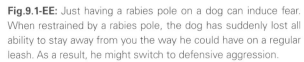

Fig.9.1-EE

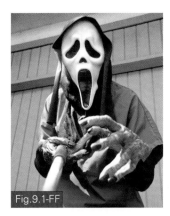

Fig.9.1-FF

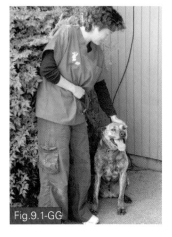

Fig.9.1-GG

Fig.9.1-EE: Just having a rabies pole on a dog can induce fear. When restrained by a rabies pole, the dog has suddenly lost all ability to stay away from you the way he could have on a regular leash. As a result, he might switch to defensive aggression.

Fig.9.1-FF: The dog's perception of the situation is that suddenly you can be 5 feet away from him and still be in his personal space.

Fig.9.1-GG: Here's the same dog on a leash instead of a rabies pole.

9.2 Placing Dogs Into Their Kennels

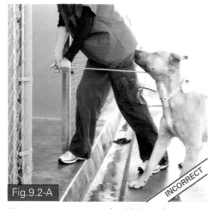

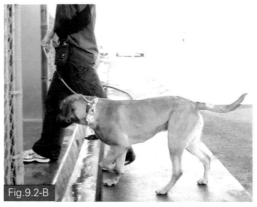

Fig.9.2-A, Incorrect: Avoid dragging a dog into a kennel by standing stationary and expecting him to go in ahead of you.

Fig.9.2-B, Correct: Instead, walk in ahead of the dog so that he follows.

9.3 Entering and Exiting Kennels Safely

Sometimes you have to go into the kennel because the dog is bouncing around too much or doesn't like when you reach for him. In these cases, you must be able to get in and out without letting the dog rush past you.

9.3.1 Entering the kennel.

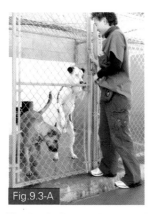

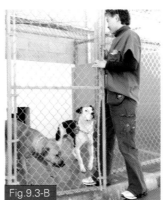

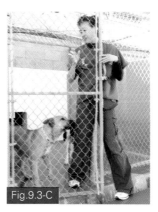

Fig.9.3-A: Stand with the side of your body toward the kennel opening. Your body should face the door hinges. Lift the latch and open the door just wide enough to fit through. You can open the door inwards or outwards. The technique for both is the same.

Fig.9.3-B, C: Step in with your lead leg first while facing inside the kennel so you can see where you're going. If the dog is crowding the door, just squeeze your way through anyway so that the dog must move out of the way.

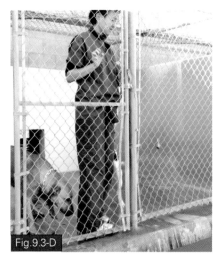

Fig.9.3-D

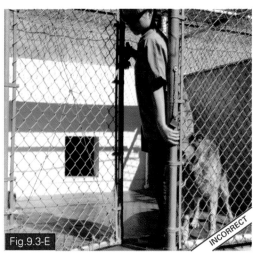

Fig.9.3-E

Fig.9.3-D: Once inside, quickly close the door behind you. It's not necessary to face the dog when you do this because you're blocking the door with your legs and body and simultaneously closing it. Done smoothly, this process should take 1-2 seconds and 2 footsteps.

Fig.9.3-E, Example 1, Incorrect: The technician should be looking into the kennel until she's in far enough to close the gate. She also opened the door wider than necessary. She is, however, blocking the dog's exit.

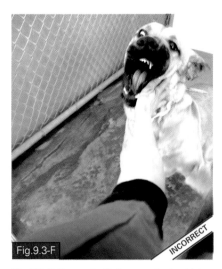

Fig.9.3-F

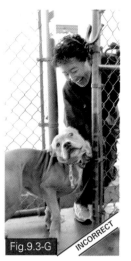

Fig.9.3-G

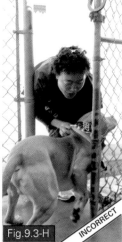

Fig.9.3-H

Fig.9.3-F, Example 2, Incorrect: Avoid trying to keep the dog in by pushing him with your hands. Some might perceive this as a threat and snap or bite.

Fig.9.3-G,H, Example 2, Incorrect: Using your hands to keep the dog inside actually makes it easier for the dog to escape. The dog can often wiggle or struggle by.

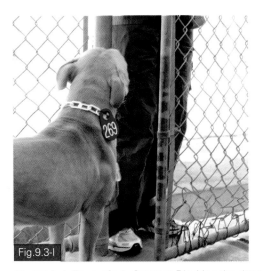
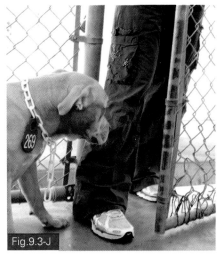

Fig.9.3-I, J: Example 2, Correct: Blocking the doorway with your body and legs provides a more secure barrier to the dog and is less threatening. The dog perceives your legs as inanimate objects that moved into his path.

9.3.2 Exiting the kennel.

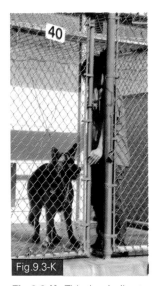
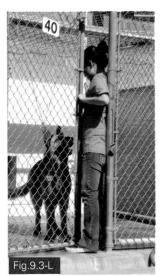
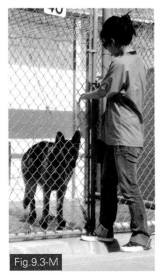

Fig.9.3-K: This is similar to going into the kennel, but in reverse. Open the door with your outside hand.

Fig.9.3-L: Step out while keeping your eye on the dog. The door should open just wide enough to let you through.

Fig.9.3-M: Once outside, close the door. Place your foot against the gate to keep it closed while you're latching it.

WHAT'S WRONG WITH THESE ENTERING AND EXITING SCENARIOS?

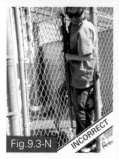
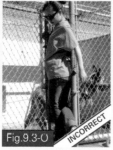
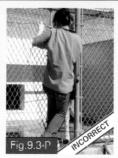
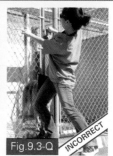

Fig.9.3-N   Fig.9.3-O   Fig.9.3-P   Fig.9.3-Q

Fig.9.3-N, Example 1, Incorrect: The technician is looking out of the kennel as she's exiting. She should keep her eye on the dog as she's leaving.

Fig.9.3-O, Example 2, Incorrect: Here, she crosses her feet to step out. She should step out with her outside foot first. She's also looking in the wrong direction.

Fig.9.3-P, Example 3a, Incorrect: Because her feet crossed over, the gate must open wider. Now it's harder to block the dog if he tries to get out.

Fig.9.3-Q, Example 3b, Incorrect: Continuing her exit, she becomes off balance. As ridiculous as this looks, this is just a reenactment of something this technician actually did earlier.

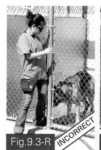
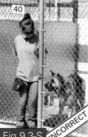
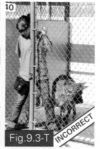

Fig.9.3-R   Fig.9.3-S   Fig.9.3-T

Fig.9.3-R, Example 4a, Incorrect: Here, because the dog is on the right side of the gate, the technician tries to face the dog to enter the kennel. She is not facing the door hinges.

Fig.9.3-S, Example 4b, Incorrect: As a result, she has to hold the door behind her back.

Fig.9.3-T, Example 4c, Incorrect: She also ends up looking away from the dog when she enters because it's difficult to control the door when it's behind her.

Fig.9.3-U, Example 4d, Incorrect: Once in, she must turn her back on the dog before she has good control of the door.

Fig.9.3-V, Example 4e, Incorrect: This process is awkward.

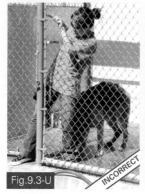
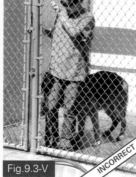

Fig.9.3-U   Fig.9.3-V

9.4 Taking Off the Leash

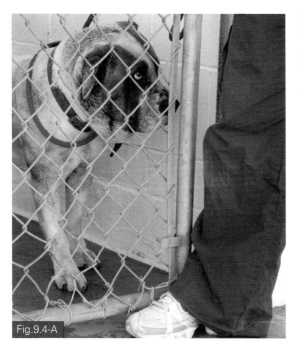

Fig.9.4-A: This involves virtually the same procedure as getting the leash on. With a fearful dog, reach toward the dog as little as possible because doing so can cause the dog to feel more threatened, leading to a snap or bite.

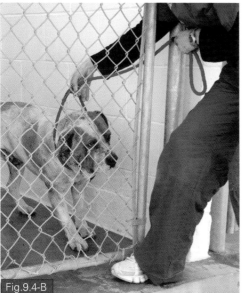

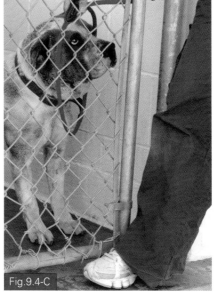

Fig.9.4-B, C: Here, I do have to reach over his head to loosen the leash. I try to do so smoothly so I don't induce a fear response. If the leash is firm enough, just push it through the metal ring. Or for such dogs you can use an Easy Slip lead (Premier Pet, Midlothian, Virginia), pictured in Figures 9.4-D,E,F.

Premier Pet (Midlothian, Virginia) makes the Easy Slip Lead, a leash with a release string that enables you to loosen the collar without reaching down for the dog.

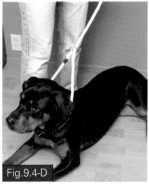
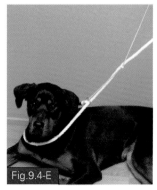
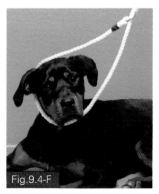

Fig.9.4-D, E, F: The Easy Slip Lead is simple to remove. The yellow string can be used to widen the noose enough to slip the lead over the dog's head to remove it.

9.5 Walking Dogs

Avoid letting the dog drag you around, pull anxiously or pace back and forth. Even when walking, you should keep the dog calm rather than letting him become anxious or aroused.

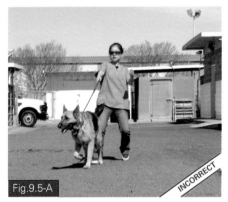
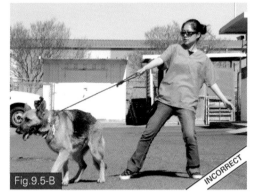

Fig.9.5-A, Incorrect: Don't allow the dog to drag you around. Pacing, dragging and scrambling can put the dog in an aroused state or into escape mode. If uncontrolled, he could also walk too close to other patients.

Fig.9.5-B, Incorrect: Letting him walk this way tells him something about your handling abilities—that you are unable to provide guidance and help him control his emotional state.

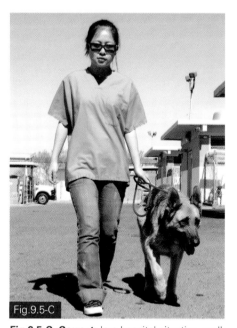

Fig.9.5-C

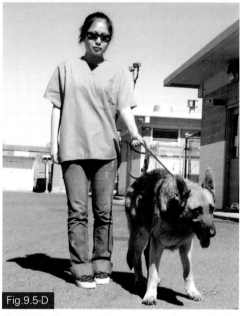

Fig.9.5-D

Fig.9.5-C, Correct: In a hospital situation, walk dogs on a short leash.

Fig.9.5-D, Correct: If the dog walks fast and pulls, stop and stand still until he is more controlled. Then walk forward again. You might have to stop several times along the way.

9.6 Picking Up Dogs

9.6.1 Lifting small dogs. *(Video 5)*

Method 1

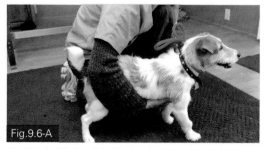

Fig.9.6-A

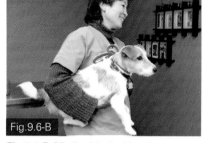

Fig.9.6-B

Fig.9.6-A, Method 1: Hold onto the collar or leash so that the dog cannot move away from you. Reach over his back and place your hand under the dog's chest and between the front legs. Your fingers should be flat on the chest and your thumb should be on the lateral side of the dog's outside upper leg. This keeps him from trying to back out. Now hold the dog against your side and pick him up.

Fig.9.6-B, Method 1: At this point, you can carry him one-handed against your side.

Method 2

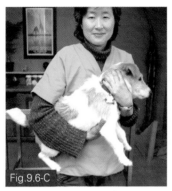

Fig.9.6-C

Fig.9.6-C, Method 2 (dogs who may struggle): If you think the dog will struggle when being carried, hold the dog's neck close to your body using a "C" hold (refer to Chapter 11) with your free hand. To do this, place your hand around the outside of the dog's neck and your thumb under the neck. Then pull the neck close to your body if the dog starts to wiggle.

Method 3

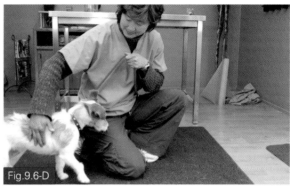

Fig.9.6-D

Fig.9.6-D, Method 3 (fearful dogs or dogs who might bite): To safely pick up fearful dogs or those who might bite when reached for, guide the dog's head forward and away from you with the leash. Then pull him up to your side (or back up so that you're in position beside him) and put your arm around him. This keeps the head safely away from you while you reach over the dog to pick him up. Consider having the owner place a muzzle on the dog first, or put a temporary leash muzzle on him just to pick him up. Muzzling, however, can be stressful to the dog and make some more fearful, whereas confidently picking up the dog in a way that protects you from being bitten can often keep the dog calm.

Method 4

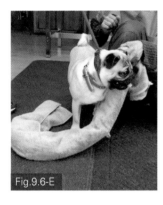

Fig.9.6-E

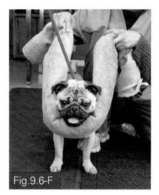

Fig.9.6-F

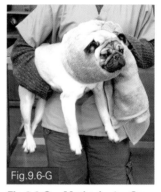

Fig.9.6-G

Fig.9.6-F, Method 4: A technician can hold the dog's leash and even distract him with food while you encircle the dog's head with a rolled towel.

Fig.9.6-G, Method 4: Once the head is wrapped, grasp the towel where the two ends meet. Grasp tight enough so it's snug around the dog's head, allowing you to control the head and keep the dog from turning and biting.

Method 5

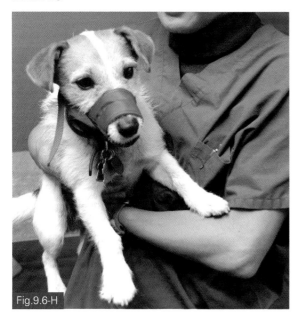

Fig.9.6-H

Fig.9.6-H, Method 5: Fearful or aggressive dogs can also be muzzled prior to being picked up, if they tolerate muzzles well. If a dog needs to be muzzled, the owner should counter-condition him to the muzzle at home. Doing so will associate muzzling with good things (see Chapter 18) so that muzzling in the hospital won't present a bad experience, and the dog can be easily muzzled again in the future.

9.6.2 Lifting medium-size dogs.

Method 1

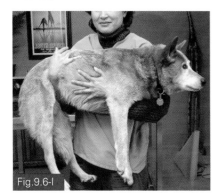

Fig.9.6-I

Fig.9.6-I, Method 1: First control the dog's movement by grasping either the collar or the leash close to the collar. Place one arm under the abdomen and the other in front of the dogs' chest, reaching between the legs and then under the chest. For most dogs, this is the most balanced hold, but it does not control the head. So while you can control struggling dogs with this method, you cannot restrain the head and prevent fearful dogs from snapping at you.

Method 2

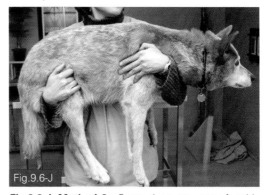

Fig.9.6-J

Fig.9.6-J, Method 2: Some dogs are uncomfortable with pressure under their abdomen. For these dogs, placing one arm around the rear and one around the front of the chest can be more comfortable. However, if they are inclined to struggle, they can do so with this method. Make the hold more secure by grasping the front aspect of the upper thigh with the hand controlling the rear end. This can help keep the dog from flailing with that hind leg. Since you don't have control of the head with this method, the dog could snap at you.

Method 3   **Method 4**

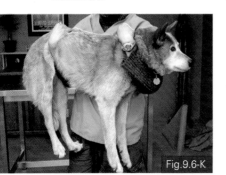
Fig.9.6-K

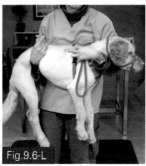
Fig.9.6-L

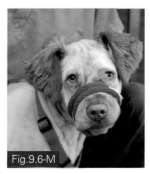
Fig.9.6-M

Fig. 9.6-K, Method 3: For dogs with unknown temperament or those who snap at you when being lifted (but not necessarily at any other time), first gain control of the head by wrapping your arm around the neck. Only use this lift if you know you can control the head this way. Place the second arm under the abdomen. This hold is uncomfortable for some dogs because you are lifting the front end by placing pressure on the neck.

Fig.9.6-L,M, Method 4: For these dogs, you can also take the precaution of placing a leash muzzle on the dog (refer to Chapter 14 for instructions) for the short lift and transport period.

WHAT'S WRONG WITH THESE SCENARIOS?

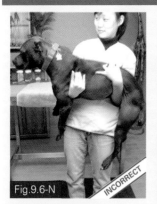
Fig.9.6-N   INCORRECT

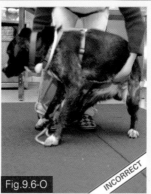
Fig.9.6-O   INCORRECT

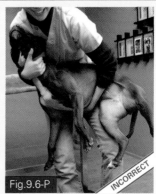
Fig.9.6-P   INCORRECT

Fig.9.6-N, Example 1, Incorrect: This method of placing one arm behind the front legs and one in front of the back legs can work for dogs who are small enough. It provides little control if the dog struggles, though. Additionally, it does not control the head.

Fig.9.6-O, Example 2a, Incorrect: Placing one arm around the neck to control the head while wrapping the other under the abdomen from over the back can work for getting some dogs off tables. But it is not suitable for picking up dogs and lifting them.

Fig.9.6-P, Example 2b, Incorrect: This method does not provide good control if the dog struggles. Here the dog is struggling and the technician is about to drop her.

9.6.3 Lifting large dogs.

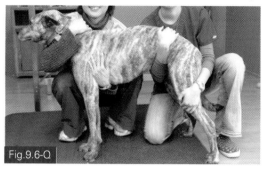

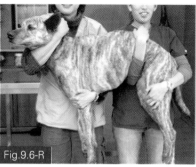

Fig.9.6-Q, Method 1: The person at the front of the dog should wrap her arm around the dog's neck to control the head. The other arm should go under the chest just behind the front leg. The technician at the rear should place one hand under the abdomen as caudally as possible. Her free hand holds the patellar region to keep the leg straight so that the dog does not kick and struggle with that leg.

Fig.9.6-R, Method 1: The two should lift in a coordinated fashion so that the dog is level. Once elevated, if the dog's chest is heavy or large relative to the person holding the front end, she can grip the front of the dog's upper leg in the bicep region. This is comfortable for the dog and takes the weight off the holder's arms.

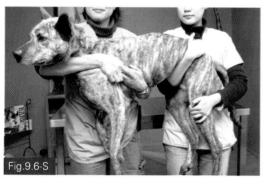

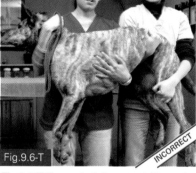

Fig.9.6-S, Method 2: Another way to stabilize the dog's front end (which is heavier than the back end) is to lock your hands together. If the dog starts to struggle, reposition your arms around his neck.

Fig.9.6-T, Example 1, Incorrect: The technician in front is supporting the dog behind the rib cage instead of holding her arm just caudal to the front legs. As a result, she's carrying most of the dog's weight.

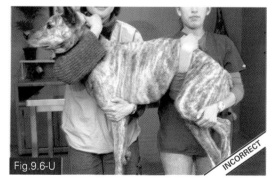

Fig.9.6-U, Example 2, Incorrect: Here, the technician at the rear is holding the back leg bent. The purpose of the hand on the patella is to help stabilize the dog by straightening the leg. She should have her hand up higher so that the leg is straight.

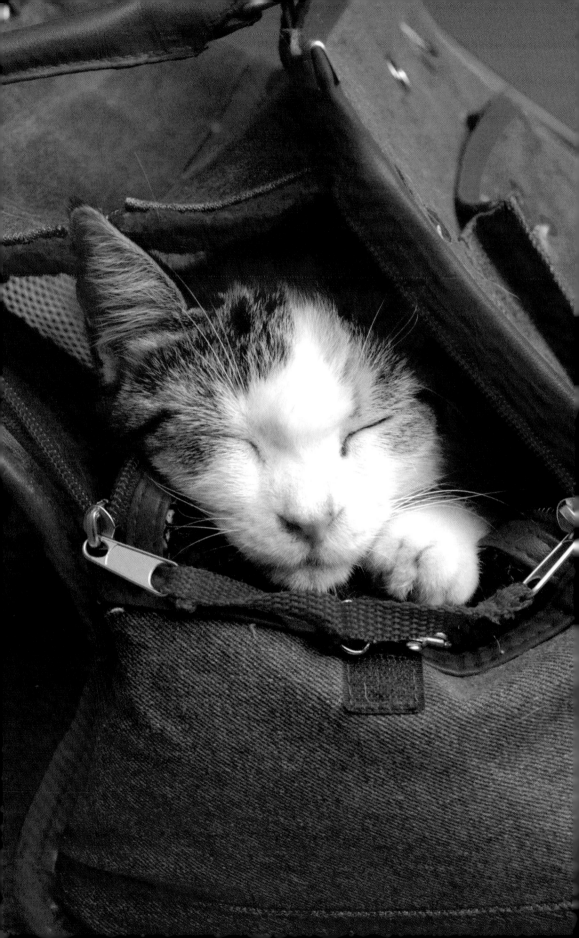

CHAPTER 10.
TRANSPORTING CATS
Within the Hospital

"Well, Mia's usually calm at the hospital, but her last visit was different. The receptionists and hospital staff were nice enough, but we had a new technician this time. The first thing he did was dump Mia out of her carrier," says the woman waiting in line at the supermarket. "They didn't even give her a chance to walk out on her own. I could tell she was nervous because she was hunched in a little ball. She usually lies quietly at the vet but doesn't hunker down. Then the new veterinarian walked in and immediately scruffed her to hold her still, even though she was already holding still. It made her hiss even though she's usually calm at the hospital. Once I got her home, she was upset for the rest of the afternoon. I had to keep her separated from the other cats because she started hissing at them, too."

Every interaction you have with your feline patient will tell the cat something about you. Even something as simple as getting her out of a carrier and putting her back in will affect her perception. To gain the cat's trust and cooperation, you must be aware of every action you take when near the cat.

10.1 Removing Cats From Travel Carriers

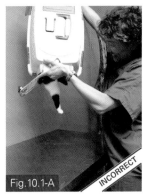

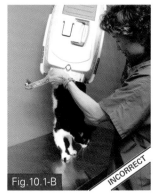

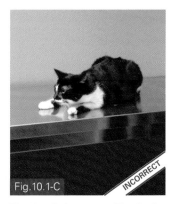

Fig.10.1-A, B, Incorrect: Avoid dumping a cat out of the carrier. This can cause heightened fear or agitation, which will increase the likelihood of later aggression. It's also an indicator to the cat of how you will handle her during the rest of her stay. You can always ask the owner to get the cat out if she's in the exam room.

Fig.10.1-C, Incorrect: Here's the cat after she was dumped out. Her body language (ears back, crouching and body weight more toward the back end) indicates that she's fearful and ready to bolt off the table.

Method 1

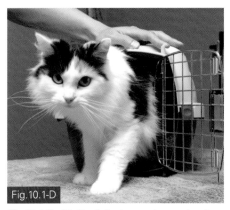

Fig.10.1-D, Method 1: Leave the carrier door open and let the cat walk out on her own.

Method 2

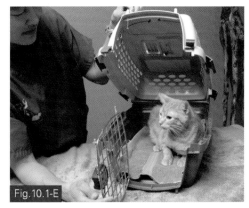

Fig.10.1-E, Method 2: Take the carrier apart and lift the top off. Be sure to avoid dropping the door, as this will scare the cat. The cat can then be examined in the carrier or on the table—wherever she is comfortable.

Method 3

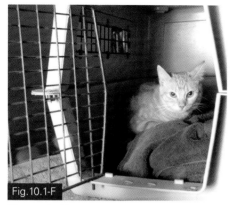

Fig.10.1-F, Method 3: If you're unable to take the carrier apart, use a towel to get the cat out. This option works if the carrier is large enough to fit the cat and your arms through the opening. If you need to use this method, it's a good idea to recommend to the client that they obtain a carrier that easily opens from the top.

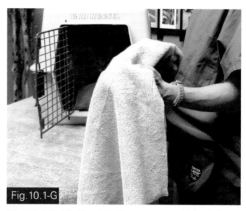

Fig.10.1-G, Method 3: Choose a towel that's large enough to cover the cat and thick enough to protect you if the cat tries to claw or bite. If the cat is giving signals that she might become aggressive, you might want to use two towels or one towel plus protective gloves.

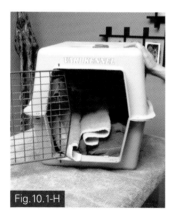

Fig.10.1-H, Method 3: Place the towel inside the carrier and over the cat.

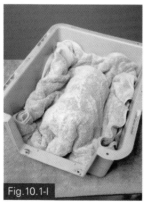

Fig.10.1-I, Method 3: Push the edges of the towel down over the cat so that it wraps around the end of the cat. In this way, pulling the towel brings the cat closer to you.

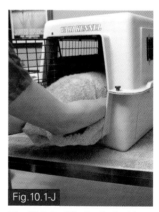

Fig.10.1-J, Method 3: Next, guide the cat toward you. You might need to scoop up the cat and lift her a little. Once out, either leave the towel on for the examination or take it off.

10.2 Lifting Cats From Disposable Carriers

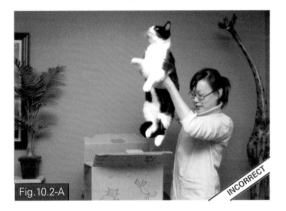

Fig.10.2-A

Fig.10.2-A, Incorrect: Avoid lifting a cat solely by the scruff. While some cats relax with, or accept scruffing, others can become aggressive. Furthermore, some may be stressed by scruffing even though they do not struggle. This anxiety will affect their overall impression of their hospital stay and can lead to difficulty managing the cat later on.

INCORRECT

Method 1

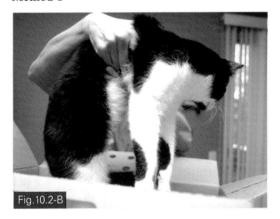

Fig.10.2-B

Fig.10.2-B, Method 1: If the cat is calm and friendly, lift her out without scruffing. Place your hands around her body behind the front legs.

Method 2

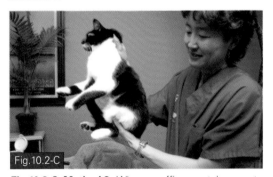

Fig.10.2-C

Fig.10.2-C, Method 2: When scruffing a cat, be sure to support the rear end. Generally cats do not need to be held in this manner. This hold provides less support than method 3 where the cat is held close to your body.

Method 3

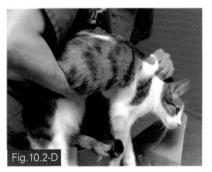

Fig.10.2-D

Fig.10.2-D, Method 3: Alternatively, scruff the cat loosely with one hand and place the other hand under the abdomen to support the body weight. Be ready to scruff more firmly if the cat bolts.

Method 4

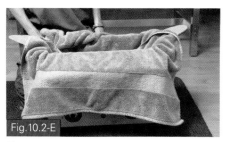

Fig.10.2-E, Method 4: With a cat who appears fearful or aggressive, place a towel over her.

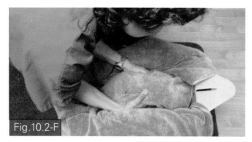

Fig.10.2-F, Method 4: Press the sides of the towel snugly around the cat. Then grasp the cat behind the front legs.

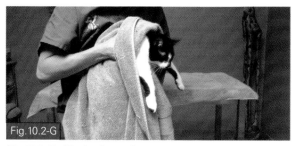

Fig.10.2-G, Method 4: Some cats remain relaxed when grasped behind their front legs and can be lifted in this manner onto the table. (Here, the towel is pulled back to show the cat remaining calm.)

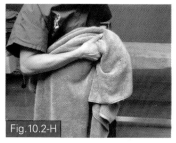

Fig.10.2-H, Method 4: Keep the towel over the cat's head until she's on the table.

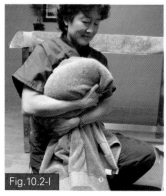

Fig.10.2-I, Method 4: If the cat is not relaxed, quickly wrap the towel around the entire cat so that it comes together under the cat. Then lift the cat onto the table. Notice that the entire cat, including her rear end, is above my supporting arms.

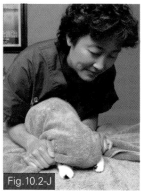

Fig.10.2-J, Method 4: Keep the towel over the cat's head with your arms holding it down along her side until the cat relaxes.

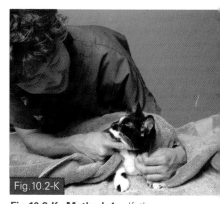

Fig.10.2-K, Method 4: If the cat seems relaxed, lift the towel from her head and interact with her.

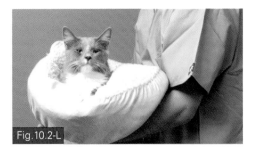

Fig.10.2-L: Tailor your method to the cat. This friendly and calm cat does not ambulate well. The technician is familiar with the cat's personality. He has decided to transport the cat in her bed from the cage to the treatment table several feet away. That way, the technician does not need to disturb the sick cat by lifting her out of her bed.

10.3 Carrying Cats

Method 1

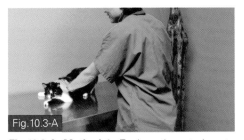

Fig.10.3-A, Method 1: To draw the cat close to you, place one hand loosely on the scruff so that she can't move away. Be ready to hold the scruff more firmly if the cat tries to bolt.

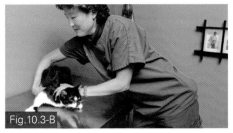

Fig.10.3-B, Method 1: Reach your other arm over the cat. With your hand behind her elbow so she can't back away, place your arm along her side. Use your entire arm to draw the cat closer.

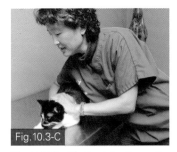

Fig.10.3-C, Method 1: Draw the cat against the side of your body.

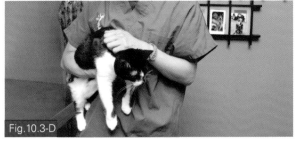

Fig.10.3-D, Method 1: Now the hand of the arm that's extending over the cat can reach under the chest so that the cat's elbow still sits between your thumb and index finger. Her inside leg can be held between your second (index finger) and third fingers. Your hand and arm support the cat's weight and hold her against your body.

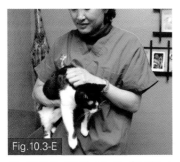

Fig.10.3-E, Method 1: Continue holding the cat's scruff lightly in your other hand. Tighten your grip if the cat tries to struggle.

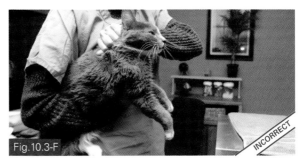

Fig.10.3-F, Incorrect: Avoid automatically placing a death grip on the cat. This position is uncomfortable for the cat, and holding in this manner indicates to the cat how the rest of your handling will be. Only grip tightly if the cat is showing signs of bolting. Always be ready to tighten your grip though.

Method 2

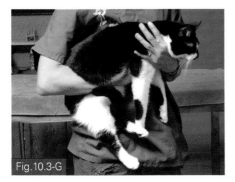

Fig.10.3-G, Method 2: Many cats are relaxed when carried and do not need to be scruffed. For these cats, place your hand in a "U" hold under the neck so that the neck sits in the webbing between your thumb and index finger.

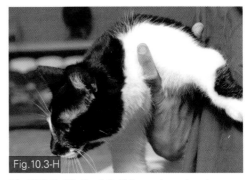

Fig.10.3-H, Method 2: If the cat reaches her paw over your hand and places her paw on you, remove it by rotating your supporting hand. The leg should already be between your second (index finger) and third finger.

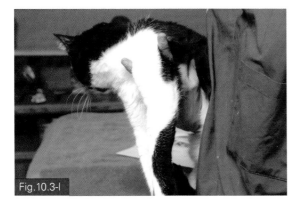

Fig.10.3-I, Method 2: Moving these fingers forward will cause the cat's leg to move forward so that it is no longer on you.

Method 3

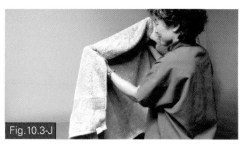

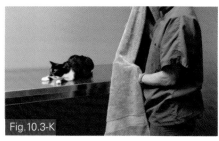

Fig.10.3-J, Method 3: For cats who are fearful or even fractious, remove them from the cage by placing a large towel (e.g., a 30 x 50-inch thick bath towel) over them. Hold your arms parallel and several inches from the end of the towel. This is important, because you'll need enough towel to wrap around the front of the cat's head. *(Video 1)*

Fig.10.3-K, Method 3: If you're afraid the cat might bite, use two thick towels or one towel along with leather gloves, whichever provides you with better dexterity and ability to restrain the cat. Having a second person on hand with a towel or gloves is a good idea in case you need help.

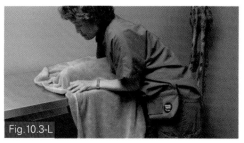

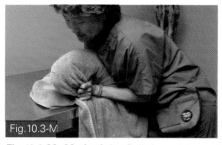

Fig.10.3-L, Method 3: In one rapid movement, place the towel over the cat. Immediately place both arms on each side of the cat like a chute so that the towel is held down snuggly. Simultaneously pull the front portion over the end of the cat so that she can't escape in that direction.

Fig.10.3-M, Method 3: Pull the cat toward you, making sure to keep your elbows as close to you as possible to block off a rearward escape. Make sure the towel is wrapped over the cat's head.

Fig.10.3-N, Method 3: Next, wrap all ends of the towel together under the cat so that there's no room for the cat to struggle. Now the cat can be placed on a table or into her carrier.

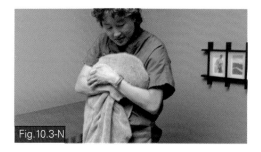

Another option for removing cats from cages for procedures such as injection with a tranquilizer is to use the EZ Nabber (Campbell Pet Company, Vancouver, Washington). If the cat is being removed to go home, try just placing the carrier up to or into her cage. Cats will often choose to hide in the carrier.

10.4 Placing Cats in Carriers

Method 1

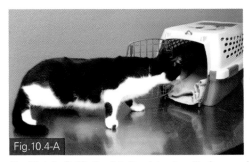

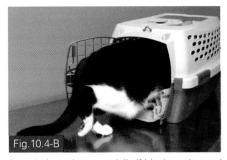

Fig.10.4-A, B, Method 1: Fearful cats will often go right into their carrier, especially if it's the only good hiding spot nearby, even if they dislike going into their carrier at home.

Method 2

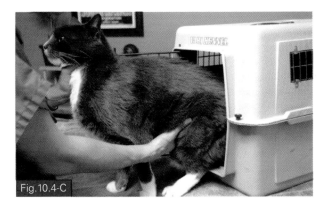

Fig.10.4-C, Method 2: For cats who won't readily go into their carrier head first, try guiding them in backwards.

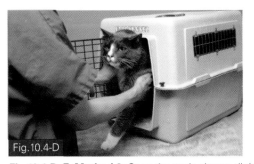

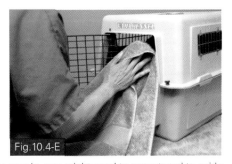

Fig.10.4-D, E, Method 2: Once the cat is almost all the way in, you might need to use a towel to guide her in the rest of the way.

Restraint Techniques

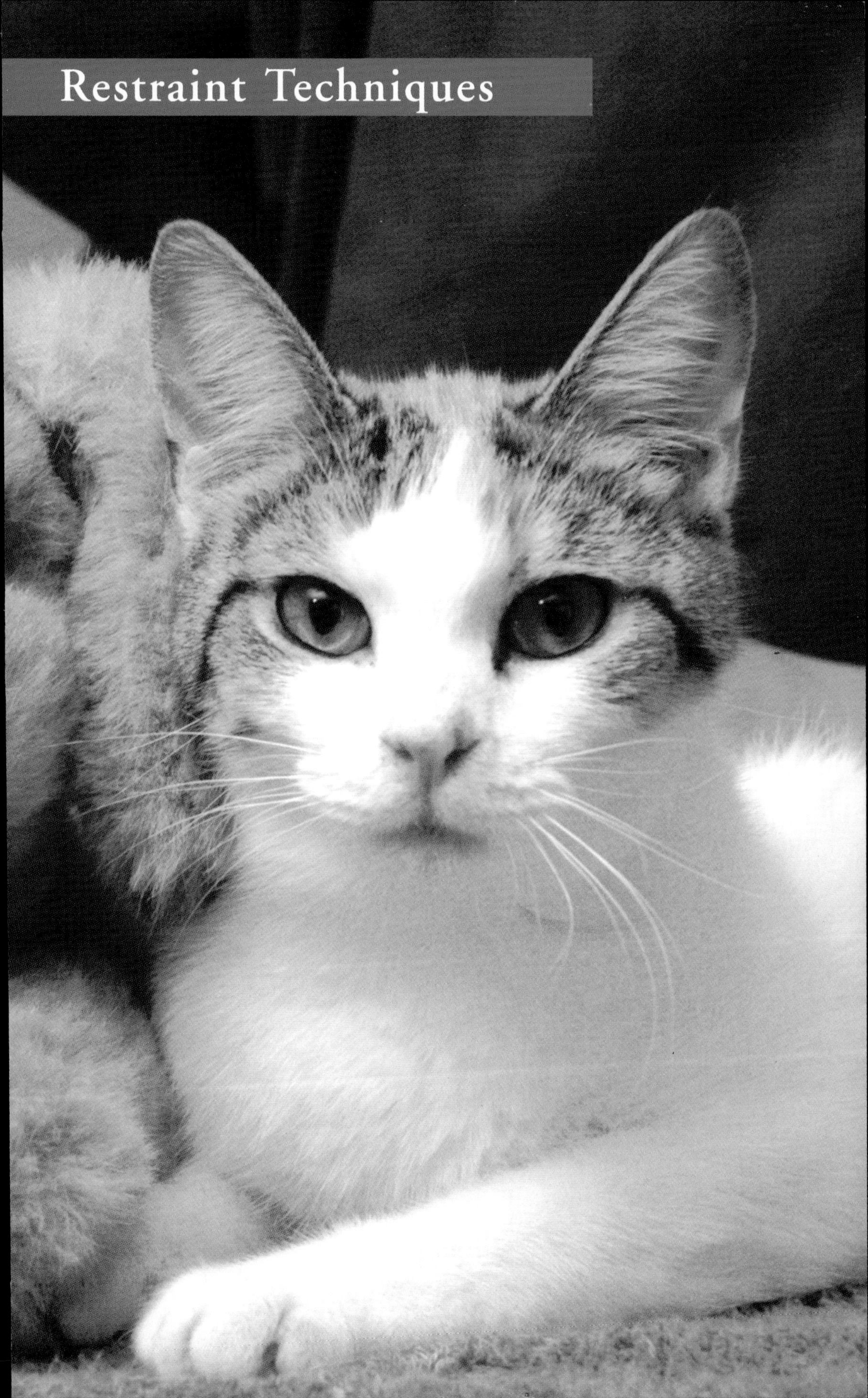

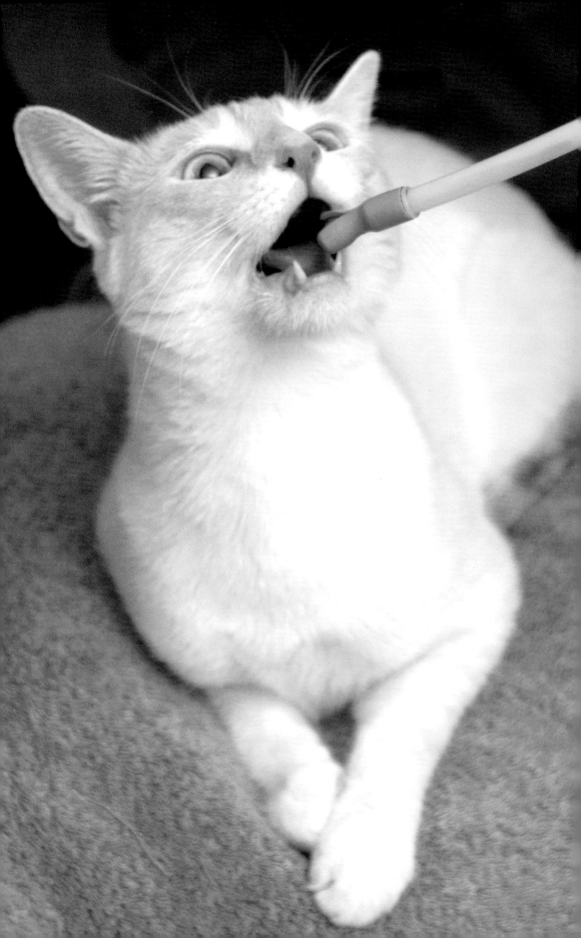

CHAPTER 11.
GENERAL
HANDLING
Principles

If an animal is comfortable with the environment, the handlers and the positions in which he is being held, he's more likely to remain calm and cooperative for the procedures. For this reason, it's more effective to focus on our interactions with the animal and his response to the handling rather than to try restraining the animal by grasping him in the strongest, most secure hold possible. Handling that is harsh, overly restrictive or simply improper for the individual pet can make that pet struggle more or become worse with repeated handling and on later visits. Even the most well-socialized and cooperative pets can become difficult or aggressive if restrained in a manner that causes them to struggle.

191

Before handlers are taught specific restraint positions, they must first understand the important principles of handling. They should also practice some exercises that will help them adapt to the many animals and situations they'll face. This chapter explores 10 principles of handling dogs and cats and offers examples that highlight each principle. For some principles, practice exercises are also given.

TEN PRINCIPLES OF HANDLING

Principle 1: Start with a comfortable environment.

Principle 2: Keep the animal from pacing, moving nervously or excitedly, squirming or suddenly trying to escape.

Principle 3: Support the animal well by having your hands, arms and body positioned appropriately. The pet should not feel as if he will fall or is off balance.

Principle 4: Be aware that physically positioning animals or asking them to perform behaviors when they are nervous, scared or confused can cause them to resist handling. Thus, when they act confused or scared, it's important to move deliberately and slowly to avoid a reflex resistance or escape behavior.

Principle 5: Know how to place your hands and body to control movement in any direction.

Principle 6: Wait until the pet is relaxed before starting a procedure.

Principle 7: Use the minimum restraint needed for the individual.

Principle 8: Avoid prolonged (more than 2 seconds) or repeated fighting or struggling.

Principle 9: Use distractions and rewards when appropriate.

Principle 10: Adjust your handling based on the animal and his response to restraint, and learn to adjust your sample-taking technique.

11.1 Principle 1: Start With a Comfortable Environment

Little changes in the hospital set-up can have a big effect on the pet's emotional state.

Try to keep the animal comfortable to help decrease fear.

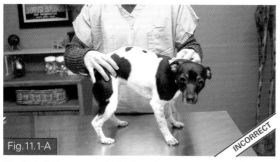

Fig.11.1-A, Incorrect: This dog does not want to sit or lie down because she's uncomfortable on the cold table. *(Video 1)*

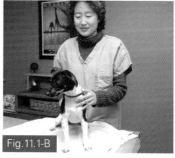

Fig.11.1-B, Correct: Make the area comfortable. Once a towel is added, this dog automatically sits.

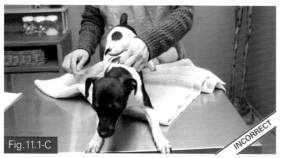

Fig.11.1-C, Incorrect: For dogs who squirm a lot, the towel can be slippery on the metal table.

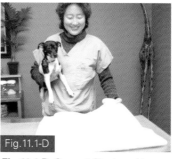

Fig.11.1-D, Correct: The towel is now on top of a nonslip piece of plastic that's easy to clean.

Fig.11.1-E: This dog is usually friendly and outgoing with people and dogs, but in the hospital setting she's fearful.

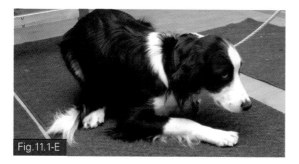

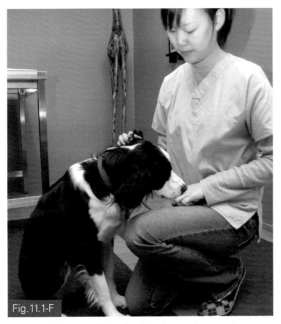

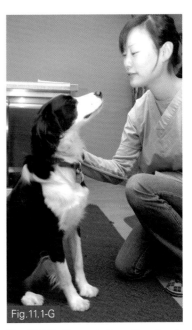

Fig.11.1-F, Correct: Take the time (several seconds or several minutes) to greet the pet properly. Prior to restraint or performing an exam or procedure, the technician should give treats, let the dog approach at his own rate and then pet the dog while giving additional treats. Try to get the dog into a happy, even playful emotional state.

Fig.11.1-G, Correct: Now the dog is relaxed and will be more likely to cooperate for the procedures and to improve behaviorally on his next visit.

Avoid situations that make the dog or cat feel unsafe

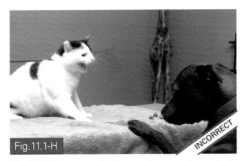

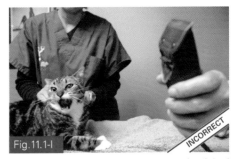

Fig.11.1-H, Incorrect: Most cats are not comfortable with dogs, especially unfamiliar ones. For them, seeing a dog is like you seeing Bigfoot walk outside your hospital room. Dogs, too, might be fearful of other dogs and unfamiliar people. Be aware of this when moving animals around the hospital and choosing where to perform treatments.

Fig.11.1-I, Incorrect: Many cats are fearful of clippers and other loud sounds. Whenever clippers are activated in a treatment room, the user should first check to see whether cats—or fearful dogs—are nearby. Ideally, fearful or nervous cats should be treated in a quiet room with no other animals.

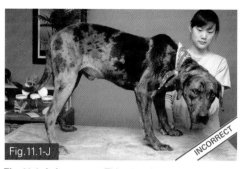

Fig.11.1-J

Fig.11.1-J, Incorrect: This dog is nervous on the table. Some technicians and veterinarians choose to put dogs on a table because the animal might hold still better when he is fearful. But this strategy can backfire.

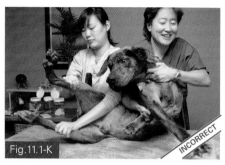

Fig.11.1-K

Fig.11.1-K, Incorrect: Due to his fear, this dog tenaciously resists being put into lateral recumbency.

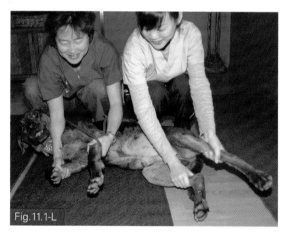

Fig.11.1-L

Fig.11.1-L, Correct: The dog is fine being restrained on the floor because he's not fearful here. It is best to use good technique to control energetic animals, rather than put them into a fearful state in the hope that they will freeze or move less.

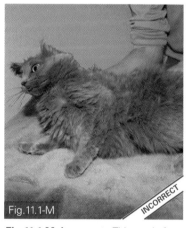

Fig.11.1-M

Fig.11.1-M, Incorrect: This cat is fearful and ready to bolt. She's about to explode.

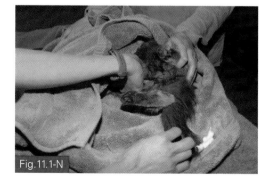

Fig.11.1-N

Fig.11.1-N, Correct: When wrapped loosely but securely in a towel with her head also covered, she feels safe and does not try to escape. We can perform a full exam from the neck back, take blood from the medial saphenous vein and collect urine via cystocentesis, while she remains relaxed the entire time.

11.2 Principle 2: Control the Pet's Movement

Keep animals from pacing, moving in a hyperactive manner, squirming or suddenly bolting. *(Video 2)* Avoid letting the dog or cat move around frantically or out of control. Anxious, nervous pets, especially dogs, can become more nervous and even frantic as they pace and strain to get away. Dogs who are simply excited can become out of control, and those with a tendency to become mouthy or to nip will be more likely to do so in this state. The dog should stand, sit or lie down calmly and move in a calm, relaxed manner. Controlling the dog skillfully in a calm, clear manner that he understands will help the dog trust you and look to you for future guidance. The following set of photos shows dogs who are overly excited or anxious and are pacing or hyperactive.

Control the dog's movement by first shortening the leash and then having her sit or lie down, if needed.

Example 1

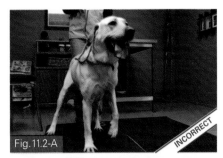

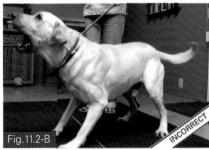

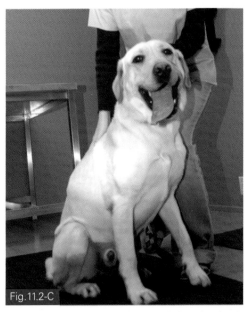

Fig.11.2-A, B, Example 1, Incorrect: This dog is moving back and forth in constant motion. He is working himself into a more aroused state and could be upsetting other patients.

Fig.11.2-C, Example 1, Correct: With the leash shortened so that he can't pace, the dog automatically sits.

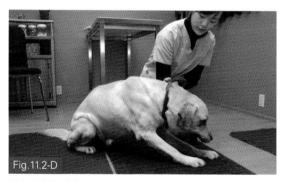

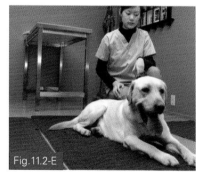

Fig.11.2-D, E, Example 1, Correct: He lies down with just a point to the ground, without even a verbal cue. Pets are more likely to behave appropriately when you can clearly and calmly communicate what you want.

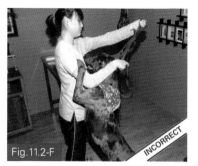

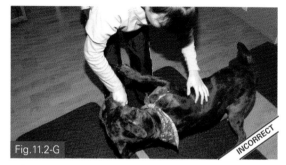

Fig.11.2-F, Example 1, Incorrect: This unruly dog is able to run and jump because the leash is too loose.

Fig.11.2-G, Example 1, Incorrect: Unlike the overly active yellow Labrador Retriever, this dog is out of control even with a tighter leash. Here, he's trying to grab the leash in his mouth.

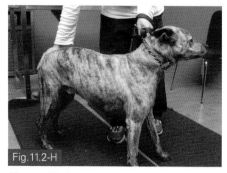

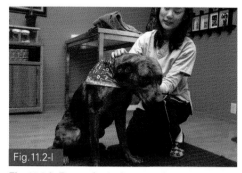

Fig.11.2-H, Example 1, Correct: To control this dog she needs to stabilize the rear end by placing her hand on the dog's hip in addition to holding the dog's collar.

Fig.11.2-I, Example 1, Correct: Once the dog is standing still he's much calmer and the technician is easily able to get him to sit. Sitting helps keep him calm. (See Chapter 12 for several methods for getting dogs to sit.)

It's a good idea to reward dogs for sitting and remaining seated.

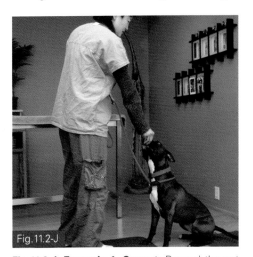

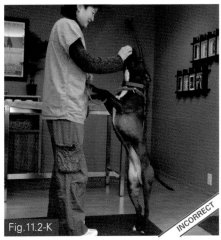

Fig.11.2-J, Example 1, Correct: Reward the pet for calm behavior using small treats. Five small treats are better than one big treat. Give one reward for sitting, followed by additional rewards for continuing to sit calmly. If you don't have the skill to deliver treats in a manner that keeps the dog calm, then stop giving treats or have someone else give them.

Fig.11.2-K, Example 1, Incorrect: Be careful to give treats in a manner that rewards the dog for calm behavior. Here, I hold the treat up high, causing the dog to jump. I should keep the treat hidden until I decide to give it to her, at which time I must give it quickly and present it directly to her mouth so that she doesn't have to jump to get it. (see Chapter 12, Section 12.3)

Don't let the dog wiggle just because you think he's friendly.

Remember, every interaction you have with the pet tells him something about you and whether you're able to provide clear guidance.

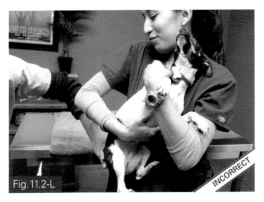

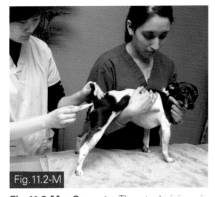

Fig.11.2-L, Incorrect: Here, the dog is being held in a way that allows her to struggle a lot. The dog is happy and excited, but the behavior can quickly deteriorate to nipping if she dislikes the handling. In fact, this dog has a history of being mouthy when restrained.

Fig.11.2-M, Correct: The technician is better able to keep the dog calm and controlled on the exam table.

Keep your hands on the pet or leash at all times, and always be ready for him to bolt or suddenly jump or fall off the table. Be alert and in control of the pet even when you're just standing around relaxed, or when the animal is sick and can't move well.

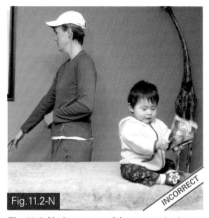

Fig.11.2-N

INCORRECT

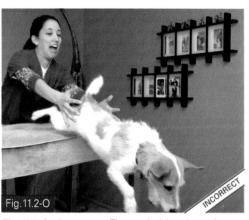

Fig.11.2-O

INCORRECT

Fig.11.2-N, Incorrect: Most people know that when you put a toddler or even a poorly mobile infant on a table, you should always keep a hand on her and watch carefully to prevent accidents. The same applies to dogs and cats, even those who are tranquilized or ill.

Fig.11.2-O, Incorrect: The technician here is not paying attention and the dog jumps off the table. This could cause injury or lead to the escape of an animal. **Never let dogs or cats escape off a table**.

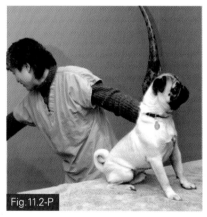

Fig.11.2-P

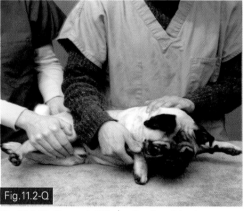

Fig.11.2-Q

Fig.11.2-P, Correct: To keep this dog from bolting when I reach for a dog treat, I keep my hand on his collar.

Fig.11.2-Q, Correct: When allowing this dog to get up, we'll keep our hands on him to prevent him from leaping off the table or scrambling around once standing.

11.3. Principle 3: Support the Animal Well

Provide support for the patient by having your hands, arms and body positioned appropriately. For instance, many people place pets onto their side by flipping them in a judo-like throw. This makes the pet anxious and gives him a bad hospital experience. If you are supporting the pet well, he should not flop around when changing from one position to another. In fact, when moving the animal around and changing positions, you should be able to do so in slow motion and freeze at any instant, and the dog or cat should be in complete balance (not flailing).

Avoid flipping dogs and cats when repositioning them. *(Video 3)*

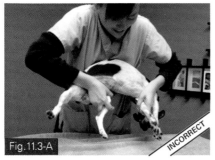 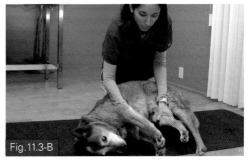

Fig. 11.3-A, Incorrect: Avoid flipping dogs and cats into position in judo-like throws. Flying and landing with a thud on their side will scare many animals. After this, they might not trust you.

Fig. 11.3-B, Correct: Instead, support the dog so that she doesn't think she's off balance or falling. Here, the technician slides the dog down the front of her legs and can stop the progression and hold the dog stationary if necessary before reaching the final position. Practice this technique on calm dogs first.

Support the animal by placing your arms and body in the right positions to prevent movement in all directions. Then meet the animal's pressure instead if he tries to wiggle or struggle rather than immediately letting him loose or continuously holding him in a death grip.

Never let a pet thunk or flop or whack his head when you are positioning him on his side or back. What would you think if your doctor handled you or a family member in such an unskilled manner?

Supporting the animal well doesn't mean holding him in a death grip. Your arms and body just need to be positioned appropriately so that you can apply the needed pressure. Think of the safety bars on a roller coaster; they secure you in place but don't excessively push you into the seat. Even if you're upside down, the bars meet the pressure of your body to keep you in place rather than flying open to let you fall. Similarly, when restraining an animal, you must meet the animal's pressure instead of letting the animal pull your arm out of place or drag you around.

> Supporting the animal well doesn't mean holding him in a death grip. Your arms and body just need to be positioned appropriately so that you can apply the needed pressure when the animal tries to move.

The greater the surface area in contact with you, the more securely you are held in place.

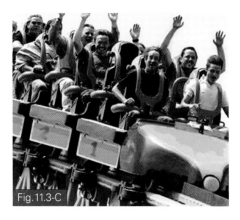

Fig.11.3-C

Fig.11.3-C: On a roller coaster, the seat secures your bottom and back. The bars prevent you from moving up or forward. The bars do not squish you into the seat, but they keep you secure. The greater the surface area in contact with you, the more securely you are held in place. If the bars were narrower or the seats were made of wire bars, you might feel less secure.

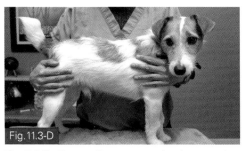

Fig.11.3-D

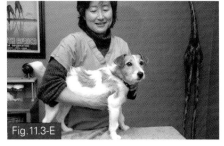

Fig.11.3-E

Fig.11.3-D, Correct: To prevent a dog from moving away from you, put one hand on the chest and one on the rear end. This is appropriate in cases where the dog is not likely to move around a lot.

Fig.11.3-E, Correct: Here, I have more contact with the dog and consequently more control. I am hugging him close to my body, and my arm along the opposite side helps prevent him from moving away. The hand in front helps keep him from moving forward.

Secure the animal on all sides. Again, the more contact you have, the more secure the animal will be.

Exercise 1: Rotating Objects Around Their Center

To support animals, it's important to understand how objects move. The goal when changing body positions is to keep the animal balanced and centered. This often requires you to use both hands in concert. After showing a couple of examples with inanimate objects (below), we'll apply this concept to rolling a dog onto his hip. Like rolling a ball, you will use both hands in concert to roll the dog.

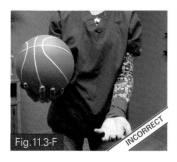

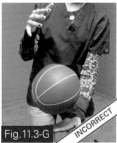

Fig.11.3-F, G, Example 1, Incorrect: Obviously, this is not the most secure way to rotate a ball 180 degrees. Losing contact with the ball might cause you to drop it.

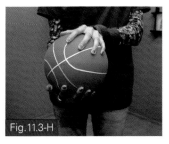

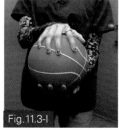

Fig.11.3-H, I, Example 1, Correct: A more secure method is to keep both hands on the ball while rotating it. This way, the ball is supported on two sides at all times; it's not likely to be dropped. Also, the amount of rotation can be carefully controlled.

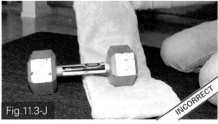

Fig.11.3-J, Example 2, Incorrect: It's hard to roll an object if its entire weight is on the floor.

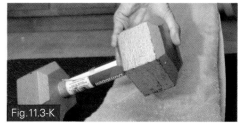

Fig.11.3-K, Example 2, Correct: But if you lift the object off the floor, it's easier to roll. So when working with a dog, be sure to lift the weight off the dog's rear slightly to more easily roll him onto his hip.

Example 3: Rotating a dog's hip.

This method of rotating works for both small and large dogs. To do this exercise, use a calm dog that will lie down readily and stay lying down. If needed, a second handler can place a hand over the dog's shoulder or restrain it in some other manner to keep the dog down.

(Video 4)

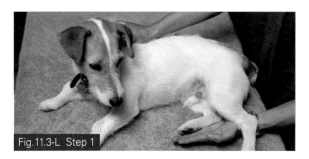

Fig.11.3-L Step 1: Start with the dog on his right hip so you can rotate him onto his left hip in this exercise. First tuck the right leg under him by placing your left hand next to the right foot and leg (up to the ankle), and slide the foot under the dog.

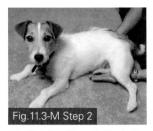
Fig.11.3-M Step 2

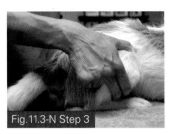
Fig.11.3-N Step 3

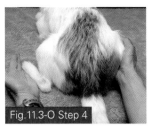
Fig.11.3-O Step 4

Fig.11.3-M, Step 2: Push the right foot far enough under for you to grasp the right knee without having to reach under the dog (see next photo). The dog in this photo needs to have his right foot pushed farther under his body.

Fig.11.3-N, Step 3: Grasp the right leg just below the knee using your right hand. You might need to reach slightly under the dog to do this, depending on how far you previously pushed the foot under the dog. **Do not try to rotate the dog yet. You must have the left hand in place first.**

Fig.11.3-O, Step 4: To tuck the left leg under the dog, place the left hand just lateral to and slightly under the side of the left foot. Now you can push this leg under while simultaneously using the right hand to rotate the right side up.

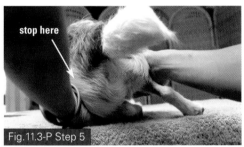
stop here
Fig.11.3-P Step 5

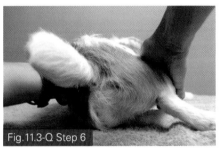
Fig.11.3-Q Step 6

Fig.11.3-P, Step 5: Remember, it's like rotating a ball. The hands work in concert. And, as with the dumbbell, you might need to elevate the dog slightly (almost imperceptibly) to rotate the legs under. This dog's hip is already rotated far enough. Do not rotate farther or you will cause the dog to get up.

Fig.11.3-Q, Step 6: Remove your left hand from below the dog as soon as the hip is rotated. Your hand should never be completely under the dog. Note that the left leg does not protrude much from under the dog.

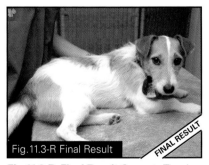
Fig.11.3-R Final Result
FINAL RESULT

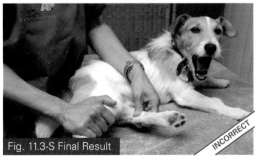
Fig. 11.3-S Final Result
INCORRECT

Fig.11.3-R, Final Result Correct: The dog is now comfortably lying on his left hip.

Fig.11.3-S, Final Result, Incorrect: The left leg DOES NOT need to be pulled out like this. In fact, doing so can cause the dog to become anxious.

Exercise 2: Keep Objects in the Same Location

Just like the roller coaster safety bars must support the pressure of the person so that the person does not fly out of the seat, the technician must meet the animal's pressure to keep the animal from squirming loose and falling or escaping. The goal of the Exercise 2 variations is to keep the ball in the same location no matter how hard or in what direction the coach tries to push the ball loose. Between the coach's attempts, the technician should relax to prevent fatigue, yet she should be ready for the next directional change of the ball.

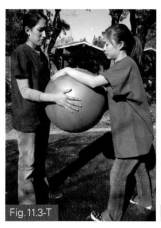 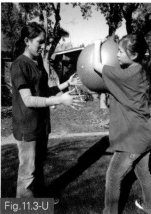 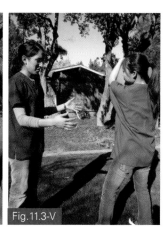

Fig.11.3-T

Fig.11.3-U

Fig.11.3-V

Fig.11.3-T,U,V, Part 1: If you're holding a ball and someone comes over and grabs it out of your hands, the next time you have the ball and the person approaches, you'll know to hold onto it more firmly. Similarly, when an animal first starts to struggle, your first reaction should be to hold him securely so that he doesn't escape (and bite someone, run loose in or out of the hospital, or jump off the table and injure himself). While this book demonstrates many different ways to hold an animal, you should have a good understanding of how to use your body so that you can adapt to the animal, rather than trying to memorize a large number of restraint methods.

> Just like the roller coaster safety bars must support the pressure of the person so that the person does not fly out of the seat, the technician must meet the animal's pressure to keep the animal from squirming loose and falling or escaping

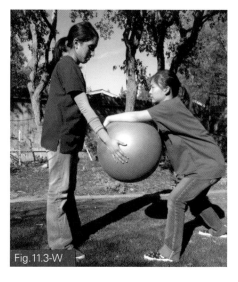

Fig.11.3-W

Fig.11.3-W, Part 2: Have two technicians practice trying to pull the ball from one another. In this contest, which technician do you think is going to win? Probably the one on the right because she has a better grip. She's hugging the ball close to her so that she can grab it with her entire arm. In general, the greater the surface area in contact with an object or animal (in the right locations), the better you can secure and support it.

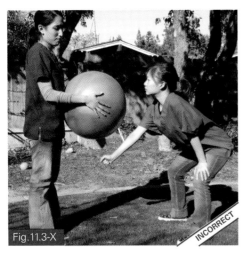

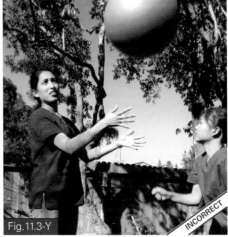

Fig.11.3-X, Y, Part 3, Incorrect: Now have one technician hold the ball as if she is going to rotate the ball in the same manner as in Exercise 1. Have a second technician hit the bottom of the ball while the first technician tries to keep it in exactly the same place. The first technician (the one holding the ball) is not allowed to move her hands.

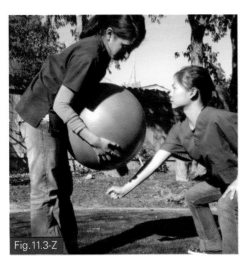

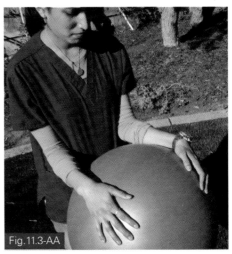

Fig.11.3-Z, Part 3, Correct: This time, the technician blocks the ball from flying out the top by leaning over it. Notice that she's right against it. If there's room between her body and the ball, then there's room for the ball to get loose. Now, what happens if the rules change and the technician is no longer allowed to lean over the ball, yet she must support the ball evenly?

Fig.11.3-AA, Part 3 (variation): This is the only other solution. She must block the top. Grabbing around the sides is not an efficient way to keep something from flying out the top. Notice that her entire forearm is in contact with the ball.

Now apply this concept to a dog.

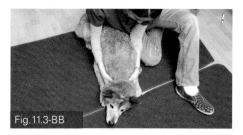 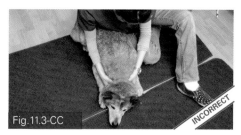

Fig. 11.3-BB, Part 5, Correct: Here's how this exercise can be applied. Some dogs do not like having someone lean over them. The technician is using the same hold on the dog as she did on the ball (refer to Figure 11.3-AA) to keep the dog from getting up.

Fig.11.3-CC, Part 5, Incorrect: Notice that here, she does not have good contact on one side; there's space between her left arm and the dog. The dog could wiggle free and get up if he tried because the technician is not supporting him evenly.

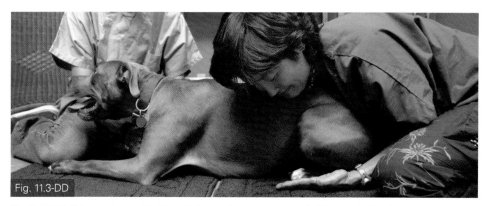

Fig.11.3-DD: This can be applied to rotating a dog's hips, as well. When rotating the hips, you might need to lean over the dog from the rear to keep him from getting up.

Exercise 3: Practice rotating objects and animals around their center axes.

The objective is to keep the object or animal balanced the whole time.

First practice with an animate object

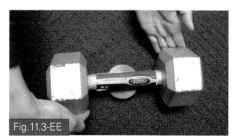 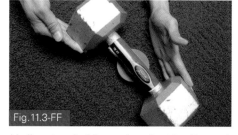

Fig. 11.3-EE, FF, Example 1, Correct: To keep the dumbbell centered while moving, direct it with equal pressure from both sides.

First practice with an animate object

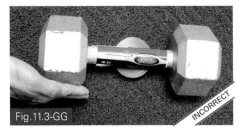 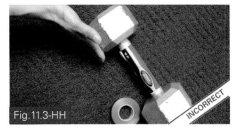

Fig. 11.3-GG, HH, Example 2, Incorrect: Using just one hand here will knock the dumbbell off its center axis.

Then practice with a dog

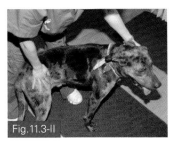 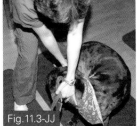 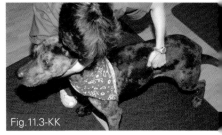

Fig.11.3-II, Step 1: The next three photos show a **balanced change of direction**. A clear way of directing the dog is to place one hand on the side of the head just caudal to (behind) the ear and the other on the opposite hip. Guide the head away from your body so that the dog doesn't turn his head into your leg. Push his hip in the opposite direction to keep the dog centered during the turn.

Fig.11.3-JJ, Step 2: The turn is almost complete.

Fig.11.3-KK, Step 3: When the dog is facing the new direction, keep one hand on the hip or flank and the other on the collar or around the neck, depending on what works best for the dog.

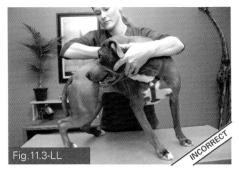 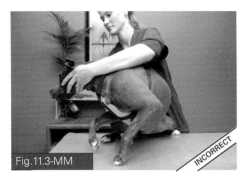

Fig.11.3-LL, Incorrect: Some people physically turn a dog around by taking his head and guiding just the head to face the opposite direction.

Fig.11.3-MM, Incorrect: This dog is confused and is therefore resisting as the technician guides only his head and not his hind end. The same dog was cooperative for a centered turn.

Exercise 4: Applying the principle of rotation around an axis to positioning dogs into a sit.

The principle of rotation around an axis can be applied to positioning dogs into a sit.

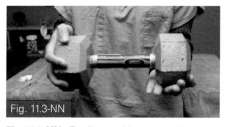

Fig.11.3-NN: To tilt an object at a 45-degree angle, as you would a dog whom you're placing into a sit, you would raise one hand while the other lowers.

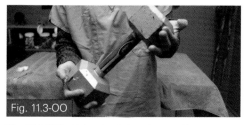

Fig.11.3-OO: Using both hands provides support and changes the angle of the object.

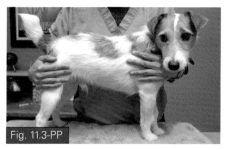

Fig.11.3-PP, Step 1: Similarly, to physically have a dog sit, shift the weight off the front end and toward the rear end. For small dogs, start with one hand on the chest and the other on the rear.

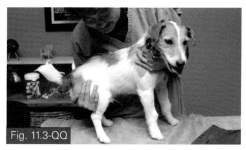

Fig.11.3-QQ, Step 2: Slightly raise your arm and hand in front while pushing caudally on the chest, at the same time bending the rear legs. Notice I'm leaning toward the rear end to help shift the dog's weight back.

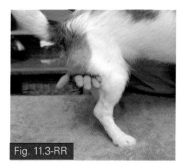

Fig.11.3-RR: To bend the rear legs, place pressure on the backs of the knees. Think of doing a karate chop— but gently and in slow motion—right in the groove where the femur and the tibia meet.

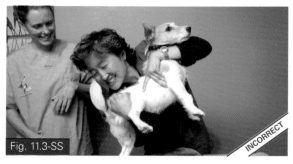

Fig.11.3-SS, Incorrect: This shows what happens if you place pressure in the wrong location; it causes the dog to struggle and become distressed. If you were the recipient of this type of handling, you probably would not trust the person thereafter.

Exercise 5: Placing Animals on Their Backs in Your Lap

In this exercise, we'll practice placing an animal onto his back in your lap with the animal starting in a standing position. To do this requires you to keep the dog's front and rear supported. We'll start with the dog's left side against the handler and the dog's head facing the holder's left shoulder. *(Video 5)*

Keep the pet balanced around its center at all times.

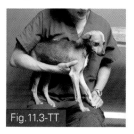
Fig.11.3-TT

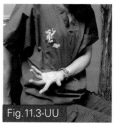
Fig.11.3-UU

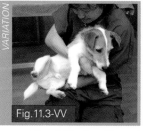
Fig.11.3-VV

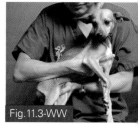
Fig.11.3-WW

Fig.11.3-TT, Step 1: Support the dog with your right arm and hand. The hand is under the chest. The thumb is on the outside of the front leg to prevent the dog from backing up. The dog should be snug against you.

Fig.11.3-UU, Step 2: This photo is illustrating without the dog the arm position you'll use. Reach back with the left hand to support the dog's left hip. Keep your arm against your side so that it's between you and the dog. For very small dogs, your right hand can remain in position on the chest.

Fig.11.3-VV, Step 2 (variation): For slightly larger dogs, you might need to grasp the left leg with your right hand as close to the elbow as possible rather than keeping your right hand on the chest.

Fig.11.3-WW, Step 3: With your arms in the position described in Step 2, rotate the dog onto her back. Because you will be sliding her into your lap, raise her front end while you rotate her body. Be sure to move both hands in a coordinated fashion.

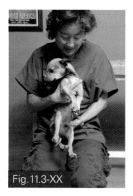
Fig.11.3-XX

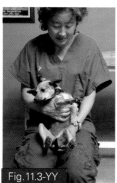
Fig.11.3-YY

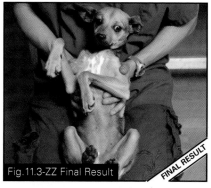
Fig.11.3-ZZ Final Result

FINAL RESULT

Fig.11.3-XX, Step 4: Now the dog is vertical with her back against you. Your hand still supports her hip. Next, slide her into your lap.

Fig.11.3-YY, Step 5: When placing the dog in your lap, make sure her rear end is tucked under and her back is curved. Then slide her farther down into your lap so that most of her body is horizontal.

Fig.11.3-ZZ, Final Step: Stabilize the dog by holding each of her forearms with one hand. Your hands should be above the dog's elbows.

Avoid doing it like this where the dog's body is unevenly supported.

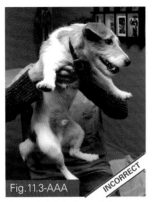
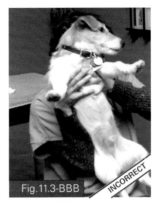
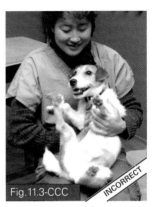

Fig.11.3-AAA, Step 5, Incorrect: The dog is unbalanced, yet this is how people frequently try to reposition dogs. The dog's front end is supported but the hind end is not. Dogs who are used to being held this way might not resist. But those who aren't might struggle, causing them to become anxious.

Fig.11.3-BBB, Step 5, Incorrect: At this stage, many dogs will start to kick with their hind legs because they are unbalanced.

Fig.11.3-CCC, Step 5, Incorrect: Here, he finally starts struggling. If he had been better supported earlier, he would not be struggling now.

11.4 Principle 4: Avoid Causing Resistance in the Pet

Be aware that physically positioning animals or asking them to perform behaviors when they are nervous, scared or confused can cause them to resist handling. *(Video 6)* This is illustrated by the following example—Imagine that someone wants you to sit in a chair, so they forcefully push you into one, like this (Figures 11.4-A,B,C):

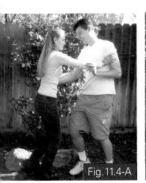
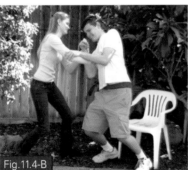
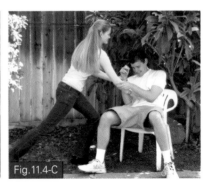

Your natural response would be to resist. Similarly, while pets might know how to perform behaviors such as sit or lie down in their home environment, in new environments they may be scared, distracted or confused. Consequently, they're less likely to understand what's being asked of them. It's important to go slowly and move deliberately so that it's clear what you want when physically positioning them. In this way, you don't cause them to resist handling or try to escape.

For instance, if someone were to physically guide you to move across the room and sit in a chair, they should guide you gently. Once you are near the chair, they should stop for an instant before guiding you to sit. (Figures 11.4-D,E,F)

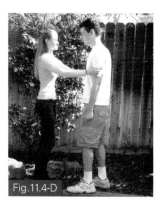 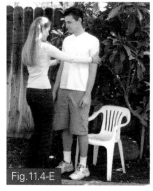 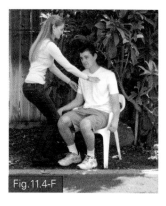

Similarly, if you need to place a dog who's nervously squirming into a sit position, first you must have him stand still. Once he's in a stable stand, then you can guide him into a sit. You can also ask the dog to "sit" once in a calm voice. Avoid commanding the dog over and over ("sit, sit, Sit, Sit, SIT!") like a military chant, or you'll likely cause the dog to be more excited or anxious.

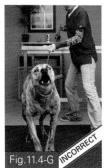 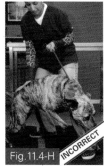 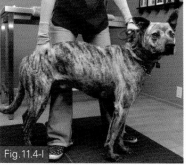 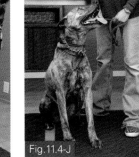

Fig.11.4-G, H, Incorrect: This dog is nervous and his movement is out of control. At this point, would you really expect him to sit if asked?

Fig.11.4-I, Correct: The technician shortened the leash to control the dog's movement and is gently using her hands on the dog's collar and hind end to stabilize him in a standing position. The dog is much calmer in this position.

Fig.11.4-J, Correct: Now that he's calm, he readily sits when the technician says "sit" in a calm, encouraging tone of voice. Some dogs will sit automatically once they are calm.

11.5 Principle 5: Know How to Place Your Hands and Body

Know how to place your hands and body to control movement. Remember the rollercoaster. (Figure 11.3-C) In general, the greater the surface area of your body that's in direct contact with the animal, the better control you have. To understand how to control movement, try these exercises. Start with a well-socialized dog who will not become stressed if you place him into various positions. Have one person handle the dog and a second person coach and test the handler by luring the dog with a treat or toy, or by pushing the dog into different positions.

Exercise 1: Practice hand and body positions used to prevent the dog from moving forward.

The coach should use a toy or treat to encourage the dog to try to move forward. If that doesn't work, the coach can also push the dog forward from behind. Evaluate which methods shown below appear to provide the best control, and practice switching among restraint positions quickly.

Methods 1 and 2 for preventing forward movement (chest holds)

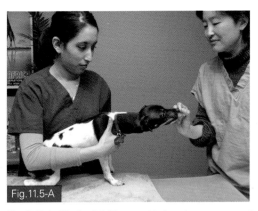 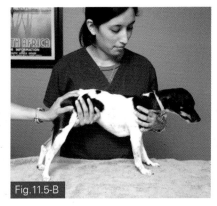

Fig.11.5-A, Method 1: The outside hand wraps around the dog's outside shoulder so that he cannot move forward. To test the effectiveness of this hold, the coach is luring the dog forward with a treat. An added benefit is that the outside arm also prevents the dog from moving away.

Fig.11.5-B, Method 2: One hand lies flat across the front of the chest to prevent forward movement and one supports the hind end from underneath. To test the effectiveness of the hold, the coach has her hand on the dog's rear end and is pushing the dog forward.

Method 3 for preventing forward movement in larger dogs (chest holds)

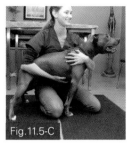
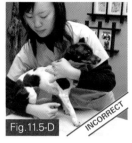
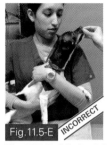
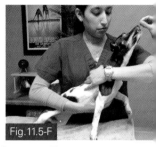

Fig.11.5-C, Method 3: With larger dogs, place your entire arm across the dog's chest or neck so that his chest and neck sit in the crook of your arm.

Fig.11.5-D, Method 3, Incorrect: The large dog method does not work well for small dogs because it does not provide good contact between your arm and the dog's neck. Look at the space between this handler's left arm and the dog.

Fig.11.5-E, Method 3, Incorrect: Because of the poor contact with the dog's chest, with this hold the dog can easily slip his leg over your arm this way. *(Video 7)*

Fig.11.5-F, Method 3 (fixing the problem): If the dog does manage to get his leg over your arm, immediately lift your left elbow so that the leg falls through and then change to a different hold. The dog's leg must be kept off your arm so that he is not in a good position to escape or struggle.

Method 4 for preventing forward movement (the U hold)

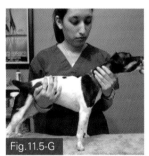
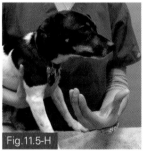
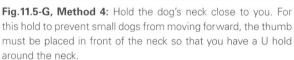
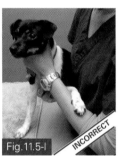
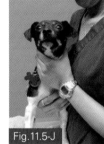

Fig.11.5-G, Method 4: Hold the dog's neck close to you. For this hold to prevent small dogs from moving forward, the thumb must be placed in front of the neck so that you have a U hold around the neck.

Fig.11.5-H, Method 4: Here's a close-up of the hand position for the U hold. Also use this to keep dogs from moving away. You can slide it around to the outside of the neck in a C hold (shown in Figure 11.5-S) to keep the dog from jumping up. Note that with this hold your hand acts like a brace or support. It does not squeeze the neck forcefully, which could affect respiration.

Fig.11.5-I, Method 4, Incorrect: This dog can still get a paw over the handler's arm because there is space between the arm and the dog.

Fig.11.5-J, Method 4, Correct: Now the technician keeps her arm right next to her body and moves the dog forward so that the dog's leg has no room to squeeze through.

Exercise 2: Practice positions to prevent the dog from jumping up.

Be able to switch quickly among these positions.

Method 1 for prevention of jumping (the collar hold)

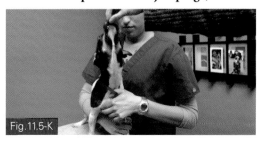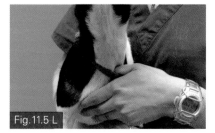

Fig.11.5-K, Method 1: Hold the collar. If the dog jumps up, he can only move about an inch. To test the holder, the coach can offer food above the dog's head. If the dog won't try to stretch or jump for the food lure, the coach can lift up on the dog's chest.

Fig.11.5-L, Method 1: Be sure to hold your hand steady if he tries to jump.

Method 2 for prevention of jumping (the ring hold)

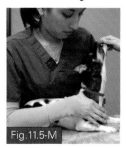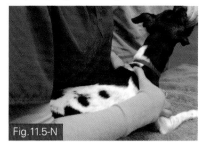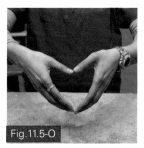

Fig.11.5-M, Method 2: For small dogs, make a ring around the neck with both hands. If the dog jumps up, your thumbs will help hold him down. Once he relaxes, ease the pressure. He only feels pressure if he tries to jump or push upward.

Fig.11.5-N, O, Method 2: This method offers the most control for keeping little dogs from jumping upward because it provides the most contact with the dog.

Method 3 for prevention of jumping (the upper leg hold) *(Video 8)*

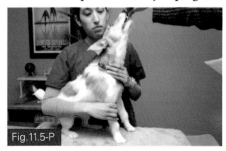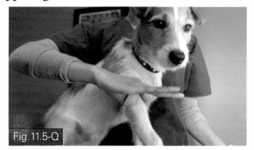

Fig.11.5-P, Method 3: You can also prevent jumping up by placing the hand of your outside arm around the proximal aspect of the leg.

Fig.11.5-Q, Method 3: The thumb and index finger should be above the elbow.

Method 4 for prevention of jumping (the C hold)

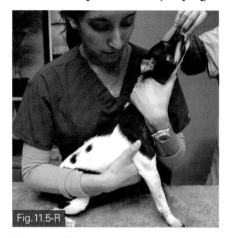

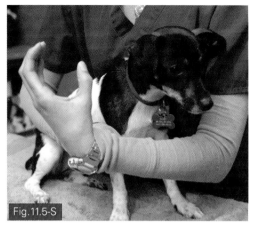

Fig.11.5-R, Method 4: For small dogs, holding the neck in a C hold (a U turned sideways) can help prevent the dog from jumping up. If needed, pull his neck close to your shoulder.

Fig.11.5-S, Method 4: Here's the "C" hold up close.

Method 5 for prevention of jumping in larger dogs (the neck hold)

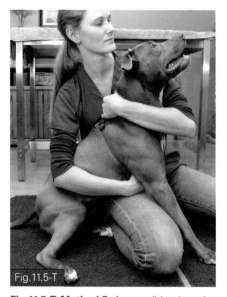

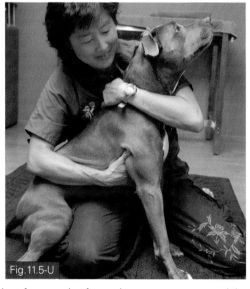

Fig.11.5-T, Method 5: As you did to keep large dogs from moving forward, wrap your arm around the dog's neck to prevent jumping. This hold would be stronger if the dog's neck were sitting in the crook of the technician's arm (as in the next photo).

Fig.11.5-U, Method 5: If the dog struggles, pull his neck close to your shoulder. This hold works best if the dog's ventral neck sits in the crook of your arm, because this provides the most surface area contact and requires less strength.

Method 6 for prevention of jumping (making a ceiling)

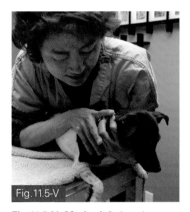

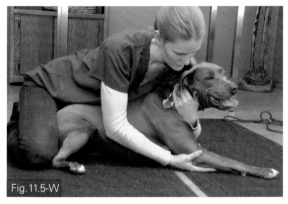

Fig.11.5-V, Method 6: Leaning over the dog or placing a hand over the shoulder can prevent him from standing. This is needed only if the dog is resisting. Once the dog is relaxed, you do not need to lean over him.

Fig.11.5-W, Method 6: Leaning works for large dogs, too, although there's no need to use this for dogs who are lying down calmly and are relaxed. Also, avoid leaning over dogs who become fearful when you try this. Once the dog is stable in the position, you do not need to continue leaning. For dogs who are not already known to be friendly for this type of handling, it's safest to use one of the more secure holds around the neck (refer to Figures 11.5-KK,LL,MM) and possibly to use a muzzle.

Exercise 3: Practice methods to prevent the dog from moving away from you.

Method 1 for preventing dogs from moving away (placing a hand on the hip)

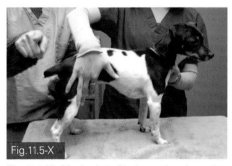

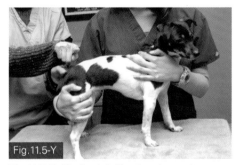

Fig.11.5-X, Method 1: Placing a hand on the dog's hip keeps him from moving his hip away. Only apply pressure when the dog tries to move away. Here, the coach is pushing the dog's rear end away.

Fig.11.5-Y, Method 1: The hand can also wrap around from the back, or even from under the dog (not pictured).

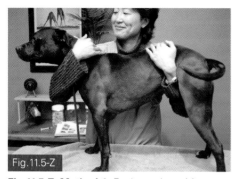

Fig.11.5-Z, Method 1: For large dogs, it's sometimes easier to place the hand across the flank by reaching either under or over the dog.

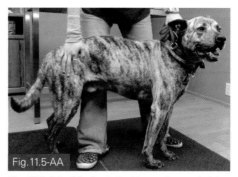

Fig.11.5-AA, Method 1: Here, the technician prevents the dog from moving away with her hand over his flank.

Method 2 for preventing dogs from moving away (the C hold for small dogs)

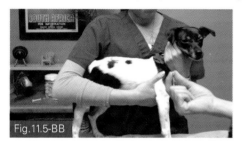

Fig.11.5-BB, Method 2: Use a C" hold on the neck to keep the dog from moving his front end away from you.

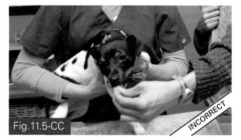

Fig.11.5-CC, Method 2, Incorrect: Be sure to hold the dog close to your shoulder so that this doesn't happen.

Method 3 for preventing dogs from moving away in medium and large dogs (the neck hold) *(Refer to Chapter 12, Video 4)*

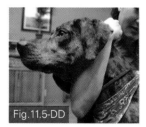

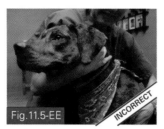

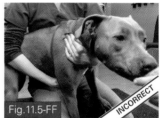

Fig.11.5-DD, Method 3: With large dogs, wrap your entire arm around the neck. Be sure to have the dog's neck in the crook of your arm so that there is more surface area in contact with the neck.

Fig.11.5-EE, Method 3, Incorrect: In these examples the dog's neck is not in the crook of my arm. As a result, I need strong biceps to keep his head pulled in against me and my arms will have to remain tense. I'll also have a slower reaction time if he starts struggling and will become tired faster.

Fig.11.5-FF, Method 3, Incorrect: Be sure to hold the dog's neck against your shoulder so this doesn't happen. If he can move his head this much, he can reach around to bite you or the veterinarian.

TIP

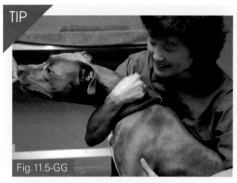

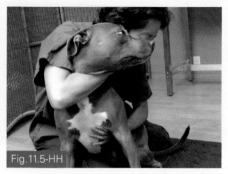

Fig.11.5-GG, HH, Method 3 (problem): In both variations, the dog can still stretch his head forward and turn the head to the side.

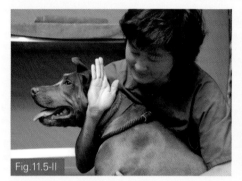

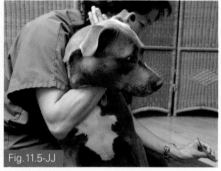

Fig.11.5-II, JJ, Method 3 (problem): For more secure restraint, hold the dog's head closer to your shoulder by turning your palm out. Be sure to keep your hand behind the dog's skull or the dog will be able to back out. The dog can still turn his head but not as far as with the previous hold.

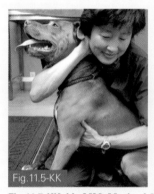

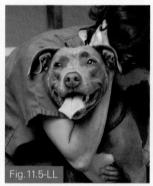

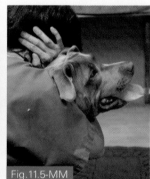

Fig.11.5-KK, LL, MM, Method 3: The hold is even more secure when you form a circle around the dog's neck with your arm by placing your hand behind your head. Again, be sure your arm is just behind the skull so that dog can't back his head out. Be sure to practice all three variations of Method 3 and compare. Have someone hold treats in a way that encourages the dog to struggle and reward the dog if he can reach far enough. Of course, only train this undesirable behavior in the dog when testing your restraint technique.

Method 4 for preventing dogs from moving away (arm on the side of the chest)

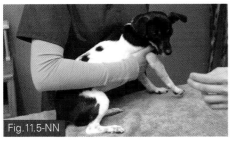 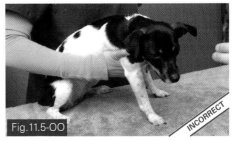

Fig.11.5-NN, Method 4: By placing the hand behind the elbow and resting the hand and arm on the dog's outer chest you can keep the dog from moving away from you by holding him close to your side.

Fig.11.5-OO, Method 4, Incorrect: This dog is not being held snugly. Use your arm to pull the dog in close to your body.

Method 5 for preventing dogs from moving away (holding the collar)

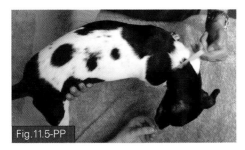

Fig.11.5-PP, Method 5: Hold the collar to prevent the dog from moving the front half of his body away.

Exercise 4: Practice methods to prevent the dog from moving backward.

Method 1 for preventing dogs from backing up

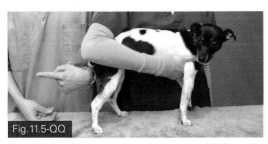 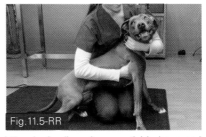

Fig.11.5-QQ, Method 1: Keeping the outside hand behind the dog's elbow is essential in large and small dogs. The hand should be open and flat to increase contact with the dog for better control. If the dog moves backward, you must draw him closer to your body so that he doesn't wiggle loose in other directions.

Fig.11.5-RR, Method 1 (large dogs): Having a hand behind the elbow is essential with large dogs. Your fingers should be in the armpit while your thumb is on the lateral aspect of the dog's arm.

Method 2 for preventing dogs from backing up (getting behind the dog)

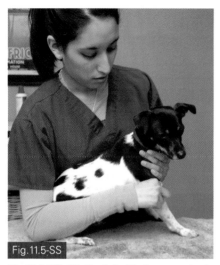

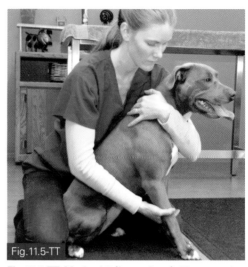

Fig.11.5-SS, Method 2: Placing your body and arm behind the dog can prevent him from backing up.

Fig.11.5-TT, Method 2 (large dogs): Place your leg or body behind the dog to prevent backing up. In this position, your body makes a wall along one side of the dog and your leg supports his rear end.

Exercise 5: Preventing dogs from sitting.

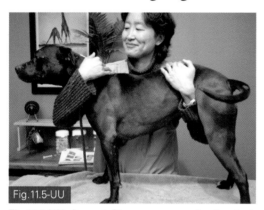

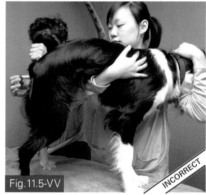

Fig.11.5-UU, Correct: Place one arm under the dog's abdomen as far back as possible to keep him from sitting. This arm also keeps the dog from pulling away.

Fig.11.5-VV, Incorrect: In this photo, the arm supporting the rear end is not far enough back. The dog could sit if he tried. The technician is trying to compensate by pulling on the dog's neck.

11.6 Principle 6: Wait Until the Pet Is Relaxed

Wait until you have the pet relaxed and under control before trying to perform any procedures.

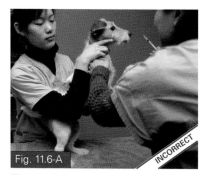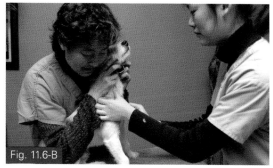

Fig. 11.6-A

Fig. 11.6-B

Fig. 11.6-A, Incorrect: The technician attempted to start the procedure before the dog was relaxed in the restraint position. As a result, the dog got nervous and tried to escape. *(Video 9).*

Fig. 11.6-B, Correct: When an animal is tense or you've had trouble getting the pet into a safe position, wait a few seconds when you have him in the correct position so that he can relax. The person performing the procedure should ask the restrainer if she's ready. If the pet does not relax, try a different technique or a quieter location or go to chemical restraint. Alternatively, set up a technician behavior modification session to countercondition the dog to the hospital, the staff and the handling procedures.

11.7 Principle 7: Use Minimal or Appropriate Restraint *(Video 10)*

Use the minimum restraint needed for the individual animal. But don't hold the animal carelessly or allow him to squirm and get loose. Rather, avoid automatically holding the pet in a death grip, squeezing his head and neck against your body in a sleeper hold, pinning him down like a wrestler trying to score a take-down, or stretching him out.

Example 1: Avoid automatically stretching animals

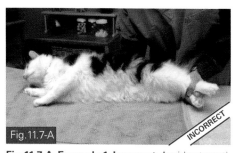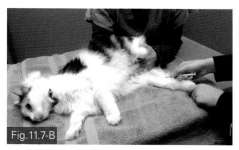

Fig. 11.7-A

Fig. 11.7-B

Fig. 11.7-A, Example 1, Incorrect: Avoid automatically stretching cats like this. Doing so can agitate the cat.

Fig. 11.7-B, Example 1, Correct: Holding just his hind legs is adequate.

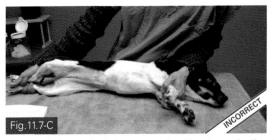

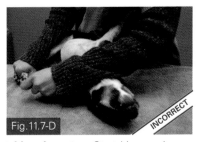

Fig.11.7-C, Example 1, Incorrect: Avoid automatically stretching dogs, too. Stretching can be uncomfortable or even painful. If the animal feels pain during restraint, he will develop a bad association with being restrained.

Fig.11.7-D, Example 1, Incorrect: Stretching caused this dog to struggle and pull his legs loose.

Example 2: Avoid uncomfortable positions.

People often restrain animals in positions that appear to provide control of the legs or head in case the animal struggles. Because these positions are uncomfortable for the animal, they can cause animals to struggle more.

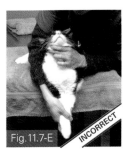
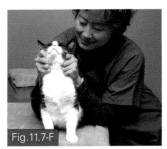
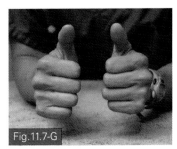

Example 11.7-E, Example 2, Incorrect: This typical cat hold attempts to prevent the cat from clawing with his front legs. Cats who want to claw or bite can still easily escape.

Example 11.7-F, G, Example 2, Correct: This position keeps cats more comfortable and more willing to hold still. My hands are just on the sides of the neck and my fingers are bent so they don't obscure the cat's jugular vein. I am not pulling on his fur. Cats rarely claw in this position, but when they do, they give ample warning by lifting and extending their legs. If you see these signs, it indicates that you should try a different restraint position or that chemical restraint is indicated. Grabbing the cat's legs and trying to restrain more firmly will most likely be ineffective.

Keep safe by controlling the dog's or cat's head when needed, but don't automatically squeeze the animal tightly. Do have your hands positioned appropriately and clearly to act as barriers to movement, and be ready to increase pressure as needed.

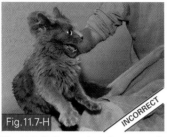 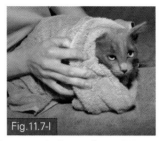 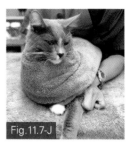

Fig.11.7-H, Example 2, Incorrect: Don't automatically scruff cats. This cat explodes and tries to escape when held by the scruff.

Fig.11.7-I, Example 2, Correct: The same cat is relaxed when wrapped in a towel.

Fig.11.7-J, Example 2 : This calm cat can be catheterized by placing a towel under his neck and extending his leg. If needed, the towel can be "scruffed" to hold the cat more securely.

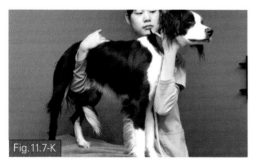 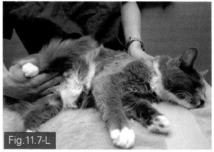

Fig.11.7-K, Example 2: In this case, there's no need to hold the dog's head against the shoulder because no procedure is occurring. A hand or arm around the neck is enough.

Fig.11.7-L, Example 2: This cat is both friendly and relaxed in the hospital setting. Additionally, he has cerebellar hypoplasia and so cannot move quickly. He does not need to be scruffed for a blood draw. A hand is kept on his neck, but with only light pressure.

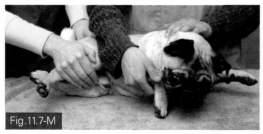 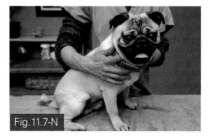

Fig.11.7-M, Example 2: The technicians allow the dog to get up but still keep their hands on him to keep him from leaping off the table or scrambling once he's sternal.

Fig.11.7-N, Example 2: Once he's sitting, one person keeps her hands on him loosely while waiting for the next procedure.

11.8 Principle 8: Avoid Prolonged Struggling

(Refer to Video 10)

Avoid prolonged (more than 2 seconds) or repeated fighting or struggling. Always be ready to tighten your hold or change your hand and body position in case the pet suddenly tries to escape or struggles. Automatically letting pets loose when they start to struggle can teach them to struggle more. Good technique can quickly secure the animal so that he stops struggling and relaxes. Average or poor technique results in the need for chemical restraint sooner. It can be difficult to know when it's appropriate to hold strongly and when to release. In general, release your hold on patients that struggle repeatedly or for prolonged periods (3 seconds in dogs and 1-2 seconds in cats). With difficult patients you will likely need to try a different plan of action.

> With good handling, the pet's behavior should improve rather than get worse
>
> _____
>
> In general, release your hold on patients that struggle repeatedly or for prolonged periods (3 seconds in dogs and 1-2 seconds in cats)

If the patient struggles for more than 3 seconds (dogs) or 1-2 seconds (cats) or struggles repeatedly try one of the following

- Fix your technique
- Switch to a different restraint position
- Get assistance: the pet may need more than one person to help restrain

- Try chemical restraint before the animal becomes too aroused
- Countercondition in the hospital or offer to send the pet home with a counterconditoning plan

---

Switch to chemical restraint before the animal becomes hyper-aroused, or else the tranquilizers will not work well. Some animals may require counterconditioning either in the hospital or at home prior to having the procedure performed.

In this series of photos, the technician is restraining the dog poorly. (Figures 11.8-A,B,C) Her right elbow is sticking out, which indicates she never had the dog restrained close to her side. When he struggles, she's unable to adapt her hold quickly enough to keep him in place. If you're unable to get the animal under control within 2 to 3 seconds, release the restraint so the dog can calm down. Be sure to get him calm and in control within 1 to 2 seconds. Do so using minimal restraint techniques with the methods described in Principle 5.

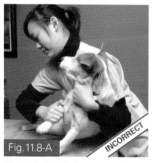
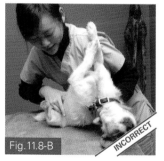
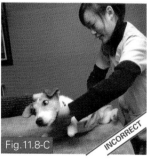

Fig.11.8-A,B,C, Incorrect: Prolonged struggling can cause the dog to become more aroused and to even bite. If the problem is your technique (note the elbows sticking out in the third picture), then either change the technique or have another technician perform the restraint. If the animal struggles several times, and other techniques such as food distractions or a quick counterconditioning session don't work, then use chemical restraint.

11.9 Principle 9: Use Distractions and Rewards

Play

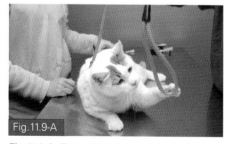

Fig.11.9-A: This cat is interested in the leash as a toy.

Use distractions, food, praise, play and petting when appropriate. The best distractions are ones that teach the pet to associate the situation with something good, making him more amenable to future procedures. Only use what works for that animal. Avoid distractions that agitate the animal. The dog or cat does not have to perform a behavior correctly for you to use motivators. The goal is to distract the animal and train a positive association (classical counterconditioning).

Petting and attention

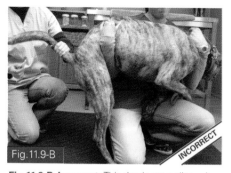

Fig.11.9-B, Incorrect: This dog is struggling when he perceives he will have his temperature taken.

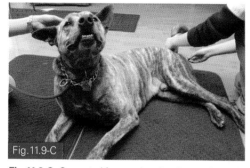

Fig.11.9-C, Correct: After petting the dog exuberantly while desensitizing his rear end to being touched, we can easily insert the thermometer with no restraint—just petting.

Treats

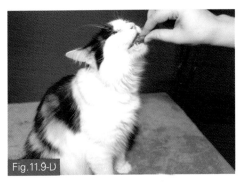

Fig.11.9-D

Fig.11.9-D: This cat takes treats between procedures. He is developing a positive association to offset any negative experience he might have had.

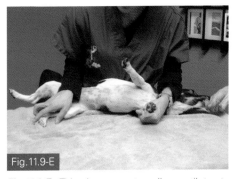

Fig.11.9-E

Fig.11.9-E: This dog was struggling until treats were offered. Be sure to put the treat right up to the pet's mouth so that he doesn't lunge to get it. *(Video 11)*

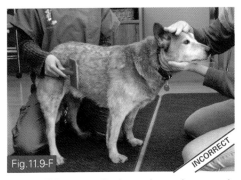

Fig.11.9-F

INCORRECT

Fig.11.9-F, Incorrect: Petting and attention are only weak motivators for this dog. He is showing little indication that he enjoys the petting.

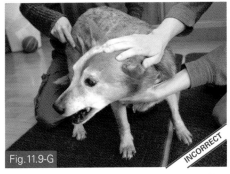

Fig.11.9-G

INCORRECT

Fig.11.9-G, Incorrect: When I start brushing him, he just struggles to get away. Since he doesn't care about petting or attention in this context, we shouldn't use them.

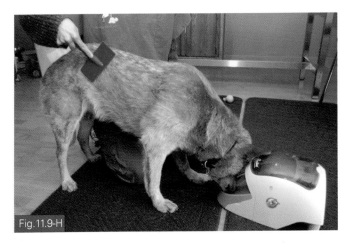

Fig.11.9-H

Fig.11.9-H, Correct: He is motivated by food, though. Here the MannersMinder is releasing kibble every 3 seconds. The dog happily eats while he's being groomed. **Use what's motivating to the individual animal.** *(Refer to Chapter 5, Video 4)*

Happy, playful tone of voice

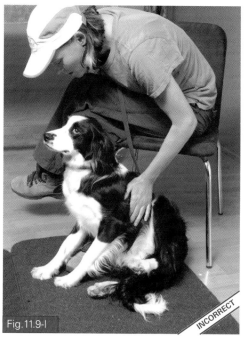

Fig.11.9-I

INCORRECT

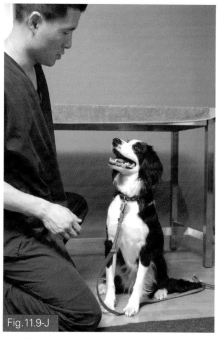

Fig.11.9-J

Fig.11.9-I, Incorrect: Talking to fearful dogs and cats often has no effect and could even make the pet more fearful. When talking to a pet, avoid speaking in a fast-paced, repetitive tempo. Imagine during a dentist appointment that the dentist keeps saying in a short, choppy manner, "It's okay. It's okay." It would give you the impression that he is nervous and it would make you more nervous. Similarly, if he said this in a slow, soothing tone, you might become more apprehensive as your mind focused on the procedures. In this photo, the person is petting the dog and the dog continues to show fearful body posture. The dog is leaning into the person for security. The woman should change her behavior if it's causing or contributing to the dog leaning against her fearfully.

Fig.11.9-J, Correct: Our goal is to change the dog's emotional state. Here, the technician used a happy tone of voice as if cheering at a soccer game. The dog responded by wagging his tail, moving away from the owner and then soliciting petting from the technician. The jolly tone of voice has distracted the dog from the possibly fearful event and changed his emotional state to happy and playful.

11.10 Principle 10: Adjust Your Handling Based on the Individual Animal

(Video 12)

Adjust your handling based on the animal and his response to restraint. Also, learn to adjust your sample-taking technique.

Case 1: A difficult cat

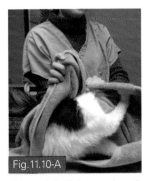

Fig.11.10-A

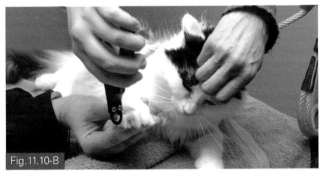

Fig.11.10-B

Fig.11.10-A: This cat doesn't like toweling or having his feet handled for a toenail trim.

Fig.11.10-B: Restraining him with a leash harness (see Chapter 15, Section 15.8) and adding a distraction of scratching his head help the cat more calmly accept the procedure. Because the cat enjoys having his head scratched, he is also developing a positive association with the procedure.

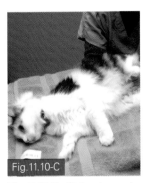

Fig.11.10-C

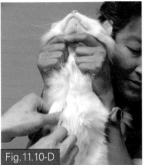

Fig.11.10-D

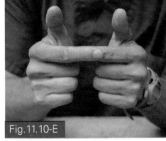

Fig.11.10-E

Fig.11.10-C: He's also calm when scruffed as long as his front feet are not being handled.

Fig.11.10-D, E: When we simply hold his head up and provide support on both sides of his body, this cat also remains relaxed for jugular venipuncture.

Case 2: Scared adolescent dog

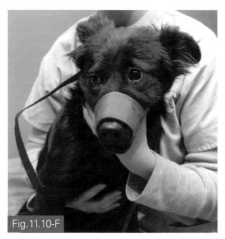

Fig.11.10-F

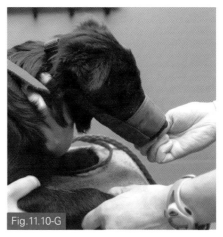

Fig.11.10-G

Fig.11.10-F: This pup looks fearful. His ears are drawn back and his brow is furrowed. For safety, we placed a muzzle on him.

Fig.11.10-G: Because he was interested in treats, we used them to countercondition him.

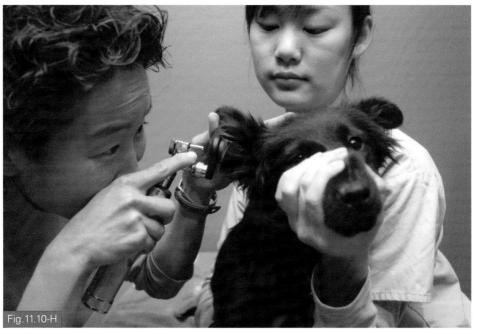

Fig.11.10-H

Fig.11.10-H: The pup is now relaxed and we no longer need the muzzle.

Case 3: An aged dog that dislikes lying on his back

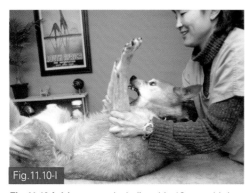

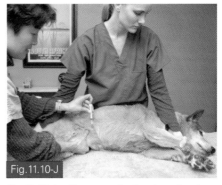

Fig.11.10-I: Many pets, including this 16-year-old dog, don't like being restrained on their back.

Fig.11.10-J: These animals benefit from having a procedure such as cystocentesis performed while they're lying on their side. Alternatively, some animals are comfortable lying on their back in a V trough.

Case 4: Cat gets a toenail trim

Many pets dislike having their nails trimmed. Technicians who are skilled at trimming nails quickly and from many different angles can greatly decrease stress in these animals.

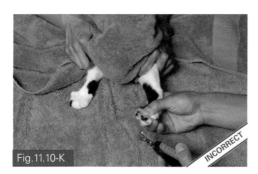

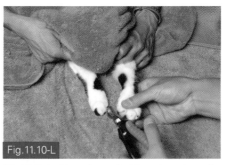

Fig.1.10-K, Incorrect: Here the paw is at an angle that's uncomfortable for the cat, so he tries to pull his paw away during the procedure.

Fig.11.10-L: Now the technician trims the nails while holding the paw in a more comfortable position and the cat remains relaxed throughout the procedure.

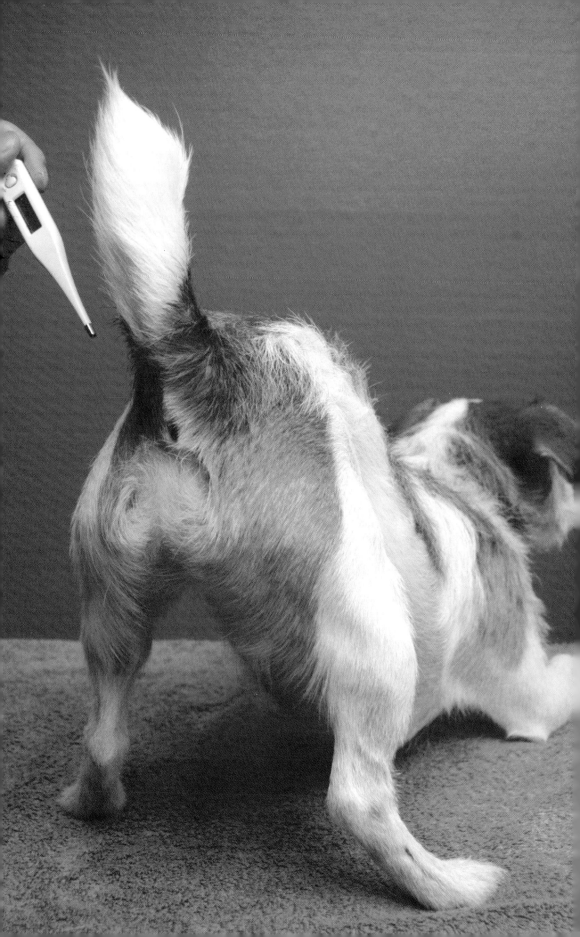

CHAPTER 12.
RESTRAINT FOR STANDARD
Positions in Dogs

Imagine that your own visit to the doctor goes like this:

The door leading from the waiting room to the exam area opens and a man the size of a small building steps through. Looking more like a villain from a James Bond movie than a nurse—even in his scrubs— he locks his gaze directly on you. "Mistajoneskamwime," he says, in an accent so thick that you can feel the words even though you can't understand them. You look around, but there's no one else in sight. So you tentatively stand and then follow when he gestures you to follow him. You enter a room with an exam table, two lonely chairs and a narrow counter holding blood collection tubes and syringes. As you're wondering where you should sit, the nurse suddenly bends over and grabs your feet out from under you so that you drop with a thud into the nearest chair. Before you can ask, "Hey, what are you doing," he grabs your arm and pulls it out. You reflexively pull your arm away and he immediately grabs it back, slaps a tourniquet on

233

and draws your blood. "Mistajoneswaitheredoctabeinsoon," he mumbles as he sticks on a bandage and then walks out.

If you experienced a visit like this, it would immediately raise red flags regarding the competency and compassion of your doctors and their staff. No wonder dogs who are handled in a similarly crude or inconsiderate manner have no confidence in your ability to guide them! Some of these dogs even respond by struggling and trying to bite. To gain the pet's confidence, it's imperative that you learn to position and restrain dogs in such a way that the dogs know what you want and feel comfortable being handled.

> In tests, 100% of people who only looked at the photos failed to imitate the photos correctly. Be sure to look at the photos, read the text and, when possible, watch the corresponding DVD clips.

12.1 Control Movement First

Before trying to restrain a dog, having her movement under control is essential. You should be able to prevent the dog from pacing back and forth or moving rapidly; these actions can lead to increased arousal, anxiety or an escape response. Controlling movement by providing clear, consistent direction will teach the dog that she can trust you to guide her. *(Video 1)*

Before attempting these techniques, work through the exercises in chapter 11.

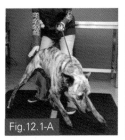 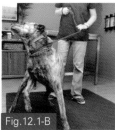 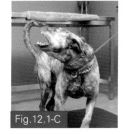 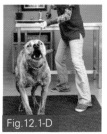

Fig.12.1-A, B: This dog is pulling and lunging excitedly.

Fig.12.1-C, D: He is overly aroused. The technician is preparing to gain better control of him.

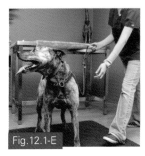 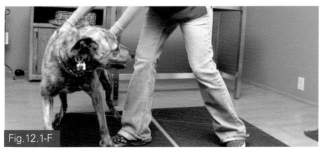

Fig.12.1-E: As soon as she drops the leash, the dog starts to walk away.

Fig.12.1-F: When she attempts to grab the dog, he turns suddenly and potentially could snap at her. It's best to avoid leaning toward or reaching for dogs. Fearful dogs might cower, or snap and bite defensively.

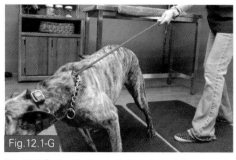

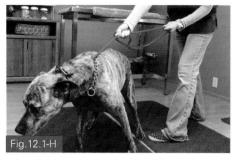

Fig.12.1-G, H: A better technique for gaining control safely is to hold onto the leash and reel the dog in. Here, the technician walks her hands down the leash.

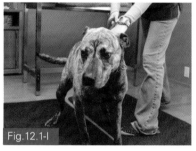

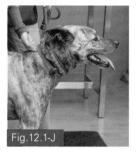

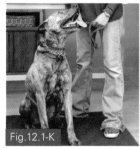

Fig.12.1-I: When she reaches the collar, she keeps tension on the leash with one hand and grasps the dog's collar with the other. Then she can loosen the leash tension.

Fig.12.1-J: Now she has the collar in one hand and the leash in the other.

Fig.12.1-K: At this point, the dog automatically sits on his own.

12.2 Restraint While in a Standing Position

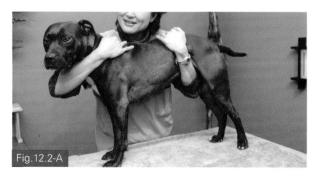

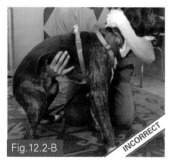

Fig.12.2-A, Method 1: Place one arm under the dog's abdomen as far back as possible to keep the dog from sitting. The other arm is around the dog's neck. If needed, draw the dog's head close to your body to hold it more securely.

Fig.12.2-B Method 1, Incorrect: The arm supporting the rear end is not far enough back. The technician is relying on pulling the head close to her shoulder to help keep the dog from leaning backward. This dog is still trying to sit.

Method 2

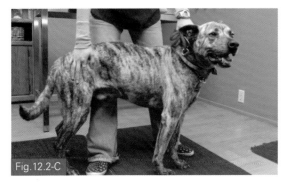

Fig.12.2-C

Fig.12.2-C, Method 2: You can also stabilize a dog in a stand just by keeping one hand on the collar and the other on the hip or flank area. Stationing the dog against your leg provides added stability. If the dog is going to be examined, the technician might need to control his head better by holding the neck close to her leg.

12.3 Positioning Dogs Into a Sit

There are several different ways to get a dog to sit at the hospital. *(Video 2)*

Method 1: Wait for the dog to automatically sit when she sees a treat.

Surprisingly, over 80% of the dogs I see in behavior consults will do this. It's an easy, hands-off technique. I use this method as a way to get the dog calm and focused. By rewarding the automatic sit, I'm rewarding calm, polite behavior without putting demands on the dog. I do not command the dog to sit. Note that commanding a child to sit in a dentist's chair would not make the chair inviting.

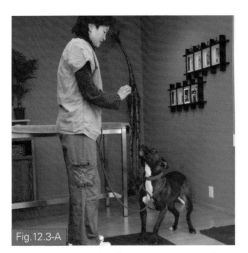

Fig.12.3-A

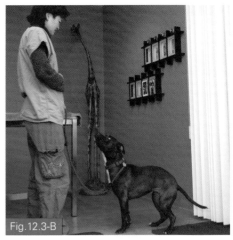

Fig.12.3-B

Fig.12.3-A, Method 1, Step 1: Many dogs will automatically sit if they see that you're holding a delicious treat. Just show the dog the treat and wait until she focuses on it.

Fig.12.3-B, Method 1, Step 2: Then hold it hidden in your hand against your belly so she can't grab it from you. Wait for her to figure out that she needs to offer a sit to get the treat. Take a history from the owners while you're waiting, if you want. If you wait more than 10 seconds and she's still looking at you, take a step away from her and show the treat again. After another 10 seconds of no sit response, say "sit" once in a whisper, as a hint. Give the dog a few more seconds to process your request.

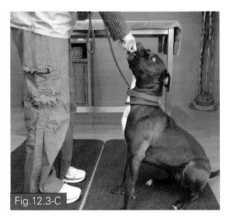

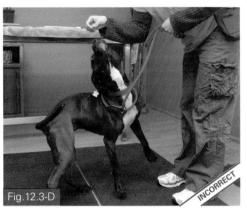

Fig.12.3-C, Method 1, Step 3: As soon as the dog sits, deliver the treat to her before she starts to get up. Then give 2-3 more treats rapidly while she's still sitting. If the dog shows interest in the food initially but then quickly loses interest and walks away or continues standing, try Method 2. Note that dogs are most likely to sit where they're comfortable (in a quiet exam room rather than a noisy treatment room, for example). So it's best to get this behavior first in a calm environment.

Fig.12.3-D, Method 1, Incorrect: Be careful to hold the treat away from the dog and deliver it all the way to her mouth. Holding it too close while you're waiting for her to sit, or delivering it too slowly or only part way to her mouth, might cause her to jump. In fact, whenever you're holding treats, be sure to use them to reward good behavior rather than accidentally luring dogs to lunge, jump or wiggle to get to the treat. Also, avoid leaning over the dog as depicted here, since this is a cue for many dogs to jump up. Leaning can also scare fearful or timid dogs.

> Whenever you're holding treats, be sure to use them to reward good behavior rather than accidentally holding them in a way that lures the dog to lunge, jump or wiggle free from restraint.

Method 2: Luring with food is another hands-off technique.

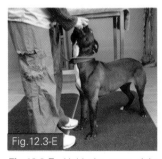

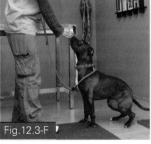

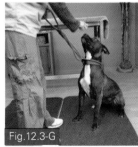

Fig.12.3-E: Hold the treat right up to the dog's nose. Then raise it above the head slightly and move it back to raise the dog's nose and shift her weight to her rear end.

Fig.12.3-F, G: Once she's sitting, give the treat and immediately give several additional treats for remaining seated. If the dog has already been rewarded with treats for sitting in the exam room or waiting room, where she was probably most comfortable, she's more likely to perform sits in the bustling treatment area using any method.

Method 3: Physical positioning is often necessary to get the pet to sit, but it can cause some pets to become confused, anxious and resistant. Hands-off methods are often better at first. **Do whatever provides the quickest and clearest guidance to the pet with the least stress**. One good strategy is to reward the dog numerous times for sitting and remaining seated while you take a history or before the exam or procedure needs to be done. Then use Method 3 or other methods of positioning. When dogs have been rewarded many times for sitting, they're more likely to respond by sitting when other methods are used.

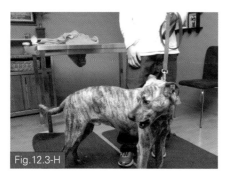 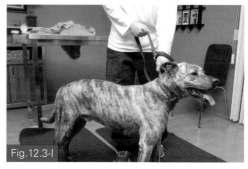

Fig.12.3-H, I, Method 3, Step 1: Grasp the leash right next to the collar, or grasp the collar so the dog can't move away from you. Remember to have the leash short enough so that you can easily reach the collar without leaning or lunging towards the dog. At this point you can try a verbal cue, "sit," using a happy, clear tone of voice before you physically position the dog. Only say "sit" once and give the dog 5 seconds to offer the sit. You can then repeat the cue if needed or just go on to Step 2.

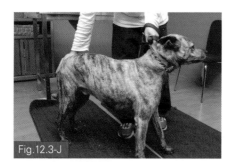 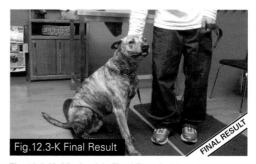

Fig.12.3-J, Method 3, Step 2: Place your free hand far back on the rear end. Use the collar to shift the dog's weight to the rear while you gently press down on the rear end. Notice that physical positioning has made this particular dog nervous. His ears are pinned back, he's tense and he has frozen (stopped panting).

Fig.12.3-K, Method 3, Final Result: Now that he's sitting and no longer being physically manipulated, he's more relaxed. Although his ears are still back, he's leaning toward the hand petting him. To decrease anxiety, be sure to provide clear direction to the dog by using the right amount of pressure in both hands. Go slowly enough when you start applying pressure so that you avoid triggering an escape or resistance response.

> When physically positioning, provide clear direction but go slowly enough when you start applying pressure so that you avoid triggering an escape or resistance response.

Method 4: Another method for physically positioning the dog into a sit is shown below. Note that even with physical positioning, a treat can be given when the dog is sitting. *(Video 3)*

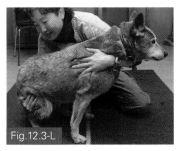 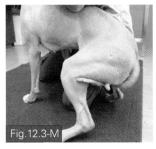 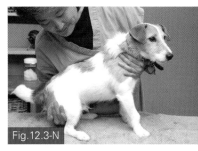

Fig.12.3-L, Method 4, Step 1: Start with one arm around the dog's chest and neck. Place the opposite hand on the caudal aspect of the knees. If the dog weaves around when she feels your arm, first give her a second to become accustomed to your hand placement. Then gently but firmly put pressure up and backward on the chest to push her weight onto her rear end. Lean toward the rear end with your body. Note that my shoulders slant down to the right.

Fig.12.3-M, Method 4, Step 2: Hand pressure should be right on the back of the knees where the femur meets the tibia. Think of a karate chop to the back of the knees—but rather than a sudden chop, just apply gradual pressure to this location while leaning the dog's weight back onto her rear.

Fig.12.3-N, Method 4 (variation): For smaller dogs, put just your hand—rather than your entire arm—on the chest. This offers greater surface area contact. Be sure to lean toward the rear yourself to get his weight far enough back for a sit.

WHAT'S WRONG WITH THESE PICTURES?

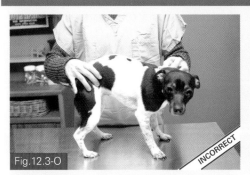 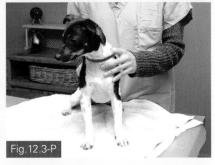

Fig.12.3-O, Example 1a, Incorrect: Here, the surface is too uncomfortable for the dog to sit on.

Fig.12.3-P, Example 1b, Correct: Once towels are added, the dog automatically sits on her own with no pressure or command.

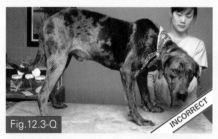 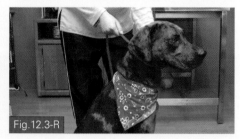

Fig.12.3-Q, Example 2a, Incorrect: This dog is uncomfortable on the table. He's more likely to willingly sit on the floor.

Fig.12.3-R, Example 2b, Correct: We were right: When placed back on the floor, he sat readily. This is a very energetic dog, making him a challenge for some to control when he's on the floor. However, putting him on a table so that he's too scared to move can backfire, causing him to struggle out of fear. This technician easily controls the dog by shortening the leash.

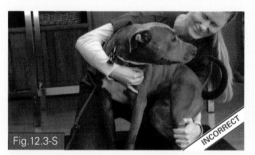 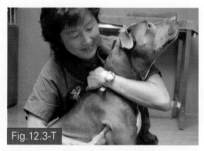

Fig.12.3-S, Example 3a, Incorrect: For some large dogs, hand pressure on the front of the chest is enough to control the front end, but this dog gets too excited. She's wiggly and gets her head loose.

Fig.12.3-T, Example 3b, Correct: For wiggly dogs, place your entire arm around the neck so that the neck sits in the crook of your arm. Now you will have better control of her front end when guiding her to sit.

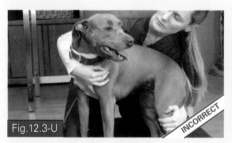 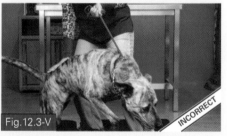

Fig.12.3-U, Example 4, Incorrect: The dog is not sitting readily because the pressure is too light on the hind leg and is placed unevenly on the two legs. The technician is pressing the leg down rather than performing a gentle "karate chop" to the back of the knee, and there's no pressure on the back of the right knee.

Fig.12.3-V, Example 5, Incorrect Here, the technician has no control of the front end. She must first get the dog into a controlled stand, then wait to make sure the dog is stable in that position. Only then can she guide the dog into a sit.

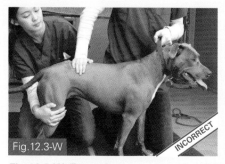 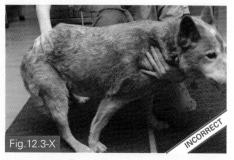

Fig.12.3-W Fig.12.3-X

Fig.12.3-W, Example 6, Incorrect: The technician on the right is pressing too far forward on the dog's hind end and the dog's weight is not distributed toward her rear end. The dog has to resist the pressure just to protect herself from injury.

Fig.12.3-X, Example 7, Incorrect: While it looks like this dog's weight is on her rear end, her front leg is positioned far back and she's fighting the pressure on her back. I need to bend her back legs so that she can sit, and use my arm on her chest to draw her weight backward.

Box 12-A: Choose the correct head restraint variation so that you can avoid being bitten. When restraining the head, choose the variation carefully. *(Video 4)*

Variation 1

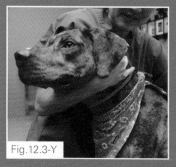 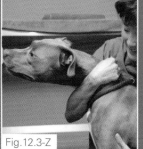 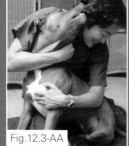

Fig.12.3-Y Fig.12.3-Z Fig.12.3-AA

Fig.12.3-Y, Head restraint, Variation 1a: Here, the dog's neck rests on my forearm. This hold requires the handler to have strong biceps, and if the dog struggles the handler will have to react quickly.

Fig.12.3-Z, AA, Head restraint, Variation 1b: Notice that this restraint only provides moderate control of the head. This dog can reach forward and can turn her head to the side—far enough to bite someone.

Variation 2

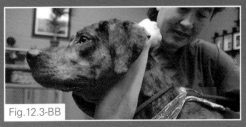

Fig.12.3-BB

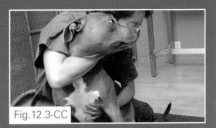

Fig.12.3-CC

Fig.12.3-BB, Head restraint, Variation 2a: In this variation, the dog's neck rests against the crook of my arm, which allows good surface area contact and requires less strength on the part of the holder. Due to the improved surface area contact, it's easier to respond when the dog suddenly starts struggling.

Fig.12.3-CC, Head restraint, Variation 2b: The dog can still turn her head almost as much as with Variation 1, though. So this is best used for dogs who are clearly happy and friendly and not likely to struggle.

Variation 3

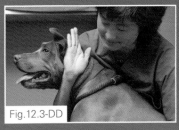

Fig.12.3-DD

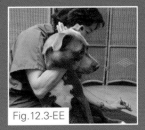

Fig.12.3-EE

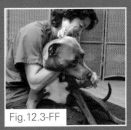

Fig.12.3-FF

Fig.12.3-DD, Head restraint, Variation 3a: Turning the palm to face outward allows the holder to snug the dog's head even closer to her shoulder, and consequently provides a more secure hold then the two previous variations. As always, the arm must be right behind the skull.

Fig.12.3-EE, FF, Head restraint, Variation 3b: Note the dog can still turn her head, but not as far as with the previous variations. However, if the dog lunges suddenly, it's still difficult to react quickly enough to keep her head against your body.

Variation 4

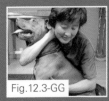

Fig.12.3-GG

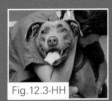

Fig.12.3-HH

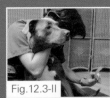

Fig.12.3-II

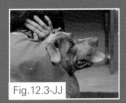

Fig.12.3-JJ

Fig.12.3-GG-JJ, Head restraint, Variation 4: This variation is the most secure and requires the least handler strength. The handler places her arm around the dog's neck and then closes the circle made by her arm by placing her hand on her own head or neck. Notice that the dog's head is always tight against my shoulder. While the dog can turn her head a little, she can't reach around to bite me and she can't pull her head away from my shoulder. Additionally, if she tries to lunge suddenly, because the loop is closed and my hand is on my head, she won't surprise me, causing my arm to be pulled away from my body.

12.4 Positioning Dogs Into a Down (Sternal Recumbency)

Method 1: Use a verbal cue or a hand signal. This is a hands-off method.

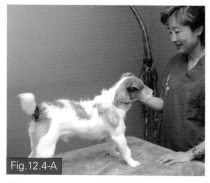

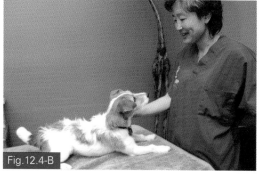

Fig.12.4-A, Method 1: Some dogs know the verbal down cue or a hand signal well enough to perform the behavior even in a hospital setting where they're nervous. These dogs might not require physical positioning.

Fig.12.4-B, Method 1: Lying down is usually easiest when the dog sits first. But some dogs, like my dog Jonesy shown here, have been rewarded a lot for downs and consequently do them directly from a stand. Point to the table or floor and say "down" once in a calm, clear voice. Give the dog 3 seconds to respond. Try one more time, if necessary, before moving on to Method 2.

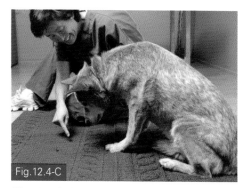

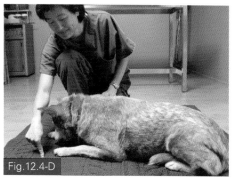

Fig.12.4-C, Method 1: The process is the same from a sit. In a calm, happy voice ask the dog to lie down by saying "down" and pointing to the surface between her front legs. Avoid rapidly saying "down, down, down, down!" Doing so can actually encourage the dog to move around more (McConnell 1990).

Fig.12.4-D, Method 1: Also avoid commanding the dog in a harsh voice. Dogs are more likely to perform the behavior correctly if a happy tone of voice is used rather than a gloomy or harsh tone (Mills et al. 2005). My 16-year-old dog, Zoe, is deaf, but she happily responds to the pointing cue alone.

Method 2: Use a food lure to move the dog into the correct position. This is also a hands-off method. *(Video 5)*

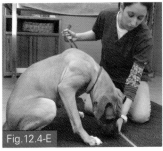
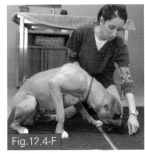
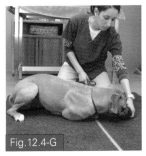

Fig.12.4-E, F, G, Method 2: Lure the dog by holding a treat on the floor directly under her nose, and then moving the treat farther away along the floor once the dog's nose is at floor level. Dogs who have learned the down this way will be familiar with the idea that they should lie down to get treats.

Method 3 (small dogs): Physically position the dog into a down. *(Video 6)*

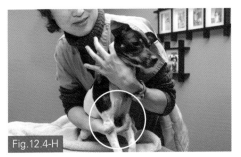
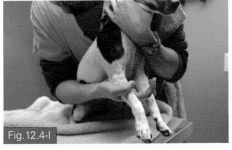

Fig.12.4-H, Method 3, Step 1: For small dogs, place your hand under the dog's chest and grasp the legs above the carpus (wrist).

Fig.12.4-I, Method 3, Step 2: Your index finger should be between the two front legs so that you have control of each leg individually.

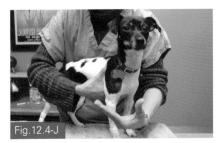
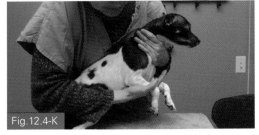

Fig.12.4-J, Method 3, Step 3: With the other hand, prevent the dog from leaping forward or turning and biting you by using a loose U hold around the dog's neck and chest.

Fig.12.4-K, Method 3, Step 4: Now lift the legs so that they bend at the elbow at a 90-degree angle. Then lower the dog's chest onto the table. There's no need to pull the dog's legs forward. You might have to lean over the dog to form a ceiling over her shoulders so that she doesn't try to get up.

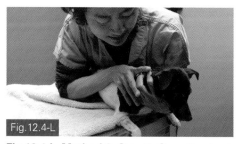

Fig.12.4-L

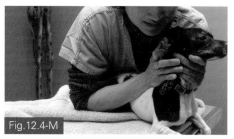

Fig.12.4-M

Fig.12.4-L, Method 3, Step 5: Once the dog is lying down, continue keeping a little pressure over the shoulders until you're sure that she is relaxed in the down position.

Fig.12.4-M, Method 3, Step 6: Change your hand position as needed once the dog is relaxed. Here, I'm preparing to hold her head up for a jugular blood draw.

Method 4 (large dogs): Physically position the dog into a down. *(Video 7)*

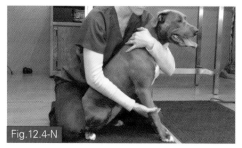

Fig.12.4-N

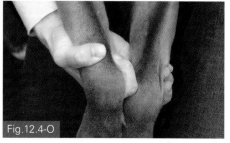

Fig.12.4-O

Fig.12.4-N, Method 4, Step 1: The method for large dogs is similar to that used for small dogs. Stabilize the rear end by placing your knee behind the dog. Wrap your arm around the neck to control the head. Stabilize one side with your body and the other side with your outside arm.

Fig.12.4-O, Method 4, Step 2: Grasp the front legs above the carpus (wrist). Be sure to have your index finger between both legs. If you cannot grasp both front legs, grasp one at a time while you lean on the dog to guide her down, or get help from another person.

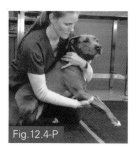

Fig.12.4-P

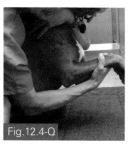

Fig.12.4-Q

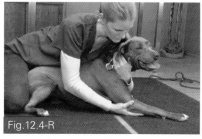

Fig.12.4-R

Fig.12.4-P, Q, Method 4, Step 3: Lift and bend the front legs at a 90-degree angle and lower the dog to the floor. Your body should form a ceiling that helps guide her to lie down. It's important to learn how to provide maximal surface area contact with dogs who might squirm and to apply pressure where needed so that you're able to guide the dog.

Fig.12.4-R, Method 4, Step 4: Your body should follow the dog into the down position and stay there until she's relaxed. When the dog is relaxed and there's no stimulus that might cause her to suddenly get up, adjust your position so that you're sitting more comfortably.

WHAT'S WRONG HERE?

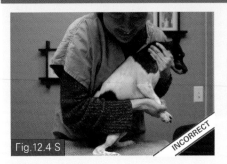

Fig.12.4 S — INCORRECT

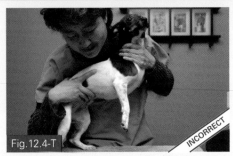

Fig.12.4-T — INCORRECT

Fig.12.4-S, Example 1a, Incorrect: Here, I hold the forepaw and pull forward rather than holding high up on the foreleg and bending the legs at the elbow. Avoid trying to keep dogs down by pulling on the distal portion of their legs. If needed, grasp above the elbow to hold the dog in place.

Fig.12.4-T, Example 1b, Incorrect: As a result of the poor leg hold, the dog struggles to escape. However, she does not escape from me because I'm holding the dog against my body so that my body forms a wall on one side, and my arms form safety bars preventing her from leaping away. Within 2 seconds, I have her sitting calmly again.

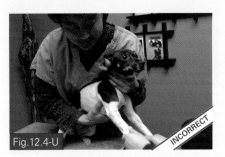

Fig.12.4-U — INCORRECT

Fig.12.4-U, Example 2, Incorrect: Here, the technician is pulling the dog's legs forward and holding too far down on the legs. This causes the dog to be off balance and she tries to get up. Notice that her rear end is elevated off the table. The more ambiguous the handling techniques are, the more the dog will struggle. Fearful dogs might become more afraid with someone manipulating them from the front.

Method 5: Physically positioning the dog into a down with two handlers. *(Video 8)*

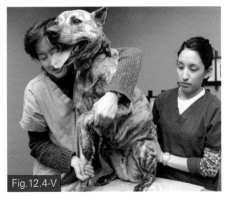

Fig.12.4-V, Method 5, Step 1: Start with the dog sitting. First grasp and bend one front leg at a 90-degree angle.

In this method, the head and neck are not controlled. Only use this technique for calm, friendly dogs who are not likely to struggle or bite. This particular dog, seen earlier in the chapter, struggles primarily when he's not held appropriately. When given clear direction, he remains calm. As a result, with these particular handlers, this technique is safe to try. If you're unsure of the temperament of the dog you are working with, try Method 6 instead. Use Method 4 if you're working with a smaller or shorter dog relative to your height.

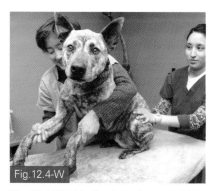

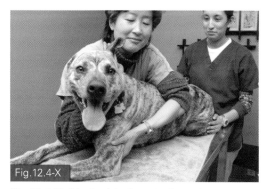

Fig.12.4-W, Method 5, Step 2: Next grasp the other leg, raise both legs at a 90-degree angle and then lower the dog. The technician in the back is preventing the dog from backing up. She must apply pressure if the dog resists. The arm over the dog's back helps support the dog.

Fig.12.4-X, Method 5, Step 3: Once the dog is lying down, control his head and neck by placing your arm around them. Pull the neck close to your body if needed. To keep the dog from rising, place your hand behind his elbow. With your palm flat, the dog's elbow sits between your thumb and index finger. The arm along the dog's side helps prevent him from moving away; lean over him if he tries to get up.

Method 6: Controlling the head with three handlers. *(Video 9)*

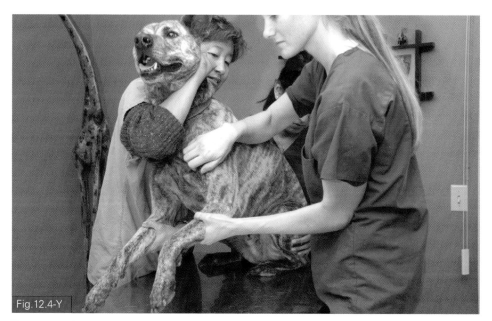

Fig.12.4-Y, Method 6: If the dog is likely to struggle, use a third helper or have the technician in the rear lift one of the legs. The handler at the front end of the dog should restrain the head by placing her arm around the neck just caudal to the skull so that the dog can't back his head out. She should choose the neck hold that is most appropriate for the dog. That is, her palm may need to be facing outward or she may need to close the loop made with her arm by putting her hand on her head if the dog is likely to struggle and get his head loose in a less secure hold.

Method 7: Controlling the head with two handlers. *(Video 10)*

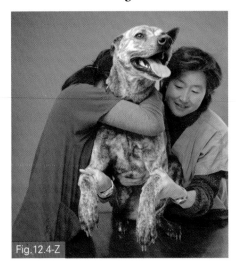

Fig.12.4-Z

Fig.12.4-Z, Method 7 (large dog): You can also use two handlers. If the dog is tall relative to the handler, the handler in the back (here, in blue) should grasp the outside front leg above the carpus (wrist) with her outside hand, and wrap her inside arm around the dog's abdomen or chest to prevent forward movement. The other handler (in red) holds the dog close to her body with one arm wrapped around his neck and the other arm coming from underneath to hold the dog's inside foreleg just proximal (nearer to the center of the body) to the carpus.

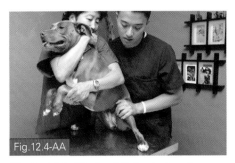

Fig.12.4-AA

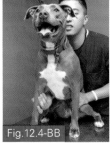

Fig.12.4-BB   Fig.12.4-CC

Fig.12.4-AA, Method 7, (variation for medium dogs): Alternatively, if the dog is short enough relative to the height of the handler in the front, the handler can place her arm over the dog and grasp the outside leg. This is more secure than the previous hold because the arm over the dog's back helps lower the dog.

Fig.12.4-BB, CC, Method 7, (variation for medium dogs): The technician in the back grasps the inside front leg.

Fig.12.4-DD, Method 7, Incorrect: The technician in the front has not bent or lifted the front inside leg. As a result, she cannot get the dog to lie down. Another common problem is grasping too far down the foreleg, which allows the dog to pull his leg away. Grasp proximal to the carpus.

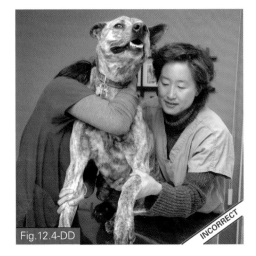

Fig.12.4-DD   INCORRECT

12.5 Achieving Lateral Recumbency From a Down

The gentlest method of placing a dog on her side is from a sternal recumbency (down) position.

Method 1: This is a one-person method that works for calm dogs who are unlikely to try to bite or get up when you rotate the hip. This method focuses on rotating the dog's hind end.

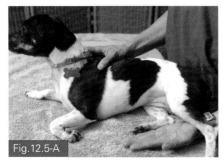

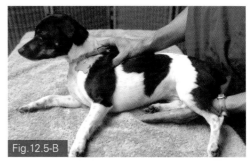

Fig.12.5-A, Method 1, Step 1: First rotate the dog onto the correct hip. We want this dog on her left hip so that she can be placed with her left side down. So first we must tuck the right leg under the dog by placing a hand next to the right foot and leg (up to the ankle) and sliding the foot under the dog. *(Chapter 11, Video 4)*

Fig.12.5-B, Method 1, Step 2: Now the dog's right foot is almost far enough under her body for you to reach with the right hand and grasp it below the knee (next photo). You must get the right foot under far enough so that you can grasp the right knee without having to reach under the dog.

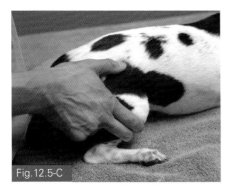

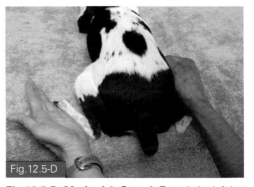

Fig.12.5-C, Method 1, Step 3: Grasp the right leg just below the knee using your right hand. You might need to reach slightly under the dog to do this, depending on how far you previously pushed this foot under the dog. Do not try to rotate the dog yet. You must have the left hand in place first.

Fig.12.5-D, Method 1, Step 4: To tuck the left leg under the dog, place the left hand just lateral to and slightly under the left foot. Now you can push this leg under while simultaneously using the right hand to rotate the right side up.

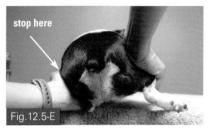

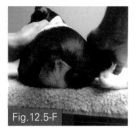

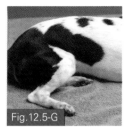

Fig.12.5-E, Method 1, Step 5: Remember that both hands must work in concert by rotating at the same time. When doing this, think about rotating a ball (see Chapter 11). Stop rotating as soon as the hip is turned. Do not rotate the hand all the way under the dog or you'll cause the dog to get up.

Fig.12.5-F, G, Method 1, Final result for back end: Now the dog is on her left hip. Note that the left leg does not protrude much from under the dog.

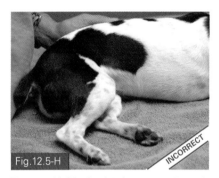

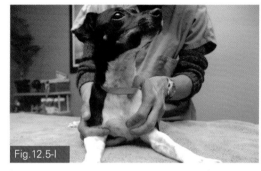

Fig.12.5-H, Method 1, Incorrect: The left leg **does not** need to be pulled out like this. In fact, pulling the leg out can cause the dog to become anxious.

Fig.12.5-I, Method 1, Step 6: Next we'll rotate the front end. Place the left hand on the dog's left shoulder and the right hand on the right shoulder so that you can rotate the dog's front half the way you would rotate a ball. On the side that will rotate downward, weave your thumb under the collar so the dog can't get up.

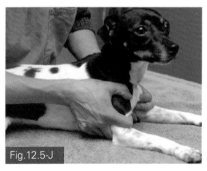

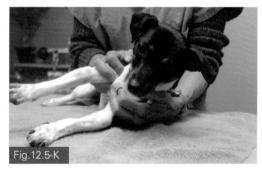

Fig.12.5-J, Method 1, Step 7: Use your fingers behind the dog's elbows to keep her from pulling her leg away from you. The hold will not be symmetric, since the thumb on one side is being used to hold the collar. (See Box 12-B for slightly larger dogs.)

Fig.12.5-K, Method 2, Step 8: Roll the front half of the dog onto her side by rotating both hands simultaneously in the same way that you would rotate a ball.

Box 12-B: Rotating the front half of a slightly larger dog. *(Video 11)*

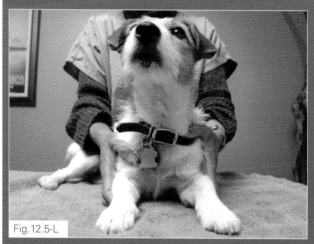

Fig.12.5-L

Fig.12.5-L, Method 1, Step 7 (slightly larger dog): The hold might be a bit different on a slightly larger dog. Again, the thumb is holding the collar on the side that will be rotated downward. The thumb of the other hand is just in front of the dog's leg.

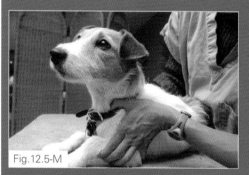

Fig.12.5-M

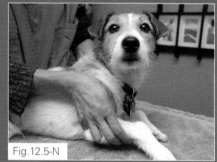

Fig.12.5-N

Fig.12.5-M, N, Method 1, Step 7 (slightly larger dog): Only the holder's pinky finger is behind the elbow. The rest of the fingers are under the leg but in front of the elbow.

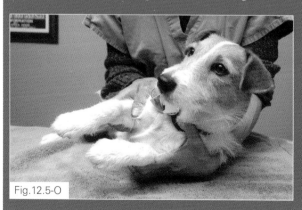

Fig.12.5-O

Fig.12.5-O, Method 1, Step 8 (slightly larger dog): Then, as with the smaller dog, rotate this dog in the same way you'd rotate a ball.

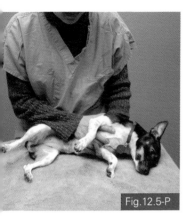
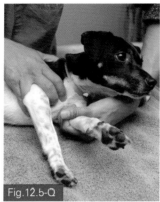
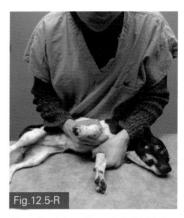

Fig.12.5-P

Fig.12.5-Q

Fig.12.5-R

Fig.12.5-P, Method 1, Step 9: The hand holding the bottom front leg should continue to hold this leg just distal to the elbow so that the dog can't pull the leg away and get up. Hold the dog for an instant calmly on her side before going on to Step 10.

Fig.12.5-Q, R Method 1, Step 10: While still holding the bottom front leg, quickly slip your bottom arm from under the dog's neck so that it rests on top of the dog's neck. Do not release your hold on the front leg while you do this. Remember that this method is for dogs who are calm and not likely to bite.

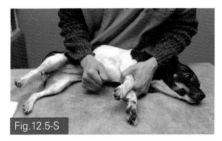
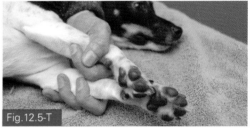

Fig.12.5-S

Fig.12.5-T

Fig.12.5-S, Method 1, Step 11: Now grasp both front legs with one hand, making sure to grasp above the carpus.

Fig.12.5-T, Method 1, Step 11 (close-up): Whenever you're grasping two legs at once with one hand, be sure your index finger is between the legs.

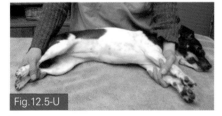
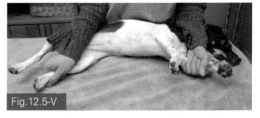

Fig.12.5-U

Fig.12.5-V

Fig.12.5-U, Method 1, Step 12: Next, grasp the back legs just below the hocks with the other hand. Be sure to keep the dog from pulling these legs away from you and getting up. Also make sure the dog's spine is resting against your abdomen to increase your control.

Fig.12.5-V, Method 1, Step 12 (variation): You can also restrain the dog by grasping just the bottom legs. The arm over the back end should extend across the dog's flank to keep her from wiggling. Both legs should be extended slightly (but not stretched) so that if the dog tries to rise, you can prevent her from pulling her legs under her.

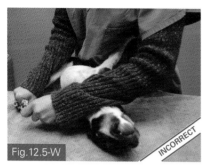

Fig.12.5-W, Method 1, Step 12, Incorrect: If the dog rolls toward you (instead of trying to escape by pulling her legs under her body), or if you suspect she might do so, then hold all four legs. Here, I'm holding only two legs and the dog has rolled.

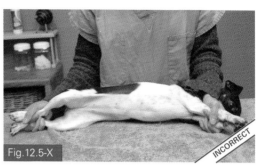

Fig.12.5-X, Method 1, Step 12, Incorrect: Avoid stretching dogs like this. Doing so can make them uncomfortable and cause pain in dogs with arthritis, thus providing a bad association with the hospital. It can also cause fear. Imagine if you were sitting in rollercoaster and the supports started stretching your arms.

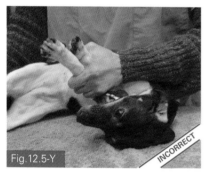

Fig.12.5-Y, Method 1, Step 12, Incorrect: This dog was comfortable on her side until I stretched her. Then she tried to bite. Notice from the previous photo that when you hold all four legs, you can't put your arm across the dog's flank to keep the body from twisting and the dog from biting.

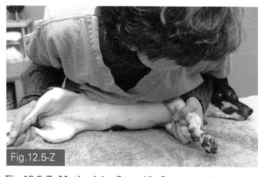

Fig.12.5-Z, Method 1, Step 12, Correct: Here, I lean gently over the dog to help push the midsection down so she can't struggle. Once she relaxes, I'll take the pressure off. Remember that if the dog struggles for more than 3 seconds, release and change the restraint method (which includes adding treats) rather than just trying to overpower the dog and causing more anxiety.

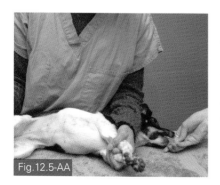

Fig.12.5-AA, Method 1, Step 12, Correct: This dog stopped struggling as soon as she was given treats. The goal of the treats is to distract her and to train her to associate restraint with good things. Don't wait until the dog is behaving well to give the treat as a reward. Rather, use treats to distract her from bad behavior and to put her into a positive emotional state. Give many of them quickly enough to keep her in this positive state. Once she's calm, you can decrease the treat rate. Treats should be given before the dog becomes too distressed to eat them.

Method 2: Hip turn using two handlers.

This method requires two people. It's used for large dogs or those who struggle. The hip is turned in the same manner as in Method 1, but the head and neck are controlled while doing this. *(Video 12)*

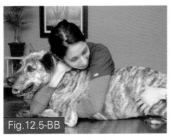

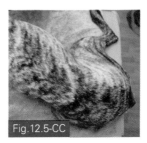

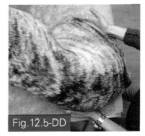

Fig.12.5-BB

Fig.12.5-CC

Fig.12.5-DD

Fig.12.5-BB, Method 2, Step 1: Start with the dog lying sternally. The technician in front should prevent the dog from getting up.

Fig.12.5-CC, DD Method 2, Step 2: First get the dog into position so that the rear end can be rotated onto the right hip. This dog's left leg is already tucked under his body (refer to Method 1 in this section for more detail on hip turns). Now use the right hand to push the right leg close to the dog.

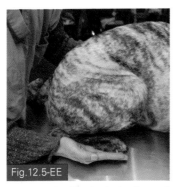

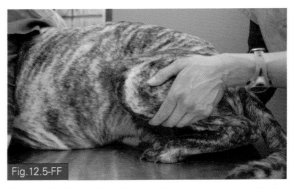

Fig.12.5-EE

Fig.12.5-FF

Fig.12.5-EE, Method 2, Step 2 (close-up): Here is a different view of Step 2, with the right hand parallel to the foot and pushing the foot toward the body. The hand is slightly under the edge of the foot. Think of doing a "karate chop" between the dog's foot and the table.

Fig.12.5-FF, Method 2, Step 3: Grasp the left knee with the left hand. The left hip will rotate upward, while pushing the opposite foot will cause that hip to rotate downward. Avoid trying to rotate the hip by just reaching under the dog and pulling the leg across. This is like trying to get someone to lie on their side by pulling a rug out from under them.

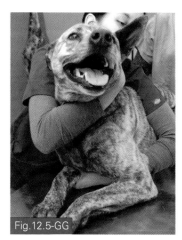

Fig.12.5-GG

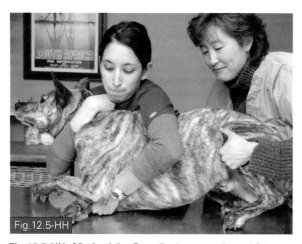

Fig.12.5-HH

Fig.12.5-GG, Method 2, Step 4: The technician controlling the front end should have her right arm around the dog's neck to control the head. Her left arm should reach over the shoulders and under the dog, and then grasp the dog's left leg. The technician in the back can push the dog's elbow forward if needed to help extend the leg.

Fig.12.5-HH, Method 2, Step 5: In a coordinated fashion, both technicians should rotate the body. The one in the front will need to bend her legs so that she can follow the dog's body down to the table. She must also pull the inside leg out from under the dog. The technician in the back will rotate the hip. Her body should be leaning against the dog's body so that he does not try to get up.

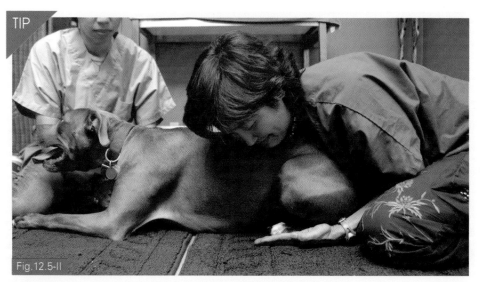

TIP

Fig.12.5-II

Fig.12.5-II, Tip: For dogs on the floor, lean over them to prevent them from rising.

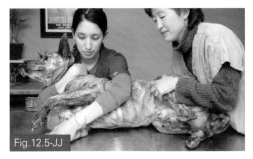

Fig.12.5-JJ, Method 2, Step 6: The front technician must extend the right leg straight so that the dog can't pull his leg back and under himself.

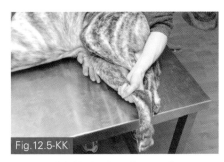

Fig.12.5-KK, Method 2, Step 7: As soon as the back end rotates, the technician handling that end should grasp the back bottom leg above the hock and hold it straight so that the dog cannot pull his leg back under his body.

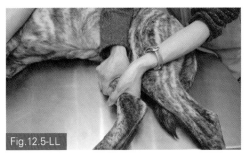

Fig.12.5-LL, Method 2, Step 8: The handler in the back must then reach around with the other arm and place it on the bottom leg. Her forearm should lie across the flank to help keep the dog from raising his midsection off the table.

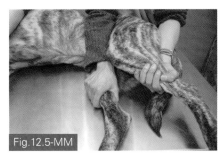

Fig.12.5-MM, Method 2, Step 9: Then she should switch the initial hand to the top leg, being sure to hold the bottom leg out straight.

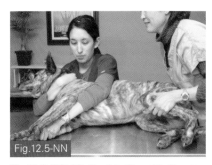

Fig.12.5-NN, Method 2, Step 10: Simultaneously, the technician controlling the front will need to change her hand positions. She should continue to keep the dog's bottom leg straight.

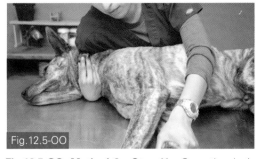

Fig.12.5-OO, Method 2, Step 11: Once the dog's head is on the table, the handler can lean on his neck with her shoulder to keep the neck and head in place while she repositions that corresponding hand and arm. She will be sliding that hand (right hand in this case) around the dog's neck so that the hand ends up on the top of the dog's neck.

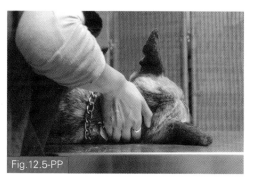

Fig.12.5-PP, Method 2, Step 12: Here she slides her hand around the dog's neck while keeping her elbow close to her side

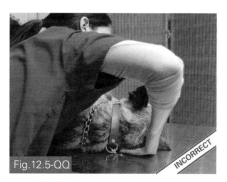

Fig.12.5-QQ, Method 2, Step 12, Incorrect: Avoid sticking the elbow out like this.

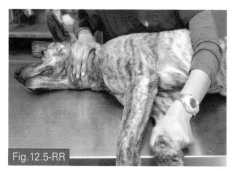

Fig.12.5-RR, Method 2, Step 13: The hand ends up resting on top of the dog's neck.

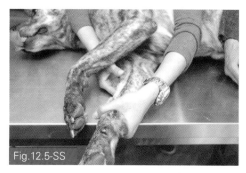

Fig.12.5-SS, Method 2, Step 14: Now the technician in front places her right forearm on the dog's neck while reaching for the bottom leg.

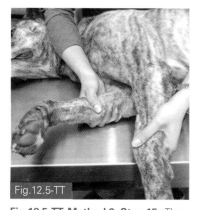

Fig.12.5-TT, Method 2, Step 15: Then she repositions the other hand on the upper leg above the carpus (wrist). Note that one arm controls both the neck and the bottom leg.

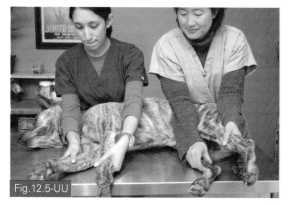

Fig.12.5-UU, Method 2, Step 16: Remember to hold the legs above the hock and well above the carpus, and keep the bottom legs straight so that the dog doesn't pull his legs underneath him.

Box 12-C: Variation on method 2

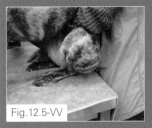

Fig.12.5-VV

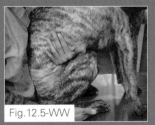

Fig.12.5-WW

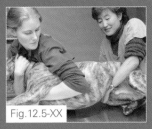

Fig.12.5-XX

Fig.12.5-VV, Method 2, Step 5 (variation): Some dogs try to leap forward or raise their rear end when you try to put them on their side. For these dogs, the rear handler should place her arm under the dog's abdomen.

Fig.12.5-WW, Method 2, Step 5 (variation): The arm should extend all the way to the other side so it can aid in rotating the dog.

Fig.12.5-XX, Method 2 (variation): The technician in the front should use the same technique as in Method 2, Step 4.

WHAT'S WRONG HERE?

Example 1

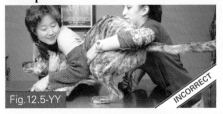

Fig.12.5-YY   INCORRECT

Example 2

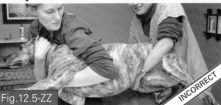

Fig.12.5-ZZ   INCORRECT

Fig.12.5-YY, Example 1, Incorrect: The dog is backing out and the technician in the back is not meeting the pressure. She tries to press the right hind foot into the table rather than pressing on the rear to keep it from rising.

Fig.12.5-ZZ, Example 2, Incorrect: To roll the dog onto his side, the front leg should be extended and the technician should be pulling it out from under him. In this photo, it's bent and forward instead of being straight and pulled out from under the body.

Example 3

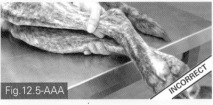

Fig.12.5-AAA   INCORRECT

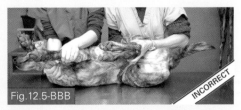

Fig.12.5-BBB   INCORRECT

Fig.12.5-AAA, Example 3a, Incorrect: Some technicians grip both hind legs in one hand and both front legs in another. Large dogs can only be restrained in this manner if they are not likely to struggle or if the holder has an incredibly strong grip.

Fig.12.5-BBB, Example 3b, Incorrect: As soon as this dog decides to struggle, the handler in the back will either let go of a leg or hold onto it by letting both legs bend, which allows the dog to move his entire body.

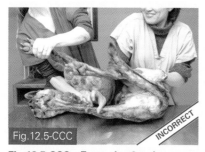

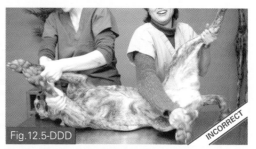

Fig.12.5-CCC, Example 3c, Incorrect: Now the front end is no longer in control and the handler in the back must try to grasp the moving hind legs separately.

Fig.12.5-DDD, Example 3d, Incorrect: The dog could now bite the technician in the front if he were so inclined. The handlers must get him under control before he starts mouthing them, or else just let him loose. If they can't control him in 2-3 seconds, they should let the dog get up so that he can calm down.

12.6 Achieving Lateral Recumbency From a Stand

Method 1: The method described here can be done by one person. But use it only with calm dogs who are unlikely to bite or with dogs who are muzzled, because the head will not be well controlled. *(Video 13)*

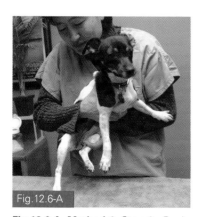

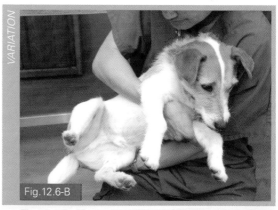

Fig.12.6-A, Method 1, Step 1: Begin with the dog facing left. Place your right arm across the dog's body with your hand under her chest.

Fig.12.6-B, Method 1, Step 1 (slightly larger dog): With slightly larger dogs, you might need to grasp the left leg as close to the elbow as possible with your right hand.

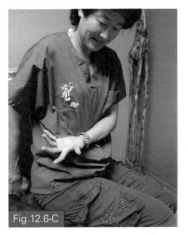
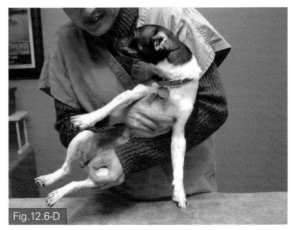

Fig.12.6-C, Method 1, Step 1 (alternate view): This shows the hand and arm position you'll need. The left hand reaches back to support the dog's left hip. Keep your left arm against your side so that it is between you and the dog.

Fig.12.6-D, Method 1, Step 2: Roll the dog over onto her side. Note that the dog's head is not restrained. Avoid this method in dogs with unknown temperaments.

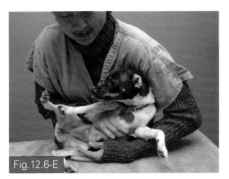
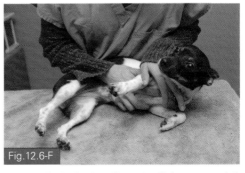

Fig.12.6-E, Method 1, Step 3: Simultaneously lower her to the table.

Fig.12.6-F, Method 1, Step 4: Release your left hand from the back leg and grab hold of the upper front leg above the elbow.

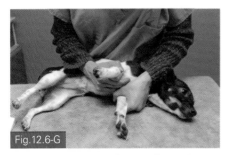
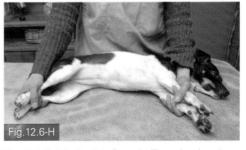

Fig.12.6-G, Method 1, Step 5: Grasp the lower leg (or both front legs) and place your arm across the dog's neck to control the head.

Fig.12.6-H, Method 1, Step 6: The other hand can grasp both hind legs or just the bottom hind leg.

Method 2: This method uses two people to place a dog on her side from a standing position. Use it for dogs who might struggle or bite. *(Video 14)*

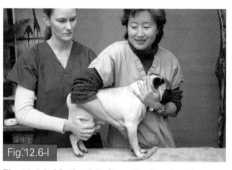

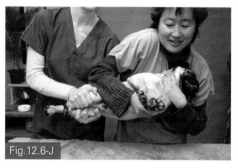

Fig.12.6-I, Method 2, Step 1: One hand secures the dog's neck and holds it close to your body. For little dogs, use a U or C hold around the neck (refer to Chapter 11). The other hand reaches across the dog and grasps the inside front leg as proximally (close to the body) as possible for best control. The second handler will take charge of the hind end by grasping the hind legs as high as possible. Small dogs can be held around the knee area.

Fig.12.6-J, Method 2, Step 2: Lift and rotate the dog so that you pull him up against your body while holding the front bottom leg straight. You should be able to suspend the dog in mid-air and he should feel secure. Make sure the hind legs are held with the knees together.

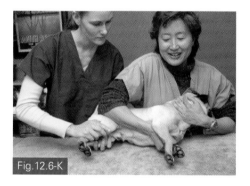

Fig.12.6-K, Method 2, Step 3: Lower the dog onto the table. To do this, the person supporting the front end can just bend her knees so that she becomes short enough to lay the dog easily onto the table. Alternatively, you can bend at the waist and lean over the dog. In this picture, my left elbow is out of place—it's sticking out instead of tucked against my side. My elbow position is correct in the series of photos below.

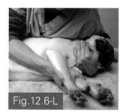
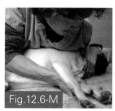
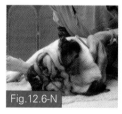
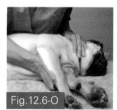

Fig.12.6-L to O, Method 2, Step 4: Be sure to keep your elbow (in this case, the left elbow) against your side so that your arm and hand continue to encircle the dog's neck. When the dog is on or almost on the table, slide the hand supporting the dog's neck around to the other side of his neck. Lean your shoulder against the dog's neck, if necessary, to help prevent him from getting up as you make this quick hand position change. Also, be sure to use your other arm across the dog's body to keep him lying down.

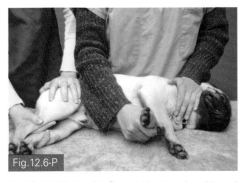

Fig.12.6-P

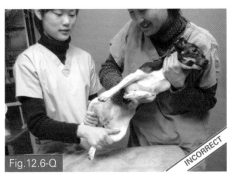

Fig.12.6-Q

INCORRECT

Fig.12.6-P, Method 2, Step 5: Your hand positioned over the dog's neck like this will help prevent him from getting up. Holding the bottom leg helps keep the dog from pulling it in and getting up.

Fig.12.6-Q, Method 2, Incorrect: This dog is tilted rather than being held level, which can cause her to feel off balance. Additionally, her back legs are split apart rather than being held together. This can lead to hip pain in arthritic dogs.

BOX 12-D: Alternate Method 2

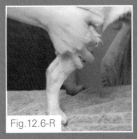

Fig.12.6-R

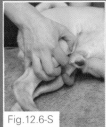

Fig.12.6-S

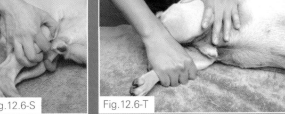

Fig.12.6-T

Fig.12.6-R, Method 2, Step 1 (alternate hind-leg hold): Another way to hold the hind limbs is to place your thumb and three fingers in front of the patellar region with the pinky finger behind the leg.

Fig.12.6-S, Method 2, Step 2 (alternate hind-leg hold): Focus on keeping the dog's knees together when you lift and rotate him onto his side.

Fig.12.6-T, Method 2, Step 3 (alternate hind-leg hold): Once he's on his side, you can hold him in the same manner as above or you can use two hands. To switch to the 2-hand hold, grasp the bottom leg with the upper hand (in this case the right hand). Then slide the left hand from the left side of the dog's body over to the right side.

Fig.12.6-U, Method 2, Step 4 (alternate hind-leg hold): Grasp the lower leg with the left hand. This frees up the right hand to grasp the upper leg. Note that the arm holding the lower leg is placed across the flank, thus helping to keep the dog in lateral recumbency.

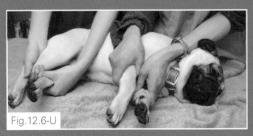

Fig.12.6-U

Method 3: Use this method to place a medium dog onto her side from a stand. Since the head is not secured, this method is for friendly dogs or those who are muzzled. *(Video 15)*

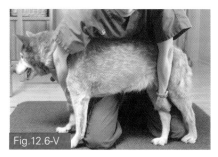

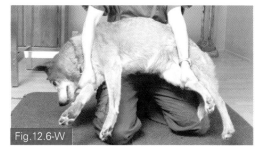

Fig.12.6-V, Method 3, Step 1: Reach over the dog and grasp the legs closest to you as high up the leg as possible. The arm near the dog's head should be in front of the outside leg.

Fig.12.6-W, Method 3, Step 2: Straighten your torso and simultaneously pull the dog's legs up so that you're hugging her body close; then you can gently let her slide down your body. Use your upper body—not your arms—to do this, and keep the dog's legs as straight as possible for improved control.

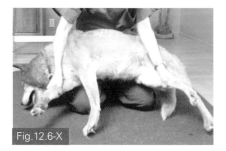

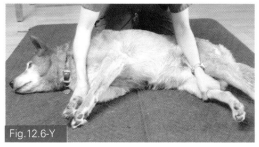

Fig.12.6-X, Method 3, Step 3: Bend your torso so the dog lowers and then slides down your legs.

Fig.12.6-Y, Method 3, Step 4: Once the dog is on her side, your arms are automatically placed correctly to restrain her there. Holding the bottom legs prevents her from pulling them away to get up. Your arm across the neck controls her head and neck.

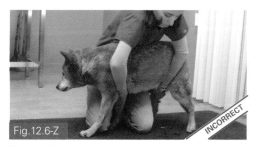

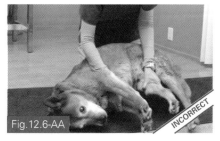

Fig.12.6-Z, AA Method 3, Step 1, Incorrect: If you begin with your front arm behind the dog's front leg instead of in front of it, then once the dog is on her side, you'll have to reposition your arm so that it will sit on the neck when she's in lateral recumbency. Consequently, this variation is not as safe for the technician. However, grasping in this manner (with your front arm behind the dog's front leg) can provide better support during the position change, depending on the dog's size.

Method 4: Here's how to maneuver a large dog from a standing position on the floor to lying on her side. *(Video 16)*

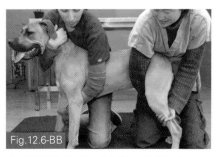

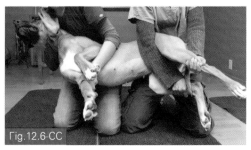

Fig.12.6-BB, Method 4, Step 1: This is similar to placing a small dog on her side using two people (Method 2, this section), except the hold on the hind legs is revised. Both handlers should grasp as far up the legs as possible.

Fig.12.6-CC, Method 4, Step 2: The handlers simultaneously pull the dog toward their bodies and rotate her. The person at the rear might have to lean back to pull the dog to her body. Notice that the handler in front is holding the palm of her right arm out to gain a more secure hold on this dog's neck.

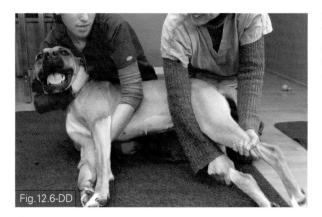

Fig.12.6-DD, Method 4, Step 3: Then the dog can slide down their bodies. The technician supporting the front continues to support the dog's neck in her arm.

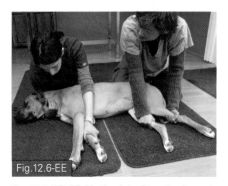

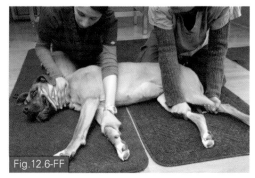

Fig.12.6-EE, FF, Method 4, Step 4: Once the dog is on the floor, the technician in the front slides her hand and arm from the bottom of the neck around to the top. She must be sure to extend the bottom front leg so that the dog does not get up.

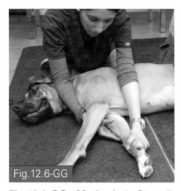

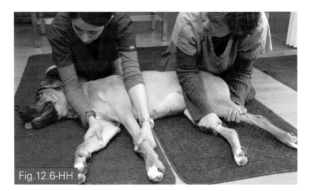

Fig.12.6-GG, Method 4, Step 5: Then she switches hands to grasp the bottom leg with the arm that's holding the neck down.

Fig.12.6-HH, Method 4, Step 6: Note that as she switches hands, her arm is placing light pressure on the neck so that the dog can't get up. If the dog tries to raise her head, the pressure on the neck will increase rather than just giving way.

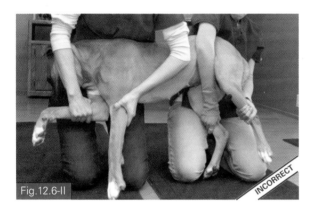

Fig.12.6-II, Method 4, Incorrect: Here, the technician in the front is bending the front leg instead of holding it straight. This allows the dog to squirm more.

Method 5: This is a variation of the previous method for large dog handling. In this case the head and neck are not being held. *(Video 17)*

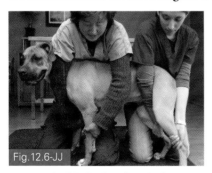

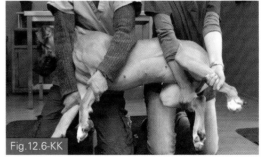

Fig.12.6-JJ, Method 5, Step 1: Grasp the front legs as far above the carpus (wrist) as possible and the hind legs just above the hock.

Fig.12.6-KK, Method 5, Step 2: Lift the dog, lean back and pull the dog up against your body. Try to hold the hind legs close together (they could be closer in this photo). Think about connecting the knees to one another.

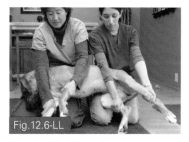

Fig.12.6-LL

Fig.12.6-LL, Method 5, Step 3: Next, slide the dog down your body.

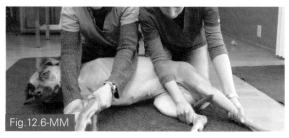

Fig.12.6-MM

Fig.12.6-MM, Method 5, Step 4: With the dog on the floor, your hands are already in position to keep her in lateral recumbency. The arm of the hand holding the front lower leg lies across the dog's neck to control the head and neck. The arm holding the lower back leg is leaning across the dog's flank to prevent her from pulling her leg in and getting up.

WHAT'S WRONG HERE?

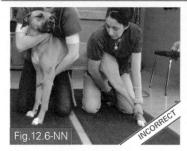

Fig.12.6-NN

INCORRECT

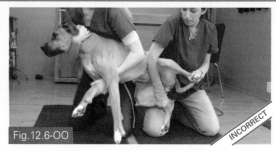

Fig.12.6-OO

INCORRECT

Fig.12.6-NN, Method 5, Incorrect: Here, the hind legs are grasped too low.

Fig.12.6-OO, Method 5, Incorrect: As a result, the technician cannot control the rear end well and the dog's hind legs split apart. Additionally, the technician did not pull the dog's rear end up against her body; consequently, the handler is only supporting the dog by her legs right now.

12.7 Placing Dogs Onto Their Backs

The gentlest way to place a dog onto her back is to first get the dog into lateral recumbency. This can be done in one step or two. Below, we show the procedure starting with the dog in a lateral position. *(Video 18)*

Method 1

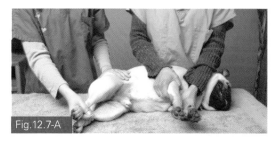

Fig.12.7-A

Fig.12.7-A, Method 1, Step 1: The dog should be placed on his side first. The person in the front grasps both front legs as high up as possible and both arms should be resting on top of the dog. The person in the back grasps both hind legs in one hand above the hocks and places the other hand on the hip.

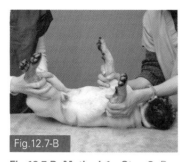

Fig.12.7-B, Method 1, Step 2: Rotate the dog onto his back while keeping the hind legs together.

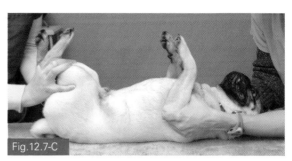

Fig.12.7-C, Method 1, Step 3: Once in dorsal recumbency, the handler in the front should reposition her hands to hold the legs proximal to the elbows. Her arms should be on each side of the head and neck, forming a trough for stabilization.

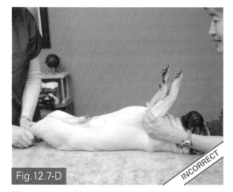

Fig.12.7-D, Method 1, Incorrect: Avoid stretching the hind legs like this, as doing so can be uncomfortable and even painful for the dog.

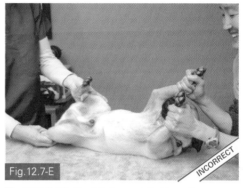

Fig.12.7-E, Method 1, Incorrect: Here, the person in the front is holding the legs too distally. As a result, the dog is able to struggle and move his front end, which allows the back end to move around more, too.

Method 2

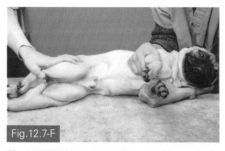

Fig.12.7-F, Method 2, Step 1: Alternatively, the handler in the front can start with one arm on each side of the dog, and the handler in the back can place one hand on each leg. The legs should be grasped in the knee region.

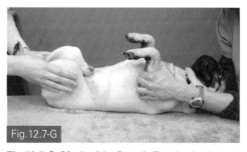

Fig.12.7-G, Method 2, Step 2: The dog is then rotated onto his back. Use Method 2 for little dogs whom you place from a stand directly onto their back.

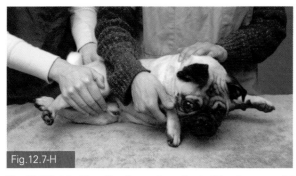

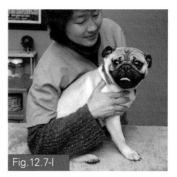

Fig.12.7-H, I, Letting the dog get up: Control the dog even at the end of the procedure. Here, as soon as we release our hold, the dog rapidly flips himself sternally. But because we kept our hands on the dog, we were able to stabilize him in a calm sit.

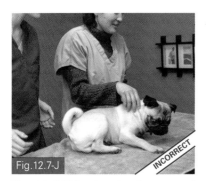

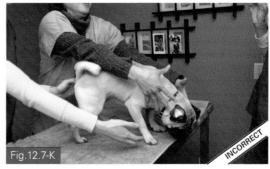

Fig.12.7-J, K, Letting the dog get up, Incorrect: Always be ready for the dog to bolt or just become frantic. Here, the handlers let go of the dog and now have little control over him. The dog almost jumps off the table because the handlers are not restraining him well. Remember, every interaction you have with an animal tells that animal something about you.

Method 3: This procedure explains how to place a large dog onto her back on the floor. Dogs are more comfortable if they are supported on both sides. *(Video 19)*

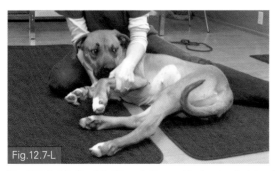

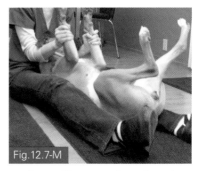

Fig.12.7-L, Method 3, Step 1: Start with the dog in lateral recumbency. Place one of your legs along the side of the dog to stabilize her. Grasp the legs near the elbows and rotate her onto her back.

Fig.12.7-M, Method 3, Step 2 : Then place your other leg out to form a trough in which she can lie.

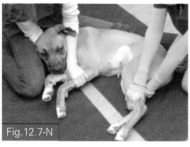
Fig.12.7-N

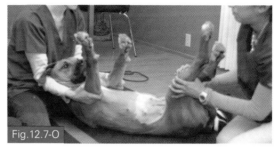
Fig.12.7-O

Fig.12.7-N, Method 3, Step 1 (variation): With two people, the technician in the back can grasp the legs above the hocks, ideally in the knee region if your hands are big enough (she's a little low here).

Fig.12.7-O, Method 3, Step 2 (variation): The technician should try to keep the back legs together. Note that the handler in the front has already repositioned her hands proximal to the dog's elbows to help stabilize the dog.

Fig.12.7-P, Method 3, Step 3 (variation): Now the dog is held stably on her back with the technician's legs on each side to form a trough. The dog's hind legs are held above the hocks and in a relaxed position. Dogs can be rolled into a commercially purchased trough in a similar manner by starting with the trough sitting on its side against the dog's back.

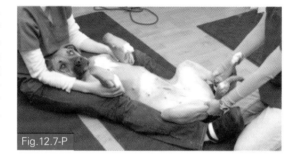
Fig.12.7-P

Method 4: Lying on back in lap. Many small dogs (and cats) are comfortable lying on their backs in your lap. For this example, start with the dog facing left. The dog's left side should be against you. *(see Chapter 11, Video 5)*

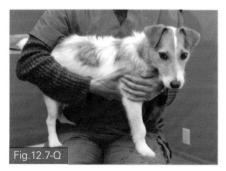
Fig.12.7-Q

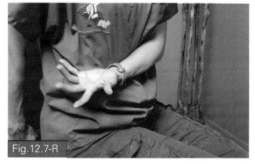
Fig.12.7-R

Fig.12.7-Q, Method 4, Step 1: Support the dog with your right arm and hand. The hand is under the chest. The thumb is on the outside of the front leg to prevent the dog from backing up. The dog should be snug against you.

Fig.12.7-R, Method 4, Step 1 (alternate view): This photo depicts what your hand and arm position should look like. The left hand reaches back and supports the dog's left hip. To do this, keep your left arm against your side so that it's between you and the dog. For very small dogs, your right hand can remain in position on the dog's chest.

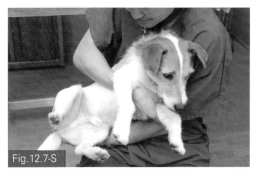

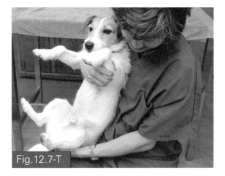

Fig.12.7-S, Method 4, Step 2: For this larger small dog, you might need to grasp the left leg above the elbow rather than keeping your hand on the dog's chest. Now rotate the dog onto his back. Because you will be sliding him into your lap, raise his front end while you rotate his body. Be sure to move both hands in a coordinated fashion.

Fig.12.7-T, Method 4, Step 3: Now the dog is vertical with his back against you and your hand still supporting his hip. Next, you'll slide him into your lap.

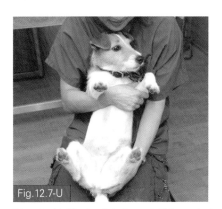

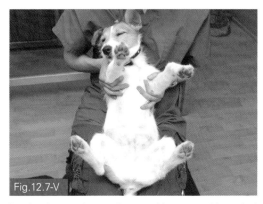

Fig.12.7-U, Method 4, Step 4: When placing the dog in your lap, make sure his rear end is tucked under and his back is curved. Then slide him farther down into your lap.

Fig.12.7-V, Method 4, Step 5: Slide him down far enough so that at least a third of his body is horizontal. Stabilize the dog by holding one front leg with each hand.

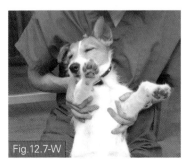

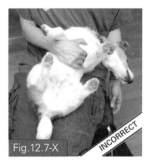

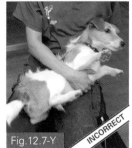

Fig.12.7-W, Method 4, Step 6 (close-up): Place your hands above the elbows for best stabilization.

Fig.12.7-X,Y, Method 4, Incorrect: Here, I have my arm on his chest instead of holding each leg individually. Consequently, it's possible for him to wiggle free.

Box 12-E: Moving the dog from dorsal recumbency to a sitting position in your lap. *(Video 20)*

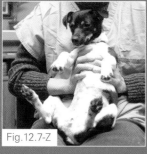

Fig.12.7-Z

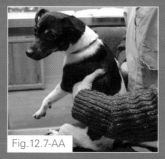

Fig.12.7-AA

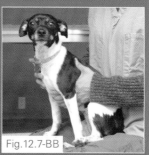

Fig.12.7-BB

Fig.12.7-Z, Method 1, Step 1: Place your fingers over the dog's chest with thumbs extending over her back.

Fig.12.7-AA, BB, Method 1, Step 2: Rotate the dog into an upright position. Do this quickly so that the dog does not feel off balance and her back retains a curve rather than straightening. End with her sitting in your lap.

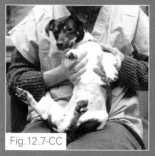

Fig.12.7-CC

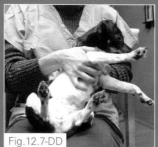

Fig.12.7-DD

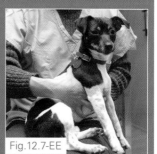

Fig.12.7-EE

Fig.12.7-CC, Method 2, Step 1: Control the body by holding a leg in each hand. Grip with the thumb and index finger above the elbow.

Fig.12.7-DD, Method 2, Step 2: Roll the dog to the side and into a sitting position.

Fig.12.7-EE, Method 2, Final Result: Now the dog is sitting nicely in your lap.

References

McConnell, P.B. 1990. Acoustic structure and receiver response in domestic dogs, *Canis familiaris*. *Animal Behaviour* 39(5):897-904.

Mills, D.S. 2005. What's in a word? Recent findings on the attributes of a command on the performance of pet dogs. *Anthrozoos* 18:208-21.

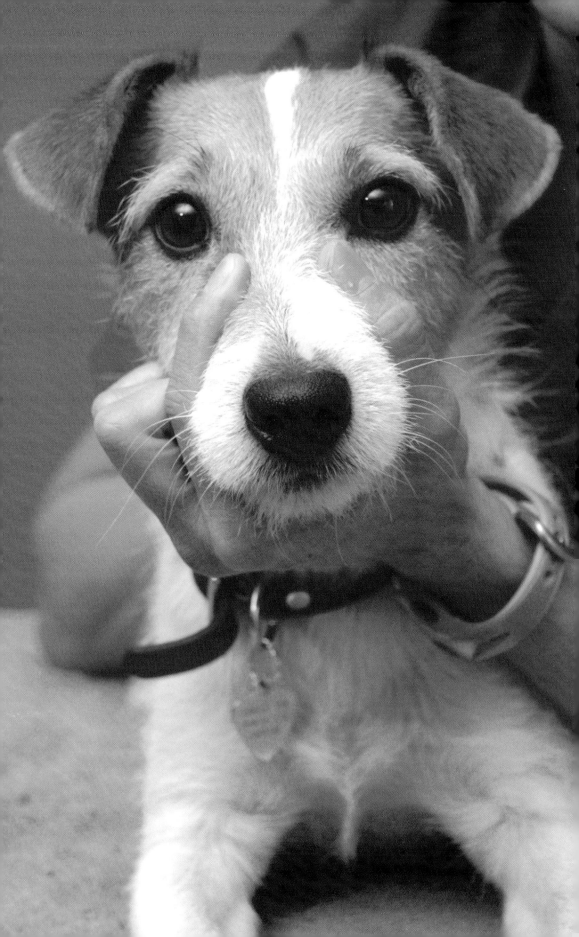

CHAPTER 13.
CANINE
RESTRAINT
For Procedures

"The veterinarian and technician took Peanut into the room and several seconds later I hear screaming," says my friend to me. "I went back in and saw them pushing on his hip to try to get him to sit or lie down or something, and Peanut has bad hips, so I'm sure it hurt." 'We need to muzzle him,' they said. 'Tell me what you want him to do,' I told them. 'We want him to lie on his side.' So I pointed at Peanut and said, 'bang bang.' And he immediately lay on his side. That's the last time I am letting Peanut out of my sight at that particular hospital."

Mediocre handling skills cause stress not only in the pets, but also in their owners. Good handling skills go a long way toward building both pet and owner confidence in the hospital.

13.1 Mouth, Eye and Ear Exams

Method 1

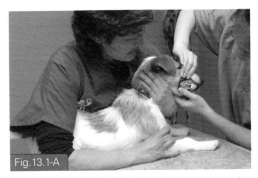

Fig.13.1-A

Fig.13.1-A, Method 1: If the dog is likely to squirm and you need to examine the **mouth**, secure the body close to you and use a C hold around the neck. Hold the neck against your shoulder if necessary. If doing so makes the dog more nervous, then you may need to countercondition him to this type of restraint or try a different technique. In this photo, because my dog, Jonesy, has a tendency to try to stand or jump up, I also hold his front leg above the right elbow.

Method 2

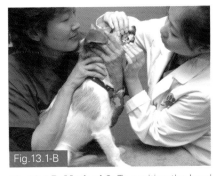

Fig.13.1-B

Fig.13.1-B, Method 2: To position the head more securely, cup the dog's jaw in your hand (i.e., use a U hold on the jaw). If the dog is comfortable and well supported, he won't struggle. Note that my outside arm is still positioned to prevent him from moving away or backing up.

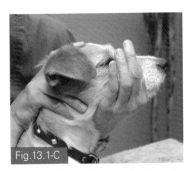

Fig.13.1-C

Fig.13.1-C, Method 2: Additionally, the hand behind his head and on the side of his neck helps keep his head positioned. If the dog is a little nervous, give treats while he's in this restraint hold so that he associates the hold with positive experiences.

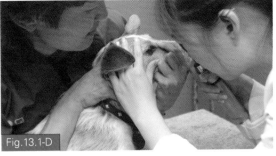

Fig.13.1-D

Fig.13.1-D, Method 2: With this hold, the **eyes, mouth and head** can be examined because the head is held securely and the body is well controlled. Dogs who are fearful at the hospital are likely to have heightened fear when a veterinarian leans close to them and stares directly into their eyes, as for an ophthalmologic exam. For these dogs, it's especially important to start counterconditioning with treats and other things they find motivating (as indicated by their reactions) well before you do the eye exam.

Method 3

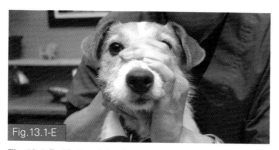

Fig.13.1-E, Method 3a: For an **ear** exam, the head frequently needs to be slightly tilted in one direction or another. In these cases, the muzzle can be grasped in one of two ways. The first variation is to place a C hold on the muzzle with fingers above the muzzle and thumb below (shown here). This hold can also be used for general head restraint; however, some dogs dislike having their muzzles grabbed.

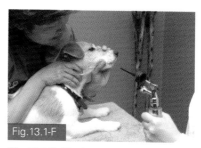

Fig.13.1-F, Method 3a: The C hold allows the holder to rotate the head. The direction of rotation depends partly on the size of the dog's head and the size of the holder's hand. Do what works best for you. Note here that my outside hand is holding the dog's neck.

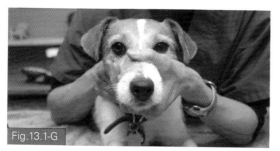

Fig.13.1-G, Method 3b: In the second variation, the fingers are below the muzzle and the thumb is above.

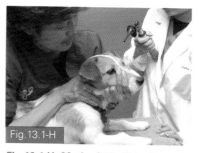

Fig.13.1-H, Method 3b: This allows for easier rotation in a different direction.

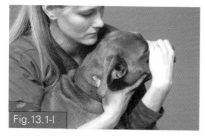

Fig.13.1-I, Method 3c: The fingers can also be wrapped around the outside of the muzzle so that the opening of the C is toward the holder's body. With the outside hand, one finger can be placed on the jaw with the thumb on the neck so that there's no pressure under the dog's ear.

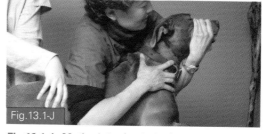

Fig.13.1-J, Method 3c (variation): Alternatively, the outside hand can be placed at the base of the neck to help hold the dog in. This way, you can pull the dog's shoulder into you, which then enables you to rotate the head so that the outside ear is up. Having the outside ear up makes it easier for the veterinarian to position an otoscope quickly and comfortably into both the lateral and vertical ear canals.

Method 4

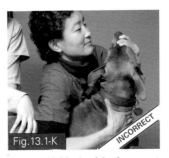

Fig.13.1-K

INCORRECT

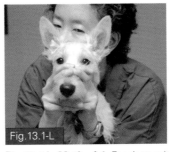

Fig.13.1-L

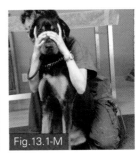

Fig.13.1-M

Fig.13.1-K, Method 3c, Incorrect: Here, I'm not drawing the dog's shoulder and neck into my body. As a result, he's able to turn his head toward me. As soon as I pull his shoulder in, I can get good control of his head (as in Fig.13.1-J).

Fig.13.1-L, Method 4: For dogs with big muzzles, this two-handed hold may be easier. Place the thumbs in the intermandibular space and the fingers above the muzzle. Your arms act as railings and hug the dog's sides. Put your head against the dog's neck so that if he suddenly tries to move his head back, it won't build up enough speed to hit you in the jaw with his skull.

Fig.13.1-M, Method 4: Large dogs can be examined on the floor. I form a wall behind the dog with my body, and my arms secure the dog's sides. My head forms a wall behind the dog's head, preventing her from moving it back.

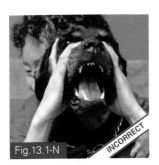

Fig.13.1-N

INCORRECT

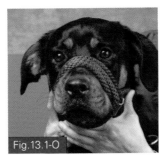

Fig.13.1-O

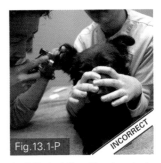

Fig.13.1-P

INCORRECT

Fig.13.1-N, Method 4, Incorrect: This dog, Mischa, begins to struggle playfully, but then the play starts escalating into aggression. Due to her size, it's hard to hold her mouth closed. Because I can't hold her mouth closed, I also can't get a good enough grip on her muzzle to control her head. In this type of situation, the handler should release the dog's head so she will stop struggling, but continue to control the body. Once the dog has calmed down, place a muzzle and then try the restraint again.

Fig.13.1-O, Method 4: In Mischa's case, we placed a leash muzzle (see Chapter 14) that holds her mouth closed, thus improving safety. With her mouth closed, I am able to control her head. After placing this leash muzzle Mischa willingly held still for an otoscopic exam. Note that a commercial muzzle could have been used as well; however many dogs become fearful or more aggressive when someone attempts to put one of these on them. In fact, Mischa had a history of not allowing the owner or veterinarians to place a muzzle on her. Her owner had to later countercondition her to wearing a commercial muzzle.

Fig.13.1-P, Method 4, Incorrect: Be sure to keep your fingers away from the dog's mouth (even if the dog is wearing a muzzle). The technician's fingers are too close here. Also, if the back of the head is not secured and the dog pulls his head away quickly, you can get hit in the jaw. Even a small dog can cause a concussion if his head hits your jaw.

Box 13-A: Counterconditioning with treats

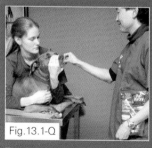

Fig.13.1-Q

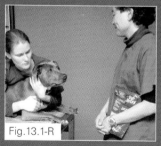

Fig.13.1-R

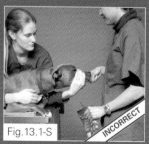

Fig.13.1-S

INCORRECT

Fig.13.1-Q: Give treats to classically countercondition enjoyment of the procedure. In general, if the dog is nervous, give treats continuously while he's in a restraint hold so that he associates the hold with positive experiences. Deliver the bite-sized treats to the dog's mouth so that he doesn't reach or move forward.

Fig.13.1-R: If you're training the dog to prepare him for a procedure, rather than actually performing the procedure, first give several treats in a row. Then stop the stream of treats and simultaneously release the dog from the hold. Repeat. The goal is to get the dog to understand that holding him by the muzzle equals food treats. When you stop giving the treats, hold the treats far enough away so that they are clearly out of the dog's reach.

Fig.13.1-S, Incorrect: Avoid holding the treat in a way that will make the dog pull out of position. Here, the dog is reaching forward for the treats because they are presented too far away from his nose.

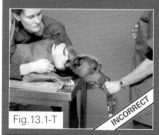

Fig.13.1-T

INCORRECT

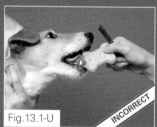

Fig.13.1-U

INCORRECT

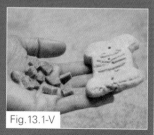

Fig.13.1-V

Fig.13.1-T, Incorrect: In addition, the treat bag is held too close to the dog's head. As a result, he struggles to get to it, even after having just received a treat.

Fig.13.1-U, Incorrect: Choose an appropriate treat size. This treat is too large. The dog will be full after just one. A jackpot of one big treat can be used if the pet is already good at performing the behavior and so doesn't need treats until after he has behaved well for the procedure, and no more treats will be needed for additional procedures.

Fig.13.1-V: Use many small treats. When counterconditioning to procedures, it's better to give 10 bite-size treats one at a time than one big treat. The goal is to keep the dog in a positive emotional state by giving the treats frequently enough. Giving treats too slowly or with too long an interval between deliveries may allow the dog to start focusing on the procedure and to slip out of the happy emotional state. The emotional state can be controlled better with multiple, small, successive treats than 1 big treat.

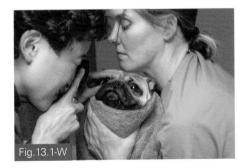

Fig.13.1-W

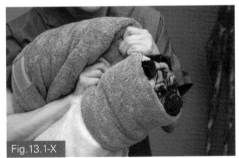

Fig.13.1-X

Fig.13.1-W, Method 5: For wiggly or aggressive dogs, a towel used as a brace around the neck can help control the head and keep the dog from turning around to bite. This is especially useful with brachycephalic dogs and for dogs that find muzzling stressful.

Fig.13.1-X, Method 5: The towel must be thick, held snugly and positioned above the atlanto-occipital joint to keep the dog from moving his head around.

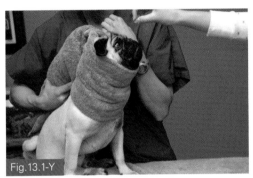

Fig.13.1-Y

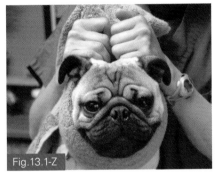

Fig.13.1-Z

Fig.13.1-Y, Method 5: The towel method can be used to stabilize the head as well as to prevent forward or upward movement. Here, it prevents the dog from jumping up to get the treat.

Fig.13.1-Z, Method 5: The towel can also be rolled, instead of folded (as in the previous photos) and then wrapped around the neck. This makes for a wrap that's rounder but covers less of the neck.

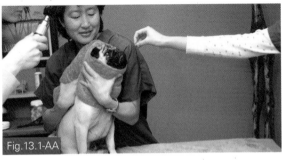

Fig.13.1-AA

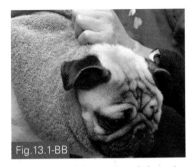

Fig.13.1-BB

Fig.13.1-AA, Method 5: For added security, place one hand under or around the neck and draw the dog's neck close to your side. Here, I'm still holding the towel snugly with one hand. This is easier with the folded towel than with the rolled towel.

Fig.13.1-BB, Method 5: Any time you use a towel to control the head, hold onto it in a manner that draws up the slack. There should be no space between the towel and the dog.

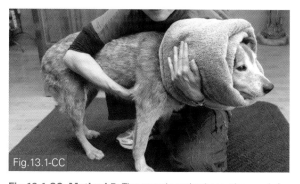

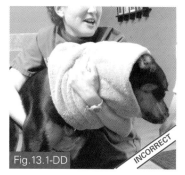

Fig.13.1-CC, Method 5: The towel method can also work for medium dogs if the towel is big enough to span the entire neck, including part of the ears. This can be useful for dogs who object to having close restraint.

Fig.13.1-DD, Method 5, Incorrect: The toweling is not secure enough in this case. The dog can still move her head and bite the vet. Other options to keep dogs from being able to reach around and bite include an Elizabethan collar or a BiteNot collar (BiteNot Products, Inc., San Francisco, California), a foam and plastic neck brace developed to prevent dogs from chewing or licking their body. Consider using them if they can be easily placed on the dog you are working with.

13.2 Intranasal Vaccines

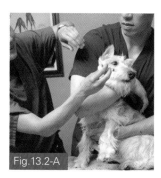

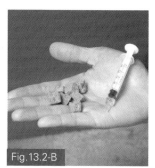

Fig.13.2-A: While some dogs accept intranasal vaccination readily, others have an extreme fear or withdrawal response. If you think the dog might resist or are just unsure about his reaction, countercondition with several treats prior to giving the vaccine.

Fig.13.2-B: In your free hand, hold the syringe plus several bite-size treats.

Fig.13.2-C: Give the dog a few treats in rapid succession while restraining the head slightly.

Fig.13.2-D: Be sure to hold the dog's head up in the position you'll use for the vaccination. Give the treats in this position to encourage the dog to keep his head here.

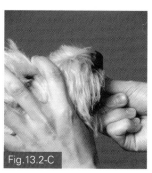

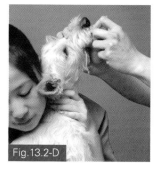

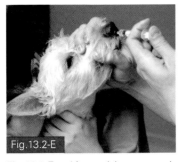

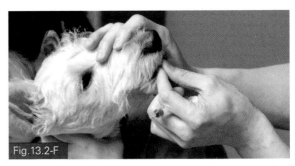

Fig.13.2-E: After giving several treats, and with the dog's head already positioned for vaccination, rapidly give the vaccine in the nostril.

Fig.13.2-F: Follow this immediately with several treats that you place directly into his mouth so that he doesn't have a chance to become upset. Even if he does become upset, it will be short-lived and the event will end on a positive note.

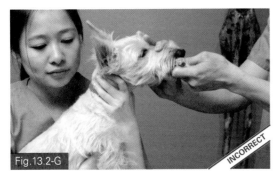

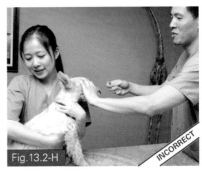

Fig.13.2-G, Incorrect: This dog's nose is too low; it should be held so that it points toward the ceiling. The technicians will have to change the direction in which the nose is pointing to give the vaccine.

Fig.13.2-H, Incorrect: The technician on the right is standing too far away and therefore has less control.

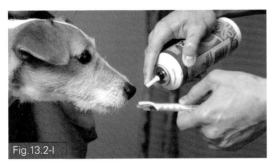

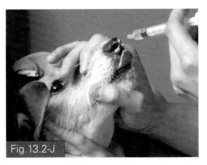

Fig.13.2-I: Another variation for giving intranasal vaccines is to put canned cheese or liver paste onto the syringe. Let the dog lick the cheese off the syringe, then rub the cheese on the dog's nose. The goal is to teach the dog that the syringe near his nose is something good.

Fig.13.2-J: While the dog is still licking the cheese, inject the vaccine into his nostril. If he responds aversely after you've administered the vaccine, immediately distract him by playing with him or giving another treat so that his adverse behavioral reaction only lasts 1-2 seconds and is followed by a positive experience. Then send him home with a counterconditioning plan.

13.3 Oral Medications

13.3.1 Giving pills.

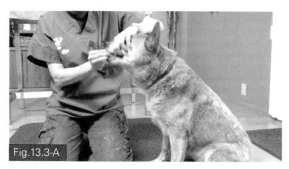

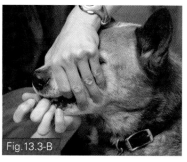

Fig.13.3-A: Grasp the dog's upper jaw behind the canines. If the dog is likely to struggle, then sit behind her or have her sit in a corner so that she can't back up (not done here).

Fig.13.3-B: Hold the pill between your index finger and thumb. Place your third or fourth finger in the region of the lower incisors, avoiding the canines.

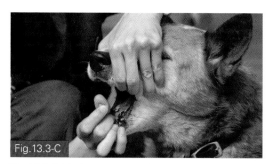

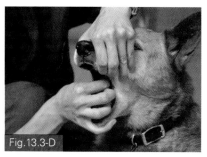

Fig.13.3-C, D: Open the mouth and place the pill at the base of her tongue before she has a chance to resist. Note that the dog's head is not tilted up at a sharp angle or stretched. Tilting up and stretching the neck can inhibit swallowing.

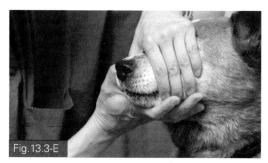

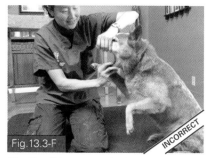

Fig.13.3-E: Next, close her mouth and rub her throat in a downward stroking motion to help encourage swallowing. Follow with some treats or water so that the pill does not get stuck, causing esophagitis.

Fig.13.3-F, Incorrect: Avoid opening the mouth this wide, or the dog will struggle.

13.3.2 Pilling difficult dogs. *(Video 1)*

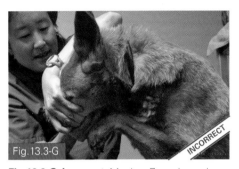

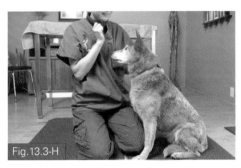

Fig.13.3-G, Incorrect: My dog, Zoe, shown here, hates being pilled. She can smell pills hidden in Pill Pockets, cheese or meat. To pill dogs like this, use several treats in a row to countercondition. Then give the pill.

Fig.13.3-H: Make sure the dog waits politely to take the treat. Hold the treat out of the dog's reach until she sits patiently.

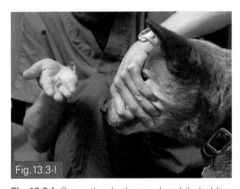

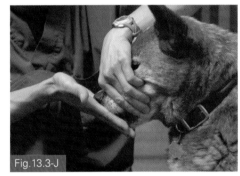

Fig.13.3-I: Grasp the dog's muzzle while holding the treat in front of her.

Fig.13.3-J: Then push the treat right up to the dog's mouth so she doesn't have to reach to get it. Repeat several times.

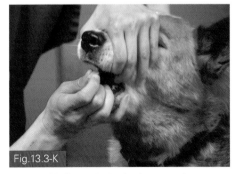

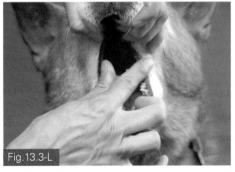

Fig.13.3-K: Once she's clearly expecting treats, work on opening her mouth. Open her mouth and toss in a treat.

Fig.13.3-L: Use the same technique you would if you were pilling.

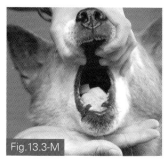

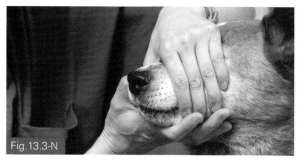

Fig.13.3-M: As soon as you toss the treat in, close her mouth.

Fig.13.3-N: Repeat this procedure several more times. Then, when she has come to expect receiving treats this way, give her the pill instead. It can be hidden in a Pill Pocket or a treat. Immediately follow with another treat so that we end with a positive experience. Remember to follow with multiple treats or a liquid chaser so the pill does not get stuck in her esophagus.

13.3.3 Administering liquids.

Liquids can be administered in the same manner as pills, except that the mouth only needs to be opened a little because the syringe can be inserted into the side of the mouth. Additionally, the head should not be tilted up; hold it level to prevent squirting liquids into the throat. Dogs who don't hold still for liquid medications can be counterconditioned quickly in the following manner.

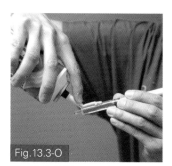

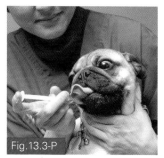

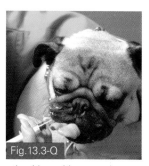

Fig.13.3-O: The goal is to teach the dog to associate the syringe in his mouth with positive experiences. Put canned cheese or a semi-moist treat on the syringe. The treat won't mask the taste, but it will put the pet in a positive emotional state.

Fig.13.3-P, Q: Restrain the dog's body against you so that the dog can't back up, and restrain his head with one hand in a U hold. With the treat on it and the medication inside, insert the syringe into the side of the mouth. While the dog is licking the treat, inject the medication. Hold the dog's head up so that he can't spit out the medication. If he acts like he doesn't like the taste, quickly shove a treat into his mouth as a positive distraction. But only do this if he will readily take the treat when you put it right up to his face. Talk to him in a happy voice if he responds by acting happy. The goal is to get him into a happy state or play mode with another treat so that we end with a positive experience. Remember to follow with multiple treats or a liquid chaser so the pill does not get stuck in his esophagus.

13.4 Jugular Venipuncture

13.4.1 Jugular venipuncture in small and and medium dogs. *(Video 2)*

Method 1

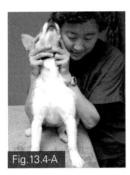 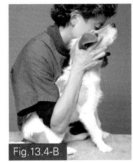 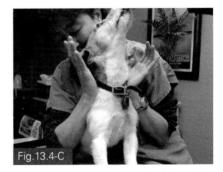

Fig.13.4-A   Fig.13.4-B   Fig.13.4-C

Fig.13.4-A, Method 1: With the dog sitting, hold his head up slightly. Your arms on both sides of his body act as railings to support the dog and prevent him from moving sideways.

Fig.13.4-B, Method 1: Block the dog from backing up by keeping your body against his back and the back of his head. Once you have the dog in position, make sure he's relaxed before beginning the procedure.

Fig.13.4-C, Method 1: If the dog tries to jump up prior to the start of the procedure, put pressure on the top of his shoulders. For the purpose of illustrating this point, I have moved my fingers away from his neck; but in reality, your hand should still be right up against his neck. The hold should be secure but relaxed, unless the dog struggles. If he does struggle, meet his pressure with equal pressure the way roller coaster safety bars only provide pressure if you're upside down or in a free fall. **A ring hold could also be used.** (Refer to Chapter 11, Figures 11.5-M,N,O)

Method 2

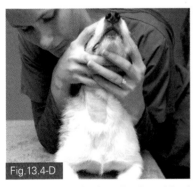 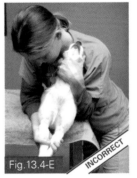 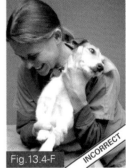

Fig.13.4-D   Fig.13.4-E *INCORRECT*   Fig.13.4-F *INCORRECT*

Fig.13.4-D, Method 2: To draw blood with the dog in sternal recumbancy align the dog's chest with the edge of the table. Then use the same hold as in Method 1. All fingers or just 2 or 3 can be placed under the chin.

Fig.13.4-E, F, Method 2, Incorrect: Stretching the dog in this manner is uncomfortable and often causes the dog to struggle more. And restraining a struggling dog by holding distally on the legs—as you do with this hold—is difficult because the dog can still move his legs.

A Note About Fasting and Lipemia

Some practitioners may be concerned about lipemia in dogs who have recently eaten fatty treats prior to blood draw. Postprandial triglycerides peak 2 to 6 hours after a meal (Watson and Barrier 1993). Giving treats immediately prior to blood draw is likely to have only a minimal effect. Additionally, if triglyceride measurements are not needed, lipemic samples can be ultracentrifuged to remove the lipids and thus remove the lipid interference. For those cases where feeding may have contributed to altered results that are preventing appropriate conclusions from being made, the sample can be retaken. The second sampling should be easier because the first one was performed with counterconditioning.

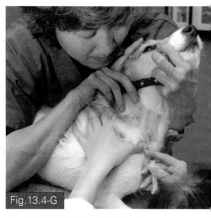

Fig.13.4-G

Fig.13.4-G, Method 2 (variation): Another option is to use the same type of hand and arm positioning as for general head restraint (Section 13.1).

Method 3

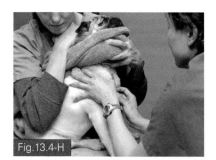

Fig.13.4-H

Fig.13.4-H, Method 3: If the dog is really wiggly, try wrapping a towel around his neck. Use a folded towel rather than a rolled one, as it is easier to raise the edge of a folded towel. The goal is to provide a comfortable position in which the dog feels secure. Give treats rapidly until immediately before the blood is drawn and then again after the needle is removed. Make sure you give the treats in a manner that prevents the dog from lunging forward to get them.

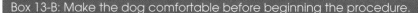

Box 13-B: Make the dog comfortable before beginning the procedure.

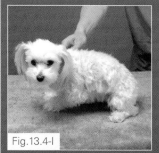

Fig.13.4-I

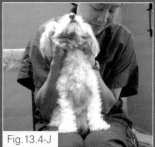

Fig.13.4-J

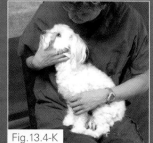

Fig.13.4-K

Fig.13.4-I, J, K: Some dogs are uncomfortable or fearful being restrained on the exam table. This dog can be restrained more comfortably in the handler's lap. The same restraint holds can be used when the dog is in your lap as when he's on the table.

Method 4

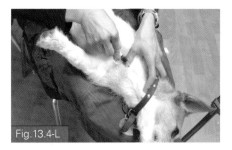

Fig.13.4-L

Fig.13.4-L, Method 4: For other dogs, unconventional positions can or must be used. My dog would not let technicians restrain him, but would allow me to draw his blood when he lay on my lap. *(Video 3)*

Box 13-C: Tips on positioning for jugular venipuncture.

Visualization or palpation of the occluded vein and its location varies from dog to dog. Start by holding the dog's head centered and the nose level or a little higher, and then adjust as needed, per the instructions of the person drawing blood.

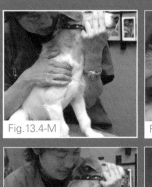

Fig.13.4-M

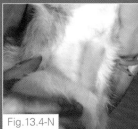

Fig.13.4-N

Fig.13.4-M: When restraining for jugular venipuncture, the direction the dog's nose points is important. Here, the dog's nose is centered and level with his eyes.

Fig.13.4-N: The dog's jugular is centered and easy to visualize. It's good for the restrainer to practice visualizing the jugular to evaluate positioning.

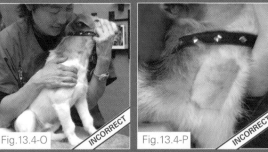

Fig.13.4-O   INCORRECT   Fig.13.4-P   INCORRECT

Fig.13.4-O, Incorrect: When the head is turned too far to the side, the vein moves to the side of the neck and flattens.

Fig.13.4-P, Incorrect: As a result, the jugular is not as visible because the vein is occluded.

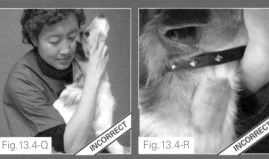

Fig.13.4-Q   INCORRECT   Fig.13.4-R   INCORRECT

Fig.13.4-Q, Incorrect: When the nose is held too high or the neck is bent backward, the jugular might flatten.

Fig.13.4-R, Incorrect: This vein is more difficult to visualize than when the head is more level.

13.4.2 Jugular venipuncture in larger dogs.

Method 1 *(Video 4)*

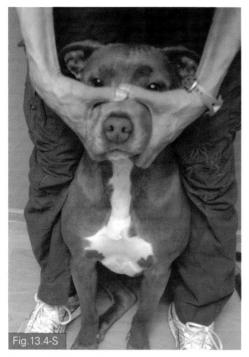

Fig.13.4-S

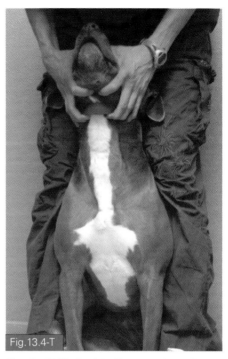

Fig.13.4-T

Fig.13.4-S, Method 1: Large dogs can be restrained in a sit. The wall acts as a barrier behind the dog and the technician's legs act as safety bars hugging the dog on both sides. Note the technicians feet are in line with her knees (unlike in Fig. 13.5-O where the dog can move her hips around causing her body to be crooked).

Fig.13.4-T, Method 1: Place your index fingers in the intermandibular space. If the dog is wearing a collar, grasp the collar too. This keeps the collar away from the venipuncture site and also provides much greater stabilization of the head. As a result, the dog is less likely to struggle. Without the collar, if the dog struggles she can easily get loose.

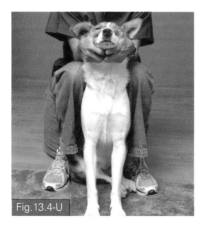

Fig.13.4-U

Fig.13.4-U: This restraint can also be performed from a sitting position if the handler is sitting on a chair with a solid base. The chair then acts as a barrier behind the dog. Notice that the technician's legs form a barrier by hugging the sides of the dog and her feet are in line with her knees. By keeping her feet in she's helping to keep the dog's hips positioned so that the dog's body is straight.

Method 2 *(Video 5)*

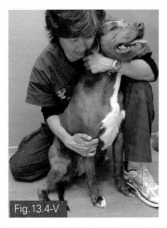
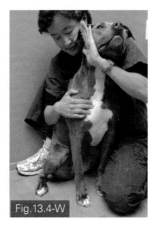
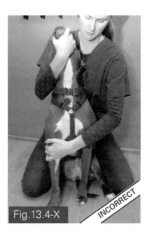

Fig.13.4-V   Fig.13.4-W   Fig.13.4-X   INCORRECT

Fig.13.4-V, Method 2: Large dogs can also be restrained using the following technique either on the table or sitting on the floor. In general, it's easier to restrain them where they feel comfortable (on the floor). Secure the dog on all sides by placing your body and foot behind her to keep her from backing up. Your other leg and body should form a wall on one side of her and your arm should form a railing on the opposite side. With one arm around her neck and the other at the point of her shoulder, the dog can't move forward. This dog is energetic and wiggly, so I hold her head close to my shoulder. If needed, I can lift my elbow under her mandible to better support her head.

Fig.13.4-W, Method 2: I can turn my hand to face outward, if necessary, so that I can draw the dog's head closer to my shoulder. Keep your hand behind the skull as you do this.

Fig.13.4-X, Method 2, Incorrect: With this hold, notice that only one side of the head is restrained and there is space between the dog's shoulder and the holder's elbow. If the dog does not struggle, the hold will work. But if a struggle does ensue, the dog will get loose. *(Video 6)*

Method 3

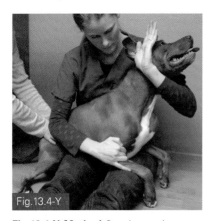
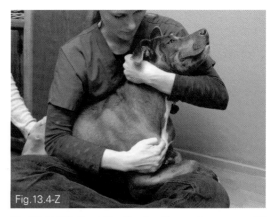

Fig.13.4-Y   Fig.13.4-Z

Fig.13.4-Y Method 3a: Large dogs can be restrained in sternal recumbency on your lap with your legs outstretched. A second technician can keep the dog from backing up, if needed.

Fig.13.4-Z Method 3b: Or sit with your legs crossed if that's more comfortable for the dog. If the dog is wiggly, then you may want to use a firmer hold around the neck than is pictured here. (See head restraint variations in Chapter 12.)

13.5 Cephalic Venipuncture and Catheterization

13.5.1 General principles for occluding the vein and stabilizing the front leg.

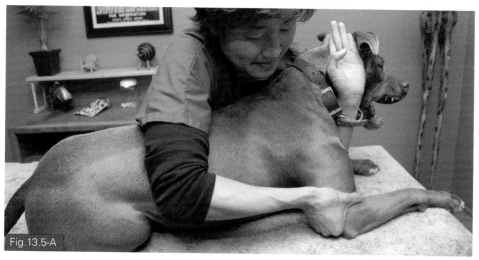

Fig.13.5-A

Fig.13.5-A: First, control the dog's head by placing your arm around her neck (or, with small dogs, use a C hold). This prevents the dog from swinging her head and biting the handler or the person taking blood. Your outside arm holds the dog in, keeps her from backing up her body and controls her leg. Recall from Chapter 11 and 12 that you may need to hold the dog in an even more secure variation to control head motion and a second handler can restrain the rear. Of course, if you're afraid she may try to bite you can also use a muzzle.

Method 1

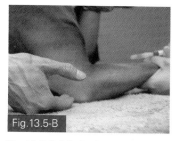

Fig.13.5-B

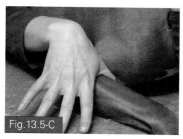

Fig.13.5-C

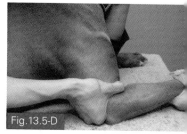

Fig.13.5-D

Fig.13.5-B, Method 1: Use your thumb to hold off the vein. The rest of your hand sits behind the elbow so that the dog cannot pull her leg back.

Fig.13.5-C, Method 1: First hold off the vein with the thumb. Then position the fingers behind and to the inside of the leg. *(next photo)*

Fig.13.5-D, Method 1: The dog's triceps should sit in the webbing between your thumb and index finger. This keeps the leg from moving backward.

Method 2

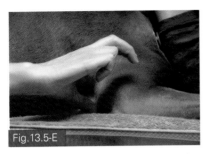

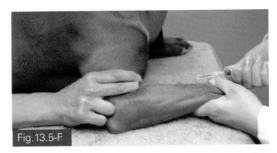

Fig.13.5-E, Method 2: Sometimes, due to the angle at which you are holding, it can be easier to grip by using the index and third finger to occlude the vein.

Fig.13.5-F, Method 2: The dog is still kept from pulling her leg away because her arm sits in the webbing between your thumb and index finger.

Method 3

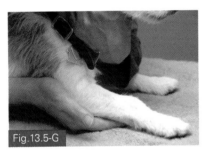

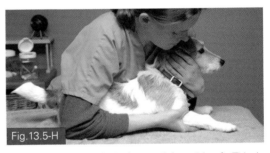

Fig.13.5-G, Method 1a: One common method of restraining the leg is similar to Method 1, except the dog's elbow sits in the palm of your hand.

Fig.13.5-H, Method 1b (potential problem): This is less effective than the previous two methods if the dog tries to move his leg.

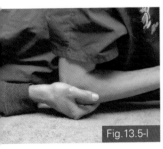

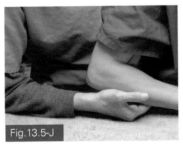

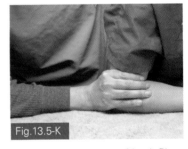

Fig.13.5-I, Exercise 1a (potential problem): To experience the problem, practice on a friend. Place your arm on the table and your hand below the elbow of your friend. Now the friend tries to move her elbow backward while you attempt to resist her movement.

Fig.13.5-J, Exercise 1b (potential problem): The elbow will easily slip past your hand.

Fig.13.5-K, Exercise 1c: However, using one of the other two methods of holding off the cephalic vein, you'll find it much easier to keep the elbow from moving.

13.5.2 Restraining the neck and body.

Method 1

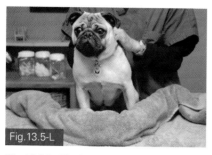

Fig.13.5-L

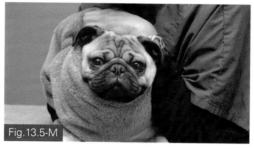

Fig.13.5-M

Fig.13.5-L, Method 1: For small dogs who might struggle, a towel wrap can be used. This works well for dogs with cardiac or pulmonary problems where struggling can cause collapse. Use a thick, rolled towel.

Fig.13.5-M, Method 1: Wrap the towel around the front of the dog high on the neck so that it extends up the neck and down to the bottom of the chest. The large surface area provides a more stable hold compared to just using your arm or hand around the neck.

Method 2

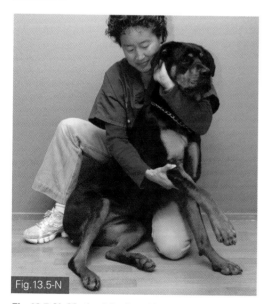

Fig.13.5-N

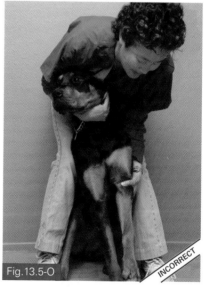

Fig.13.5-O INCORRECT

Fig.13.5-N, Method 2: As with jugular venipuncture, the dog can be on a table or large dogs can sit or lie on the floor. Choose the location where the dog is most comfortable. The restraint is similar to that used for a jugular venipuncuncture.

Fig.13.5-O, Method 2, Incorrect: When restraining dogs on the floor, avoid bending over like this, as it can cause back strain. It's also not a very secure position.

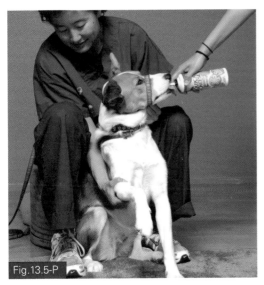

Fig. 13.5-P

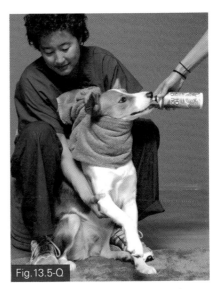

Fig. 13.5-Q

Fig.13.5-P, Method 2 (variation): Fearful dogs that do not want to have their necks hugged can be restrained with less physical contact by first sitting them near a chair with a solid base which they can't escape under. The handler can then position herself sitting behind the dog with legs forming a barrier on each side. One hand controls the head by holding the gentle leader on the side opposite the venipuncture leg. A second person simultaneously distracts/counterconditions the dog by giving treats such as canned cheese paste while the blood is drawn. (Refer to Chapter 14 for more information)

Fig.13.5-Q, Method 2, (variation): The neck can also be restrained using a towel. This restraint will not keep the dog from escaping if it struggles for more than several seconds unless the handler releases the leg and grasps the towel with both hands. But it can help keep the dog comfortable and secure so that she does not try to struggle and provides reasonable safety for both the handler and the person drawing the blood.

Method 3

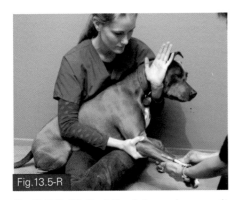

Fig. 13.5-R

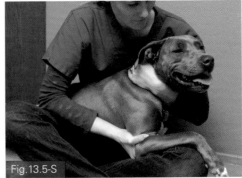

Fig. 13.5-S

Fig.13.5-R, Method 3: A large dog can sit on your lap with your legs extended. Restrain the head so that she cannot bite or snap. (See Chapter 12, head restraint variations.)

Fig.13.5-S, Method 3: Sitting with folded legs is more comfortable for the technician and provides better balance. But be sure the dog is also comfortable in this position.

Method 4

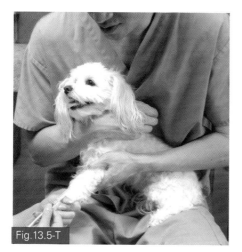

Fig.13.5-T

Fig.13.5-T, Method 4: Some nervous lapdogs are more relaxed and easier to control when sitting in your lap. The most important factor is the dog's comfort. If the dog feels comfortable and secure, then he's less likely to struggle. For small dogs, the hold this technician has around the head is not very secure. For instance, when you carry a glass or a mug, you generally do so with your hand (thumb on one side and finger on the other) rather than holding it between your arm and your body, because holding it in your hand is more secure. A C-hold provides similar improved security.

13.6 Lateral Saphenous Venipuncture

Method 1

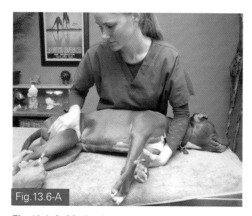

Fig.13.6-A

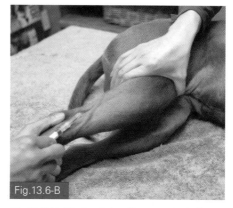

Fig.13.6-B

Fig.13.6-A, Method 1: Start with the dog in lateral recumbency. Hold the front lower leg out straight so the dog does not pull it away from you. Also, hold the back leg caudally and above the knee to occlude the lateral saphenous vein.

Fig.13.6-B, Method 1: If you occlude in the correct location, the vein should be easy to visualize. A second technician might be necessary to restrain the back end because you don't have a hold on the dog's lower back leg.

Method 2

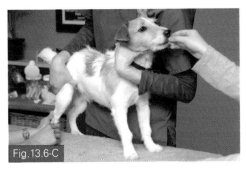

Fig.13.6-C

Fig.13.6-C, Method 2: Some dogs are calmer when standing. They might feel less vulnerable and thus more comfortable in this position. Giving treats can help distract them from the procedures. A continuous stream of goodies that the dog likes and eats works well for distraction and for keeping the dog in a positive emotional state. Notice the technician is controlling the head and neck using a C hold, and her body acts as a barrier along one side. This dog is well restrained.

Method 3

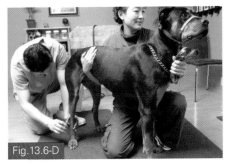

Fig.13.6-D

Fig.13.6-D, Method 3: For large dogs who are fearful and do not want to be touched, letting them stand often works well. The less threatened they feel, the more likely they will hold still. Here, I'm restraining the head by holding the leash attached to the Gentle Leader head collar. The technician taking the blood has to occlude the vein himself.

Fearful dogs may retract their leg when a handler grasps the distal portion. This can sometimes be prevented by habituating the dog to touch. The handler can place his hand proximally, in a location where the dog barely reacts, and leave it there until the dog relaxes. Then he can move the hand slowly all the way down the leg to the final position needed to restrain for venipuncture. He may have to repeat this several times until the dog remains relaxed with the hand in final restraint position distally on the leg.

Method 4

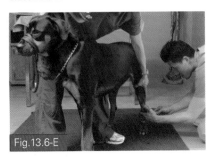

Fig.13.6-E

Fig.13.6-E, Method 4: The handler can also use a leash muzzle (see Chapter 14) to help restrain the head, and press the dog's neck against her leg for stability. This position is harder on the restrainer's back, but allows her to occlude the vein.

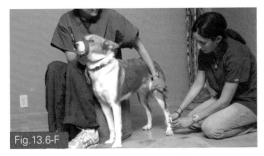

Fig.13.6-F

Fig.13.6-F, Method 4: Some dogs may feel more secure if you sit next to them. It's best if the object you sit on is solid so that the dog can firmly lean against it without feeling like he can escape by ducking under it. This position is more comfortable for the handler and it can be less threatening for the pet.

Method 5

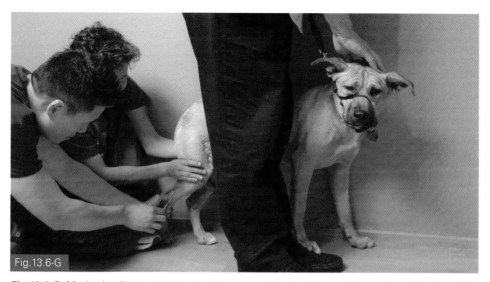

Fig.13.6-G

Fig.13.6-G, Method 5: The owner or a handler can position the dog against a wall and then keep her distracted. This handler can control the head with a Gentle Leader and also use it to help prevent the dog from moving forward or turning to snap. She can use her body to keep the dog positioned against the wall just by standing close to the dog. One technician may need to keep the dog standing while the other takes the blood. The owner could also give treats while holding the dog's leash or Gentle Leader. This should be done only if the dog trusts the owner enough to distinguish that the technician and veterinarian are the "threat" and the owner is not. Alternatively, a muzzle can be used and treats delivered with the muzzle on. *(Refer to Chapter 14, Video 12)*

13.7 Subcutaneous (SQ) and Intramuscular (IM) Injections

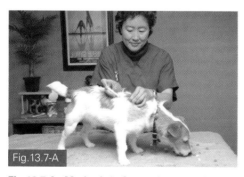

Fig.13.7-A

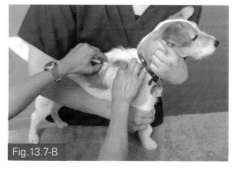

Fig.13.7-B

Fig.13.7-A, Method 1: Some dogs can be distracted enough with treats so that no restraint is needed. Be sure to inject with a decisive poke rather than inching the needle slowly through the skin.

Fig.13.7-B, Method 2: When using restraint to give injections, be sure to control the head so that the person giving the injection cannot be bitten. Notice the C hold around the dog's neck.

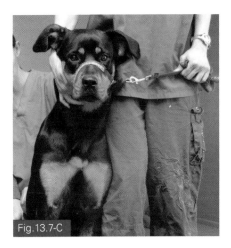

Fig.13.7-C

Fig.13.7-C, Method 3: Here, the handler restrains the head by placing a hand on the dog's neck behind the skull and guiding the head to sit against her hip and leg. Note that the technician's leg is bent, which allows it to be contoured to the dog's body so that she has better balance if the dog tries to move. She's further stabilizing the head using a Gentle Leader head halter. To stabilize correctly, allow no slack between the head collar and the hand holding the leash. Now, if the dog tries to turn toward the person giving the vaccine, her head will be stopped.

Method 4

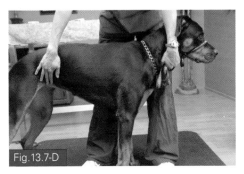

Fig.13.7-D

Fig.13.7-D, Method 4: For standing dogs, stabilize the rear end with one hand on the flank or hip and the other on the neck just behind the skull. The neck should be further stabilized against your leg. Bend your leg slightly so that if the dog knocks against it, your knee will not be injured. This dog is wearing a Gentle Leader, so you might choose a more stable hold that's also easier on your back (as depicted in the previous photo).

Method 5

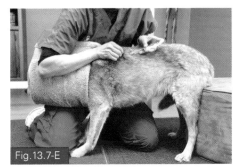

Fig.13.7-E

Fig.13.7-E, Method 5: If the dog is to be vaccinated by only one person (as is often the case in animal shelters), it's safer to place the head in a towel. This method is also a good choice for dogs with unknown temperaments as long as it does not cause them to become fearful. Restrain the head by holding your elbow close to your side, which pulls the dog against your body. The dog can't back up because there's a solid object behind her.

13.8 Cystocentesis

Method 1

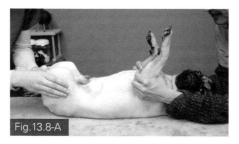
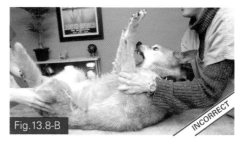

Fig.13.8-A, Method 1: The traditional manner for collecting urine via cystocentesis is to place the animal on his back. When doing so, be sure to form a trough for the dog's head and neck with your arms, and hold the front legs proximal to the elbows. The hind limbs are held above the hocks. Avoid stretching the legs, as this can cause pain in the hips.

Fig.13.8-B, Method 1, Incorrect: The dog is struggling here because, like many dogs, she does not feel comfortable being restrained on her back, even when held securely on a towel. She also dislikes being placed in trough because she's often placed unskillfully and feels off balance.

Method 2

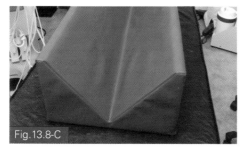
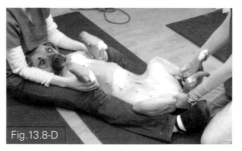

Fig.13.8-C,D, Method 2: Large dogs can be placed in a commercially purchased trough or one made by the technician's legs. The dog is resting on the floor but the technician's legs hug the sides of the dog. In general, it's easier to place dogs skillfully into a trough made by the technician's legs. The dog should wear a muzzle if you think she might be mouthy or try to bite, since the head is not controlled. If she does try to bite, use a different technique.

Method 3

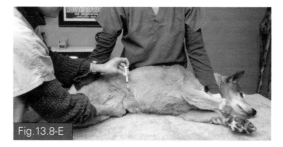

Fig.13.8-E, Method 3: For a dog who doesn't like troughs or being on her back, perform the cystocentesis on her side. Here, my dog, Zoe, is much more comfortable on her side.

Method 4

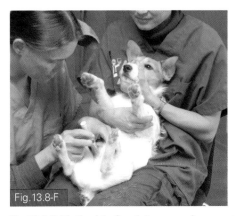
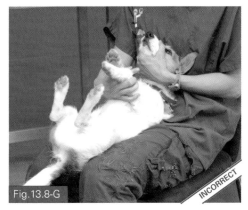

Fig.13.8-F

Fig.13.8-G

Fig.13.8-F, Method 4: Small dogs are often most comfortable in your lap. The handler's legs should be held together so that the dog does not fall through. She should stabilize the muzzle with one hand and arm, and the legs with the other. Note that my right hand is around the elbow of one front leg. To stabilize the side of the dog from the shoulder to the head, keep your elbows in. If the dog is comfortable, the hind limbs will not need to be restrained. If needed, a second helper can restrain the hind limbs.

Fig.13.8-G, Method 4, Incorrect: This dog is too low in my lap. Consequently, I cannot stabilize the neck and head well.

13.9 Toenail Trims *(Refer to Chapter 18, Video 8)*

Perform nail trims in any position in which the animal is comfortable and will hold still. A toenail trim is not an emergency procedure. Do not perform one forcibly if the patient is unwilling to hold still. Doing so can train the dog to be more fearful of people, hate the veterinary hospital, and can even escalate to aggression immediately or in the future. Consequently, forced restraint is likely to cause these dogs to become behaviorally worse than when they entered. Instead, if the dog will not hold still, inform the owner that you are concerned about the dog's behavioral health and ability to be treated in the future. Then provide them with simple counterconditioning solutions. Schedule a technician behavior health session where the technician can instruct the owners on how to perform the counterconditioning procedure (refer to Chapter 18). Some dogs can also be counterconditioned during the office visit, since the procedure may only take a few minutes.

A toenail trim is not an emergency procedure. Avoid performing one forcibly if the patient is unwilling to hold still. Instead offer the client the option of a behavior modification plan (taught in technician counterconditioning sessions). If the owner declines have them sign a consent form that states they understand the adverse effects of having procedures performed when the pet is fearful, resistant, or aggressive. For more information on technician behavior sessions refer to chapter 18. For a sample consent form go to www.nerdbook.com/lowstresshandling

Method 1

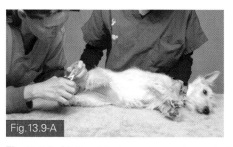

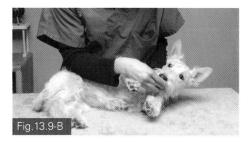

Fig.13.9-A, Method 1: Lateral recumbency is the most secure position in which to perform toenail trims. But dogs who are fearful often do not like being in lateral recumbency. This dog is small enough to restrain both front legs in one hand. I've spread treats on the table so that she can eat during the toenail trim.

Fig.13.9-B, Method 1: Prior to starting the toenail trim, I'm giving this dog a few treats. At the end of the procedure, I'll praise her exuberantly to get her into play mode and to be sure that her last experience related to the trim is a pleasant one.

Method 2   ## Method 3

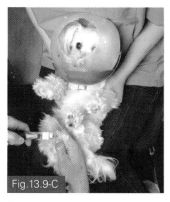

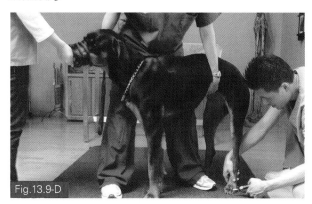

Fig.13.9-C, Method 2: Small dogs who are used to being held or cradled like a baby often do well having their toenails trimmed when they are lying on their back in your lap. This position also allows the technician performing the toenail trim good visualization so that she can perform the procedure quickly. This dog is wearing an Air Muzzle Restraint (SoftPaws.com, Three Rivers, California). An Elizabethan collar can also be used to help guard the handlers from being bitten.

Fig.13.9-D, Method 2: Some dogs do best having their nails trimmed in a standing position. Others can easily be counterconditioned to grinding the nails with a Dremel tool.

References

Watson, T.D.G., and J. Barrie. 1993. Lipoprotein metabolism and hyperlipidaemia in the dog and cat: A review. *Journal of Small Animal Practice* 34(10):479-87.

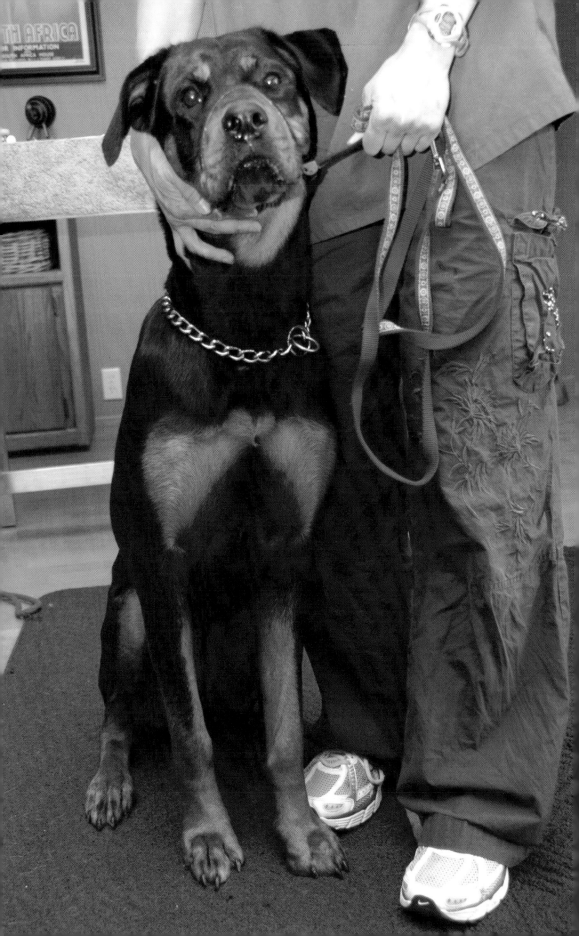

CHAPTER 14.
DEALING WITH
Difficult Dogs

When pet care professionals think of dealing with difficult dogs, their first thoughts are often about the devices and tools that can be used for restraint and how to perform the necessary procedures or apply the devices when the animal is struggling. As emphasized throughout this book, what we should be thinking is, "How can we make the animal feel comfortable and safe so that she cooperates, rather than making her feel threatened so that she thinks she has to protect herself?" The goal of low-stress handling is not to find a better way to hold down a dog. Rather, the goal is to use methods designed to keep the dog calm so that she chooses not to struggle. If the dog does struggle, the struggling should last less than 3 seconds and be repeated no more than a few times, with calm behavior in between.

301

The ultimate test of our handling is whether the dog is calmer, happier and better behaved after handling than before, and if she improves with each handling experience.

Most difficult dogs are that way because they are fearful. Still, some are difficult due to other reasons, such as having their unruly behavior reinforced in the past. Regardless of the reasons behind difficult behavior, the methods used are the same. This chapter will explain 10 methods for dealing with difficult dogs in the hospital. Staff members working with a particular dog should note in the animal's chart which techniques were successful and whether the owner was sent home with a counterconditioning plan. (For an owner information handout visit www.nerdbook.com/lowstresshandling)

"HOW CAN WE MAKE THE ANIMAL FEEL COMFORTABLE AND SAFE SO THAT SHE COOPERATES, RATHER THAN MAKING HER FEEL THREATENED SO THAT SHE THINKS SHE HAS TO PROTECT HERSELF?"

The goal of low-stress handling is for the animal's behavior to improve, rather than get worse.

14.1 Provide a Comfortable Environment

The environment sets the stage for the dog's visit. Dogs who are afraid of noises, other animals or people might experience heightened fear even before they enter the examination room. For these dogs, seeing, smelling or hearing these things at the veterinary hospital is like exposing an arachnophobic person to spiders and spider webs in a dental waiting room. In both cases, the fearful beings can easily develop an aversion to the location and then be less likely to cooperate.

Dogs with such fears should wait in the car, a comfortable exam room or some other area where they are least likely to be exposed to the sounds and sights that scare them. They can be brought in through a side or back door if needed, and their exam can be scheduled during a quiet time of day. Some animals will do better if they are greeted and even examined outside the hospital in the parking lot or car.

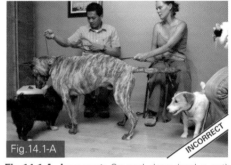

Fig.14.1-A

Fig.14.1-A, Incorrect: Several dogs (and a cat) are placed together in this waiting room. Notice that the big dog is hovering over the little black dog. Fearful dogs should wait in the car or exam room, or should be scheduled at slow times of the day. Each fearful stimulus they encounter will prime them to become even more fearful during the exam and treatment. Consequently, they will be more likely to struggle and bite.

14.1.1 The waiting room.

For fearful dogs, crowded waiting rooms can prime them to be more fearful and aggressive.

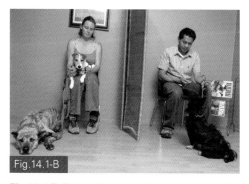

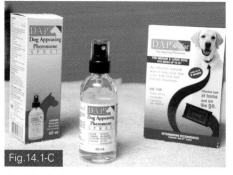

Fig.14.1-B: This waiting room is more comfortable for the animals due to the partition. The owner of the black dog can concentrate on counterconditioning with treats.

Fig.14.1-C: DAP (Dog Appeasing Pheromone, Ceva Animal Health, Lenexa, Kansas) is a synthetic pheromone that has been shown to help calm some dogs in certain situations (Tod 2005). Consider using DAP, either as a spray or diffuser, in the waiting room as well as in treatment rooms and kennel areas. Or have the owner place 6-8 squirts on a bandanna worn by the dog 15-20 minutes before entering the hospital. The dog can also wear a DAP collar.

14.1.2 Perform the exam and procedure where the dog is most comfortable.

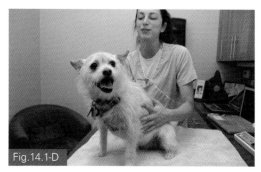

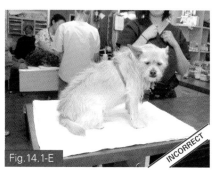

Fig.14.1-D, Correct: This dog is afraid of unfamiliar people and is considered "aggressive" at the veterinary hospital. However, she is comfortable in the exam room that has been designed to make dogs feel at home. It has chairs that look like easy chairs and a throw rug. She enjoys being petted by the technician in this environment because she's comfortable in this room and because the technician has taken time to play with her on the floor first.

Fig.14.1-E, Incorrect: Here's the same dog several minutes later in the busy treatment room. She looks like she's falling asleep. Remember that this sleepy behavior is a sign of fear. Her owner (standing in the background) cannot get her into play mode, as she was in the exam room. This dog's procedures should be performed in a quieter location, or even on the floor where she was more comfortable.

14.2 Start Counterconditioning in the Waiting Room

Counterconditioning should begin as soon as the dog enters the hospital. Known shy or fearful dogs should be brought to the clinic on an empty stomach, and the owners should bring their regular meal as well as treats. Tell the owners that the dog will be getting a meal's worth of food during the visit so that they will be sure to withhold her meal. The hospital should have tasty, bite-sized treats, too, which the front-office staff and technicians can use liberally. Start by tossing treats to the dog while looking away from her.

Of course, counterconditioning with food is not an option with dogs who are arriving for surgery or are anorexic. But for all dogs who can eat—even those who are recovering from surgery or are hospitalized and are now eating well—food can be used for counterconditioning.

Case 1: Pixie, an 8-month-old Wirehaired Pointing Griffon.

Pixie was adopted several months ago. Her owners quickly discovered that she was extremely fearful and exhibited defensive aggression. At home, when the owners tried to put on her leash or grab her collar, she would run away and then snap and growl defensively once cornered.

At the veterinary hospital, Pixie is extremely fearful and aggressive. Her regular veterinarians are unable to examine her because she snaps, whines, paces and struggles violently. When she initially presented, she was extremely lethargic so they were able to muzzle her and then hold her down forcefully. Since then, the staff has not been able to touch her or muzzle her. *(Video 1)* Pixie will not allow her owners to muzzle her either, even though she will allow them to place a Gentle Leader on her in the exam room. At this stage, the owner has already counterconditioned her to accepting the Gentle Leader, as well as to having her leash put on and her collar grabbed. Pixie now wags her tail when she sees the leash or when her collar is grabbed. Her owners have not yet counterconditioned Pixie to accept the muzzle, though.

In this case study, we demonstrate the process that can be used at a hospital to treat these behavioral issues and make dogs like Pixie manageable. This procedure should occur with all dogs who are not anorexic on presentation. With dogs who are not fearful, it can be extremely abbreviated; that is, a few treats will probably suffice.

Here, the technician, Jon, will take a history and the dog's vital signs. Pixie has seen Jon previously and was afraid of him, but she has never received treats from him before. *(Video 2)*

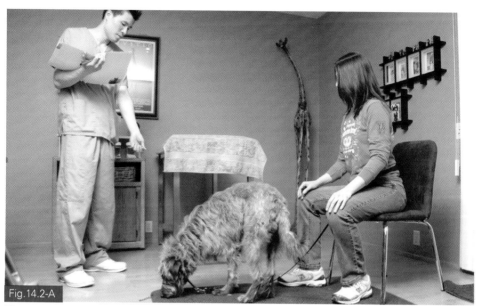

Fig.14.2-A

Fig.14.2-A: During the history-taking portion of the exam, Jon tosses treats to Pixie while avoiding eye contact. The goal is to have Pixie associate him with pleasant experiences. Nervous dogs might not take the treats immediately, but sometimes they will within several minutes. If the dog looks or acts fearful, the technician should toss treats continuously—assuming the dog is eating them—to keep the dog in a positive emotional state. It is best to toss treats so that the dog has to move around the room. This gets her away from her owner, keeps her more focused and helps her switch gears into play mode. Pixie received about 15 small treats during Jon's history-taking. Note that this dog is on leash. If you're unsure about your safety be sure the dog is on leash and the owner is keeping the leash a constant length that allows the dog to move around enough to go after the treats. Then stand out of the dog's reach.

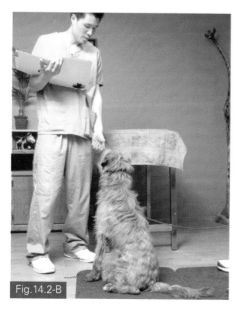

Fig.14.2-B

Fig.14.2-B: If the dog comes up to the technician, he can offer the treat out of his hand. Pixie is comfortable now, even with Jon looking at her. If the dog freezes or her ears suddenly turn out and back, she probably perceives the technician's posture or behavior as a threat, indicating that the technician should look away or nonchalantly back away. If the dog readily comes up to take treats and looks relaxed, the technician can then wait for the dog to offer a sit. (Refer to Chapter 12, Section 3 for getting dogs to sit.) Pixie sat automatically because she's learned to do this at home. She offered this behavior to Jon within the first 15 seconds of the history-taking. Jon could also ask Pixie to sit by saying "sit" in a happy tone of voice or an energetic whisper. Avoid using a commanding voice. If the dog looks confused, be sure not to look at her. **Placing perceived demands on a fearful dog often makes them more fearful and suddenly tense.**

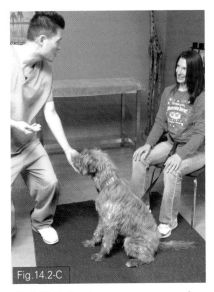

Fig.14.2-C

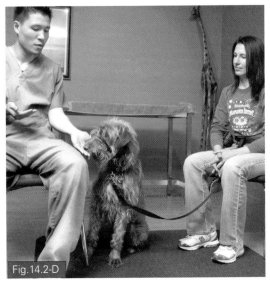

Fig.14.2-D

Fig.14.2-C: For dogs who are more fearful than Pixie, the technician should stand with his side to the dog and look away while giving treats until the dog becomes comfortable with him. Notice that Jon is bending his knees to get low enough to deliver the treat to Pixie rather than leaning over her.

Fig.14.2-D: The fact that Pixie is offering a sit for treats indicates that she is getting more comfortable. It does not mean she is safe to pet, though. Jon must be careful to remain upright instead of leaning over or toward the dog. Here, he's chosen to sit in a chair to decrease his height and look less threatening overall. The veterinarian should go through the same counterconditioning procedure. **This procedure could be as short as 1-2 minutes in some dogs.**

TIP

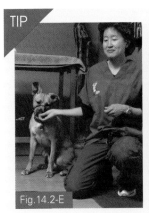

Fig.14.2-E

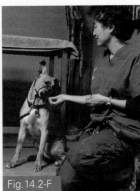

Fig.14.2-F

Fig.14.2-E, Tip: If kneeling to greet the dog, the greeter should have her side or back to the dog and should be looking away from the dog.

Fig.14.2-F, Tip: Once the dog is comfortable with this, the greeter can turn at a 45-degree angle to the dog. An exam can be done or vitals taken from this position if the person backs up a little more (See section 14.3, Case 2).

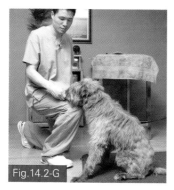

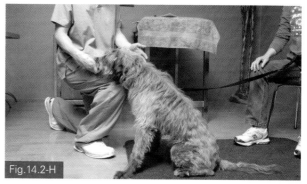

Fig.14.2-G: If the technician is going to take vital signs and basic measurements, he should countercondition the dog to every move he makes. Jon is at Pixie's level giving her treats, and Pixie is comfortably taking them. He started by kneeling sideways. When she was comfortable with that posture, he turned to face her.

Fig.14.2-H: Pixie is comfortable with Jon at her level. She's leaning into his personal space to get the treats rather than standing back and trying to stretch forward. Now Jon is counterconditioning her to being petted—he's giving treats and raising his hand at the same time. During this procedure the dog should be completely focused on the treats; i.e., her mouth should be physically touching the technician's feeding hand the entire time he is giving treats. Give enough treats so that the dog can be exposed to the outstretched petting hand for 3-5 seconds. If using semimoist treats, hold on to each one for several seconds so that the dog chews at them before she actually gets the treat.

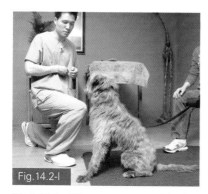

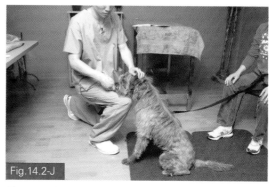

Fig.14.2-I: When counterconditioning, Jon should remove his petting hand and the treat-delivery hand at the same time. This helps Pixie make the association that petting equals treats and disappearance of the petting hand means no more treats. He should wait 3-5 seconds before he presents more treats and his petting hand again. Be careful to avoid staring or looking at the dog, unless the dog is comfortable being looked at. Here, Pixie is looking for more goodies.

Fig.14.2-J: Less than a minute later, Jon is able to pet Pixie while giving treats, even though this is his first time ever putting a dog through this counterconditioning process. It is worth taking the extra few minutes to countercondition while taking a history, because you end up with a dog who is more likely to allow examination. Pixie has a good first impression of Jon now. Note that if the dog is fearful of the reaching hand, you can first teach the dog to target to the petting hand. *(Refer to Video 4)* Once she's comfortable targeting, you can then switch to classical counterconditioning as shown in this sequence.

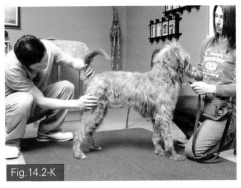

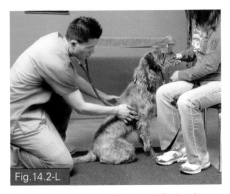

Fig.14.2-K: Jon can now examine Pixie. The owner gives a constant stream of treats while Jon is performing each procedure, and she slows the treat rate when he stops. She's holding onto Pixie's Gentle Leader so that Pixie cannot lunge and bite Jon. If Pixie were to reach the end of the leash and the Gentle Leader, her mouth would close. If you feel uncomfortable having the owner do this, the technician with whom the dog now associates food treats can restrain the dog and the veterinarian can go though the counterconditioning process and examine the dog instead. Realistically, because this dog is not afraid of her owner and the owner is not forcefully restraining her and acting as a threat, if Pixie does try to bite someone, it will be Jon.

Fig.14.2-L: Pixie is much more comfortable in the owner's presence. If she is to be handled without the owner around, then it's important to first make her feel comfortable in the presence of the owner with the handlers who will be working with her. It's also vital for the technician or veterinarian to recognize when the dog is nervous. Dogs show clear indications of fear prior to biting or snapping, but many people, including animal care professionals, frequently miss the signs.

Case 2: Shasta is a friendly dog who knows a lot of tricks. *(Videos 3 and 4)*
But she's fearful at the veterinary hospital and of some people, although not as fearful as Pixie. To most people, she is friendly.

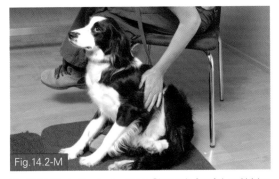

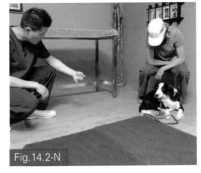

Fig.14.2-M: In the exam room, Shasta is fearful and hides under her owner's chair. The owner unintentionally reinforces this behavior by petting her. This makes her hide more, rather than changing her emotional state. If instead the petting made her come out of hiding and look happier, then the petting would be helping. The ability of animals to hide from environmental stimuli has been shown to hinder habituation to these stimuli (Price 2002).

Fig.14.2-N: Jon makes the dog more fearful by leaning toward her. Be wary of dogs who fail to show friendly behaviors. Those who show little affection or who act aloof could be fearful and consequently become fear aggressive. It's best to get the dog out of her hiding place.

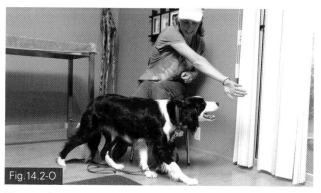

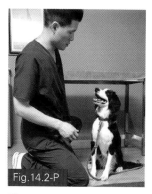

Fig.14.2-O: The owner can help by trying to get the dog into play mode (a change to a positive emotional state). If Shasta likes toys, the owner can try tossing one for her. Because Shasta knows how to target (touch her nose to the owner's hand on cue) and enjoys doing so in exchange for treats, that's what they're doing here. Now she looks happier and is out of her hiding place. The owner can physically stand up and walk her around the room while waiting to try to distract her from being fearful, too.

Fig.14.2-P: Now Jon talks to Shasta in a happy voice. Shasta responds by coming toward him and taking treats. She quickly solicits more treats and petting.

What if the dog is still aggressive?

If you've already provided a calm, comfortable environment and tossed many treats—which the dog has eaten—but are still unable to handle the dog safely (without fear of aggression), then you'll need a combination of restraint techniques, devices and counterconditioning. In addition, the owner will need to go home and practice counterconditioning to any devices (e.g., muzzles, towels) that you use on the dog so that you can use them again in the future with less stress to the dog.

The goal of low-stress restraint is to have the animal allow you to perform the procedures. Just as you would not physically restrain a crying, screaming toddler at the dentist office because it will cause him to become more fearful or resistant in the future, we should not physically struggle with these dogs at the veterinary hospital. Instead, do as much of the exam as you can, and then use chemical restraint if necessary. Send owners home with a counterconditioning plan (see Chapter 18), schedule behavior modification sessions with a technician or refer the owner to a veterinary or applied animal behaviorist.

14.3 Achieve Head and Mouth Control Using Head Halters

Muzzles alone might keep the dog's mouth closed, but they do little to control the dog's movement. If a difficult dog is already used to wearing a head halter on walks (such as the Gentle Leader or Snoot Loop), have the owners bring the dog into the hospital wearing it. If the owner has not trained the dog to wear a head halter, have them use a Wonder Walker (Premier Pet, Richmond, Virginia), which you can stock in the hospital to use for walking dogs. The Wonder Walker is like a Gentle Leader and leash combined.

Gentle Leader or Snoot Loop

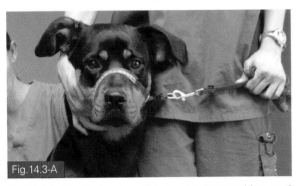

Fig.14.3-A

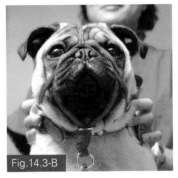

Fig.14.3-B

Fig.14.3-A, Gentle Leader: This head halter provides good control of the dog's head. For instance, the technician here is holding the leash taught. If the dog suddenly tries to turn her head to get to the person behind her, her head will be held in place due to the Gentle Leader, which wraps around her muzzle and the back of her neck. This dog is wearing a Gentle Leader Deluxe, which has soft padding on the muzzle portion.

Fig.14.3-B, Snoot Loop: Brachycephalic dogs can wear a Snoot Loop (www.snootloop.com). This product has bands that connect the nose piece to the collar so that the loop stays on short muzzles.

Box 14-A: Head halters can help close the dog's mouth if the dog snaps.

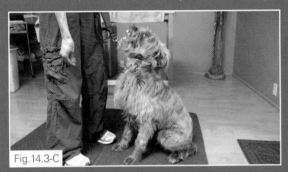

Fig.14.3-C

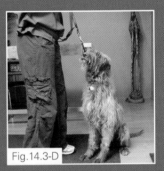

Fig.14.3-D

Fig.14.3-C, Using a head halter: Pulling on the leash tightens the nose loop so that the dog's mouth closes. Therefore, it provides some safety if you haven't yet or cannot place a muzzle. Here's Pixie, visiting us the day before the counterconditioning sequence above. She had been friendly to me at her house and in the parking lot, where she readily sat for treats. When her owners left her with us for the first time, though, she immediately became fearful. She repeatedly raised her lip if I tried to touch her and would pace frantically, if allowed.

Fig.14.3-D: With the Gentle Leader, I can guide her head up and close her mouth if she leaps up to snap at me or struggles. Then, once she is sitting or standing calmly, I can release the pressure. I must release the pressure as soon as she calms down so that she learns how to earn the release of pressure.

Wonderwalker

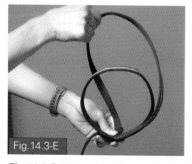 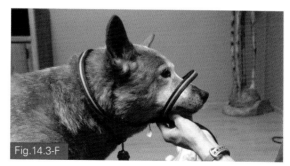

Fig.14.3-E, Wonder Walker: Wonder Walkers can be kept in the hospital for walking dogs and can also be used for dogs who do not arrive with head halters. Present the Wonder Walker like so, and instruct the owner to place the larger loop around the neck and the smaller one around the muzzle.

Fig.14.3-F: Now the dog should have two loose loops—one around the neck and one around the muzzle. Pulling on the muzzle loop tightens the neck loop. Pulling on the leash will tighten the muzzle loop.

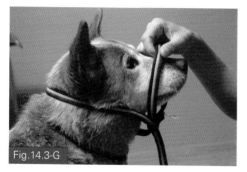 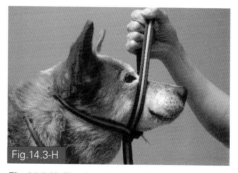

Fig.14.3-G: First pull on the muzzle loop to tighten the neck loop.

Fig.14.3-H: The loop behind the ears should be snug.

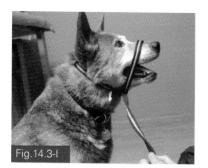 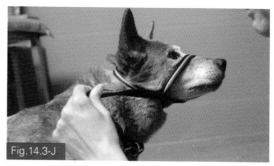

Fig.14.3-I: Next, pull the leash to tighten the muzzle loop.

Fig.14.3-J: Now it's snug around the muzzle, too. Unlike Gentle Leaders and Snoot Loops, Wonder Walkers do not loosen over the muzzle when the leash is loose. So **it's important to periodically check to make sure the muzzle loop is not too tight**.

Case 3: Examination of Pixie with a head halter (owner absent)

Here's Pixie from Case 1, during her first exam at our hospital without her owner present. *(Video 5)* This is taken the same day as the history and counterconditioning session of Case 1.

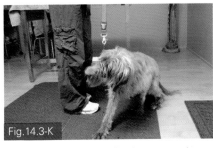

Fig.14.3-K: Pixie immediately starts trying to pace and escape because her owners have left. The first thing I do is prevent her from running around anxiously and pacing by keeping the leash short.

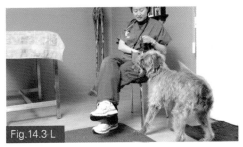

Fig.14.3-L: Next, I sit down so that I'm in a relaxed position and convey a relaxed mood. I am still holding the leash short. The head halter provides more control of her body than a collar, because it enables me to keep her head in one spot.

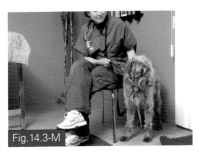

Fig.14.3-M: After a few seconds, Pixie holds still and allows me to touch her. She leans into my hand, so I know she likes the petting.

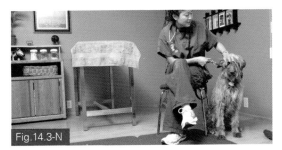

Fig.14.3-N: Then Pixie sits. With her owner gone, she is still not interested in treats, but because she likes the petting I can still provide a positive experience. Now I can start to examine her from a non-threatening position. I'm not facing her, and I'm moving slowly and smoothly.

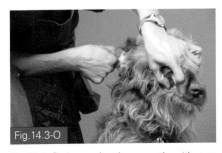

Fig.14.3-O: I examine her mouth with one hand while holding the Gentle Leader for safety purposes. If she snaps, I can pull the Gentle Leader to control her head and keep her mouth closed.

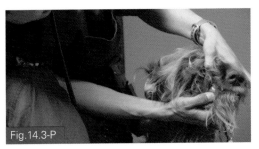

Fig.14.3-P: Because Pixie was relaxed when I looked in her mouth with one hand, I now let go of the Gentle Leader and use both hands to examine her mouth. I was also able to easily look in both ears and eyes.

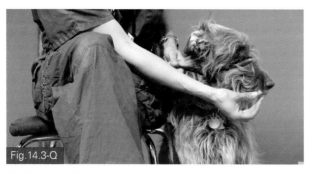
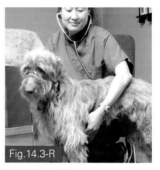

Fig.14.3-Q: I offer her a treat, but she is still not interested. Maybe I'll offer it again in a minute or 2.

Fig.14.3-R: Pixie is relaxed while I listen to her heart. I'm holding the stethoscope with one hand and her Gentle Leader with the other so that I have control of her head. She is not trying to escape or pace.

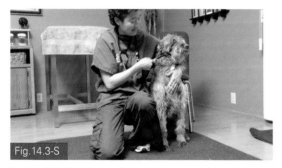
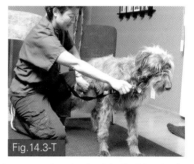

Fig.14.3-S: Now I'm getting ready to reposition Pixie so that I can examine the back half of her body. I'm petting her because her behavior indicates that the petting has a calming effect. When I pet her, she leans against me more. I'm still holding her Gentle Leader with one hand. If she showed no positive response to petting, I would stop doing it to avoid agitating her.

Fig.14.3-T: While she's standing, I hold the Gentle Leader with one hand and reach back to feel her femoral pulse with the other. She is relaxed while I'm doing this.

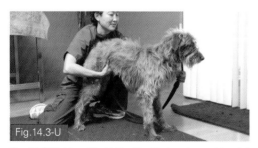
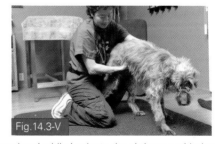

Fig.14.3-U: Now I hold the Gentle Leader and leash in one hand while I palpate the abdomen with the other hand.

Fig.14.3-V: Although she still won't take treats, she is fairly relaxed when I palpate her abdomen. So now I let go of her leash and palpate with both hands. She remains relaxed. It's important to read the dog's emotional state by observing her body language and detecting any tension.

Case 3 (continued): Examination of Pixie with a head halter and two people (owner absent).

At this point, Pixie has met me on 3 occasions and only met Jon, the technician, once. But Jon made a good first impression with her while the owners were present 30 minutes earlier . Now I will restrain Pixie for him to examine to mimic a situation at a veterinary hospital where the dog is first counterconditioned to a technician and then to the examining doctor. In this case, I'm playing the part of the technician. Because Jon has spent 10 to 15 minutes counterconditioning Pixie, she willingly allows him to examine her. *(Video 6)*

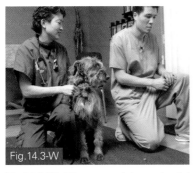

Fig.14.3-W: When examining a fearful dog, back up to the dog when approaching into her personal space. If you approach the dog while facing her, you can cause her to snap defensively.

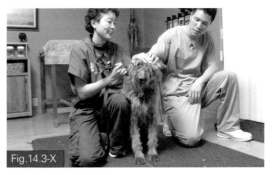

Fig.14.3-X: Perform the exam with your body facing sideways, and avoid looking directly at the dog if she shows any signs of anxiety or fear when you do. Here, Jon is examining her ears. Pixie remains relaxed. If she would eat, I'd feed her a continuous stream of treats as he was examining the ear and then stop when he removed his hands from her ear. Although she's fairly relaxed, she is still fearful, so she is not eating treats.

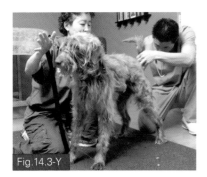

Fig.14.3-Y: The "doctor" is able to examine Pixie's rear end and insert a thermometer. Note that I have placed a hand below her abdomen to control her rear end. She is still relaxed.

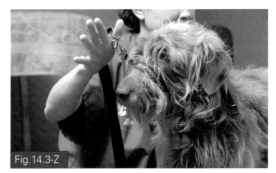

Fig.14.3-Z: I continue holding Pixie's leash and Gentle Leader. If she were a bigger, stronger dog, I would be grasping the leash tightly in my fist.

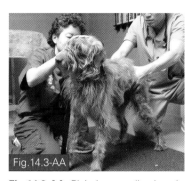

Fig.14.3-AA: Pixie is now allowing abdominal palpation.

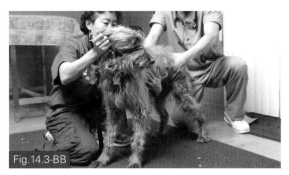

Fig.14.3-BB: Here, she looks around but she does not tense up. I hold her Gentle Leader and leash in my fist so that she can't turn her head any farther. Both the holder and the examiner must be able to recognize when the dog is tense and when she is relaxed. If she becomes tense, the examiner should stop his exam or continue more gently.

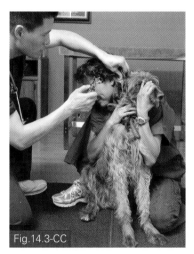

Fig.14.3-CC: On Pixie's next visit several weeks later, we went through a 20-second counterconditioning period and then examined her ears. Pixie showed no signs of fear on this visit.

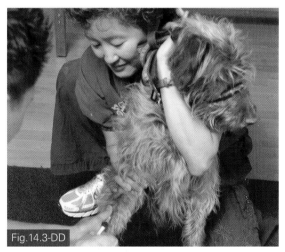

Fig.14.3-DD: We even perform cephalic venipuncture on her. We probably could have done both of these on the previous visit, but did not try because it was Jon's first time performing the counterconditioning sequence. It's as important for the technician and veterinarian to be comfortable with the procedures as the dog. Any nervousness on the part of the handlers can cause the dog to become nervous or fearful.

Case 4: Counterconditioning and restraint with a head collar.

This Rottweiler, Mischa, has a history of growling, struggling and needing to be muzzled at the veterinary hospital. Like Pixie, she is also fearful of people who suddenly approach to pet her. And she startles at sudden sounds. Most dogs who are fearful at the veterinary hospital show signs in their daily lives of being afraid of unfamiliar people, dogs or environments. Continuing to provide them with bad experiences will only strengthen their perception that people and strange environments are dangerous. *(Video 7)*

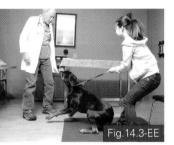 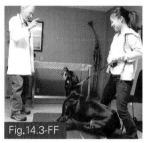 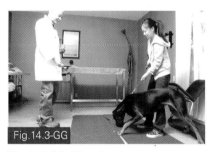

Fig.14.3-EE, FF: The veterinarian, Dr. Jim, approaches Mischa too fast and then talks to her in a gruff voice when she barks at him. Reprimanding or using a gruff voice with a fearful animal can cause the animal to feel more threatened and therefore become more aggressive out of defensiveness.

Fig.14.3-GG: Now Dr. Jim starts counterconditioning by tossing treats on the floor. To increase his safety and appear less threatening, he could sit and face sideways. He should also toss treats closer to Mischa so that the dog does not get too close to him and then suddenly look up to find him in her personal space. Notice, too, that Mischa is wearing a flat buckle collar, so the handler has very little control of her.

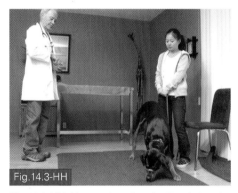 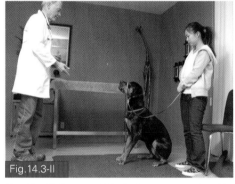

Fig.14.3-HH: Now we've placed a Gentle Leader on the dog to make things safer for the veterinarian. He has never counterconditioned a fear-aggressive dog before. Ideally the leash would be long enough so the dog can move around with little restriction until she gets to the end. The owner should keep the leash a set length.

Fig.14.3-II: Because Mischa is more comfortable now, Dr. Jim is waiting for her to sit before tossing treats. It's okay to whisper "sit" or say "sit" in a happy tone. But avoid commanding the dog to sit in a stern tone. Placing demands on a nervous dog can cause her to become more fearful and thus aggressive.

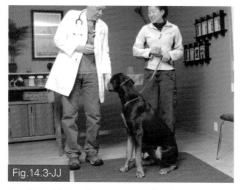

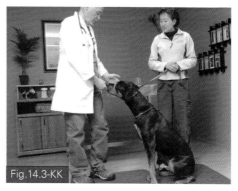

Fig.14.3-JJ: Dr. Jim can now give Mischa treats out of his hand while she's sitting. Because he's new to this process and potentially unable to read the dog's behavior, I am now holding the leash so that Mischa cannot lunge or bite. This is her first time meeting Dr. Jim, while she already knows me and has gotten many treats from me. Notice that she is relaxed and leaning forward to take treats from him.

Fig.14.3-KK: Next, Dr. Jim is counterconditioning Mischa to having his hand out. He's feeding her while he holds his left hand near her head. Her nose must physically touch his treat hand while she's getting treats out of his hand. If she removes her nose from his treat hand, he should remove both the treat hand and the "petting" hand.

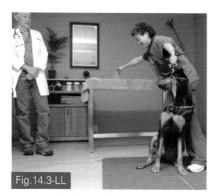

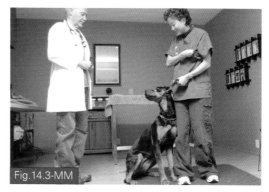

Fig.14.3-LL: Now I'm reaching to get treats. As I do this, I'm holding the leash and Gentle Leader short enough that Mischa cannot snap at the veterinarian. Dr. Jim is standing outside of the dog's personal space while I do this and avoiding a direct stare.

Fig.14.3-MM: An exam can be performed in the same manner as with Pixie, but in Mischa's case, treats will be given as each procedure is being performed. Here, the veterinarian is approaching to give her a vaccine. Because he's now behind her, she's nervous.

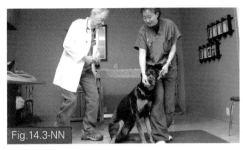

Fig.14.3-NN: I can control her head with the Gentle Leader and distract her with a treat while the veterinarian moves into position.

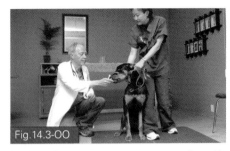

Fig.14.3-OO: Then he gives her a treat from his new position. I am still holding on so that if she lunges, she can only move about 1 inch.

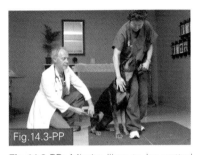

Fig.14.3-PP: Mischa likes to be petted vigorously, so I rub her on the chest and pat her head firmly. As a result, she doesn't pay much attention to Dr. Jim.

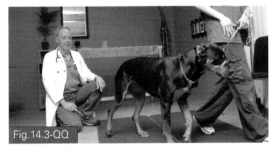

Fig.14.3-QQ: At the end of the procedure, I walk Mischa away instead of having Dr. Jim move from behind her. Movement behind her could cause her to startle and snap. Always be sure to keep control of an aggressive dog until everyone is out of her personal space.

14.4 Control the Head With Towels

Using towels to control the head of small and medium-sized dogs is often more comfortable for the dog than using a muzzle or holding the dog close to your body to restrain it. *(Videos 8 and 9)*

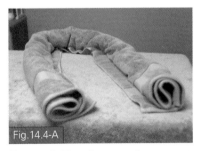

Fig.14.4-A: To make a towel wrap, start with the towel rolled lengthwise.

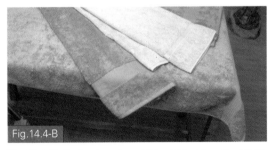

Fig.14.4-B: Or the towel could be folded lengthwise instead of rolled. Use a smaller towel for tiny dogs. The blue towel is 30 x 50 inches. You can cut towels so that you have multiple lengths.

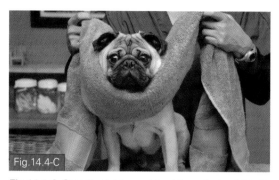
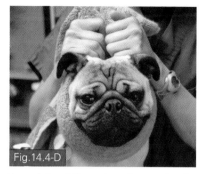

Fig.14.4-C, Step 2: Hold one side of the rolled or folded towel in each hand. Then place the towel under the dog's neck as high up as possible. At this point, if the dog tries to bolt forward you can stop him by tightening the towel around him.

Fig.14.4-D, Step 3: Hold the towel where the ends meet on the back of the dog's neck. Be sure to wrap high enough. It should be right at the base of the skull to restrain the dog. For the best head control, the towel should cover the backs of the ears.

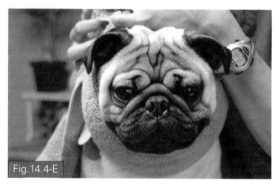
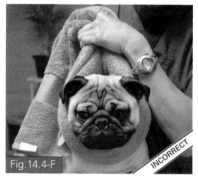

Fig.14.4-E, Step 4: Make sure there is no space between the towel and the dog.

Fig.14.4-F, Step 4, Incorrect: This is too loose; the head is not under control.

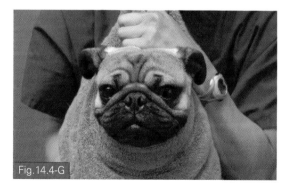
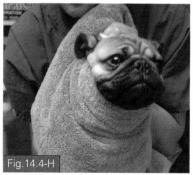

Fig.14.4-G: When the towel fits snugly like this and is placed high enough (cranial to the atlanto-occipital joint), the head can easily be directed by turning the towel in one direction or another. Here, the head is held straight.

Fig.14.4-H: In this photo, the head is tilted to the side.

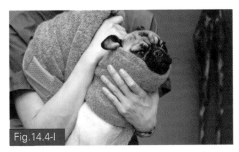

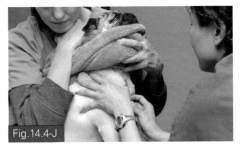

Fig.14.4-I: For fine control of the head, placing a hand under the chin and neck works best. This works better with a towel that's folded rather than rolled. If the towel is rolled, then it might be too thick to allow the technician to feel the neck. Note that this towel extends forward correctly, past the base of the skull. Secure the dog with your body on one side and your arm on the other.

Fig.14.4-J: If using a folded towel, the bottom portion can be lifted to uncover the lower neck for jugular venipuncture.

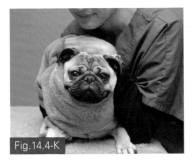

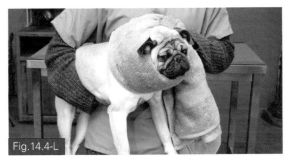

Fig.14.4-K: This wrap can also be used to control the head while performing cephalic venipuncture.

Fig.14.4-L: And it can be used to restrain the head when lifting small dogs (see Chapter 9). If needed, the owner can place the towel around the dog's neck, and then the technician can come behind the owner and dog and grasp the towel.

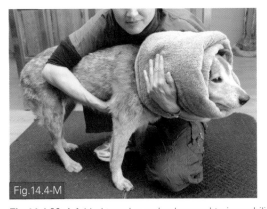

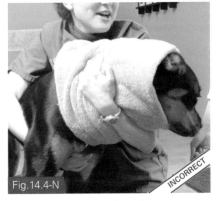

Fig.14.4-M: A folded towel can also be used to immobilize the head of some medium dogs.

Fig.14.4-N, Incorrect: This wrap is not safe for larger dogs. The towel is not wide or thick enough to restrain the dog's head. Here, we test the ability to restrain the head by baiting the dog with food. The dog can readily turn her head.

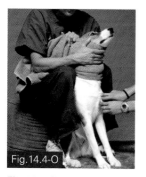
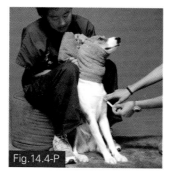
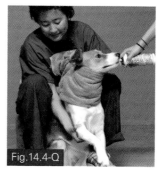

Fig.14.4-O: A towel wrap can also be used to help restrain the head for venipuncture in a medium-sized dog. Note that for the jugular venipuncture, the towel spans the neck all the way up to the ears so that the head cannot turn easily. The handler can place one hand under the base of the chin to help stabilize the head.

Fig.14.4-P: Alternatively the handler can hold the towel with both hands to ensure that the dog cannot move her head forward and reach the person drawing blood.

Fig.14.4-Q: This method can be combined with counterconditioning/distraction.

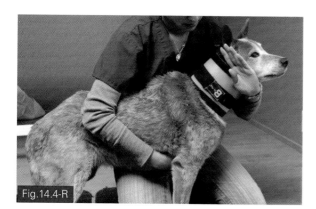

Fig.14.4-R: BiteNot collars (shown) and **Elizabethan collars** can be used in a similar manner to provide protection.

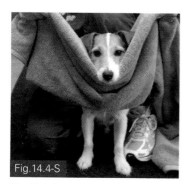
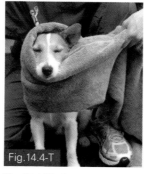
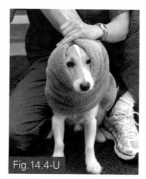

Fig.14.4-S, Toweling to control the front feet, Step 1: A towel can also be used to help control the head and front feet of little dogs who are squirmy. Start with a folded towel.

Fig.14.4-T, Step 2: Wrap the towel around the dog's head.

Fig.14.4-U, Step 3: Make sure it's snug at the top.

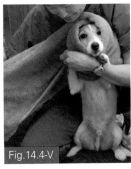 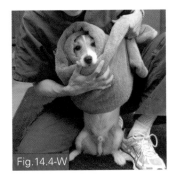 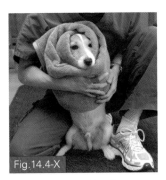

Fig.14.4-V, W, X, Step 4: Next, wrap it around again, this time including the legs up to the elbows.

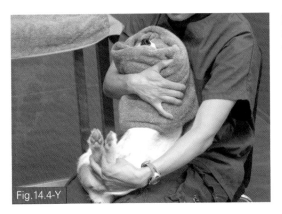

Fig.14.4-Y: Now the dog can be held calmly for ultrasound, cystocentesis or a toenail trim on the rear feet.

14.5 Use Muzzles Correctly

Veterinarians trying to avoid bites in the veterinary hospital sometimes take the extreme measure of muzzling all dogs with the assumption that muzzling will solve their injury problems. Unfortunately, even muzzled dogs can sometimes bite. People can also get bitten before the muzzle is on or while placing the muzzle. And muzzles often make dogs more fearful and aggressive, so that they become more dangerous with each visit. Consequently, although this section covers muzzles extensively, it's important to realize that muzzles must be used in conjunction with all of the other techniques covered in this book. Finally, remember that when patients stay for extended periods, muzzling may not help unless you plan to keep them muzzled the entire time.

When using a muzzle, don't wrangle it quickly onto the growling, lunging dog the way a cowboy at a rodeo ties up a calf's feet. Instead, place the muzzle so unobtrusively that the dog remains calm while you do so.

14.5.1 Making a leash muzzle.

Dogs are often more accepting of a leash muzzle, which is easy to place. In addition, a leash muzzle enables you to control the head, while a standard nylon or leather muzzle does not.

Method 1 for making a leash muzzle.

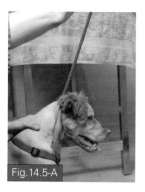

Fig.14.5-A

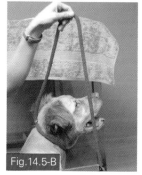

Fig.14.5-B

Fig.14.5-A, Method 1, Step 1: Using a slip lead, first pull up slack in the leash behind the dog's ears. Keep the leash in this position around the neck throughout muzzle placement, or else the leash muzzle will be too loose.

Fig.14.5-B, Method 1, Step 2: Next, make a loop. Start by holding what will be the end of the loop up high.

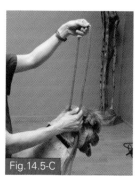

Fig.14.5-C

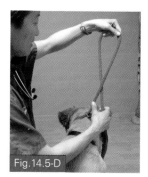

Fig.14.5-D

Fig.14.5-C, Method 1, Step 3: Hold the loose end so that the two leash portions are parallel to one another.

Fig.14.5-D, Method 1, Step 4: With the hand holding the top of the loop, twist the loop so that you form an X where the leash crosses itself.

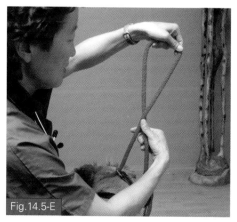

Fig.14.5-E

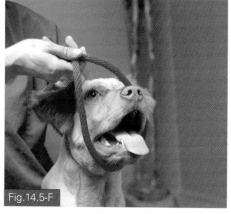

Fig.14.5-F

Fig.14.5-E, Method 1, Step 5: Use the lower hand to grasp the leash at the crossover point.

Fig.14.5-F, Method 1, Step 6: Now drop the loop over the dog's nose. The larger the loop, the easier it is to drop it over the nose on the first try. This takes practice.

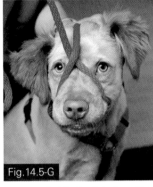 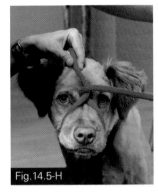 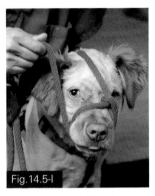

Fig.14.5-G

Fig.14.5-H

Fig.14.5-I

Fig.14.5-G, Method 1, Step 7: Once it's over the dog's nose, pull on the leash end so that the nose loop tightens around the dog's muzzle. It should also be snug at the top of the neck. You might need to have your other hand on the portion of the leash that's around the dog's neck so that the dog cannot back up. Alternatively, place your body behind the dog when doing this procedure.

Fig.14.5-H, I, Method 1, Step 8: Wrap the leash end around the nose so that it crosses the portion that comes down across the forehead. This helps prevent the leash from slipping off the nose.

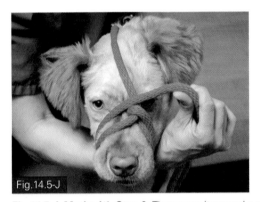 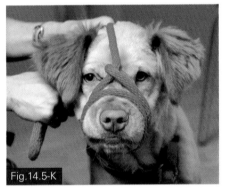

Fig.14.5-J

Fig.14.5-K

Fig.14.5-J, Method 1, Step 9: Then wrap it around a second time, making sure that it's snug.

Fig.14.5-K, Method 1, Step 10: From under the dog's muzzle, draw the end back to the portion of the leash that's around the dog's neck.

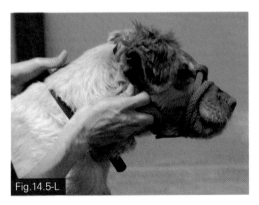

Fig.14.5-L

Fig.14.5-L, Method 1, Step 11: By holding the leash muzzle, you can control the dog's head to some extent. Realize that the control is not as good as with a head halter.

Method 2 for making a leash muzzle.

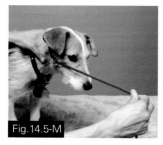 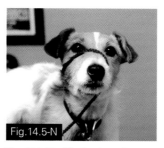 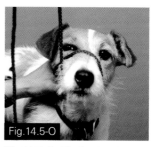

Fig.14.5-M, Method 2, Step 1: Start with the slip leash as high up on the neck as it will go.

Fig.14.5-N, Method 2, Step 2: Wrap the leash around the dog's nose.

Fig.14.5-O, Method 2, Step 3: Make sure that it's snug and that the portion around the neck is still high up on the neck, right behind the ears.

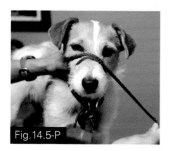 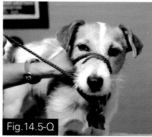 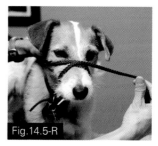

Fig.14.5-P,Q,R, Method 2, Step 4:: Wrap the leash around the nose a second time. Again, make sure it's snug but comfortable. The second loop provides added security. A third loop can be placed if the leash is long enough.

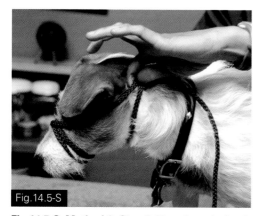 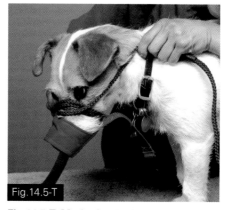

Fig.14.5-S, Method 2, Step 5: Now draw the leash to the portion around the neck and hold the two pieces together. This muzzle is good for short procedures such as lifting a dog onto a table or inserting a thermometer.

Fig.14.5-T, Method 2: It also allows for easy placement of a standard muzzle.

14.5.2 Leather or nylon muzzles.

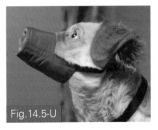
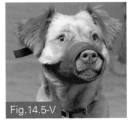
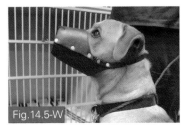

Figures 14.5-U,V: Both leather and nylon muzzles keep the dog's mouth closed. Shown here is a nylon muzzle.

Figure 14.5-W: Leather muzzles are easier to get on because they retain their shape.

14.5.3 Basket muzzles.

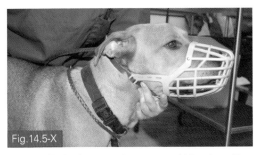
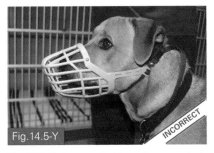

Fig.14.5-X: Basket muzzles prevent biting but allow the dog to open her mouth. Treats can be given if a small hole is cut in the front. This muzzle can be kept on for extended periods of time, if necessary.

Fig.14.5-Y, Incorrect: Here, the muzzle is not on tight enough. It should rest on the dog's nose just in front of the eyes, with little room between the tip of the dog's nose and the front of the muzzle.

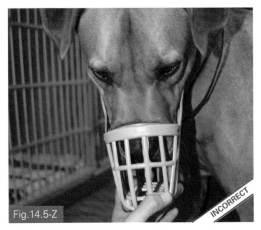
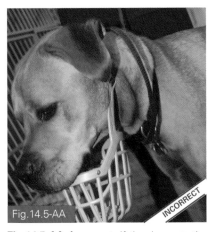

Fig.14.5-Z, Incorrect: Because this muzzle is not on tight enough, it slips off the nose when moderate pressure is applied.

Fig.14.5-AA, Incorrect: If the dog gets the muzzle off, you might not have another opportunity to get it back on.

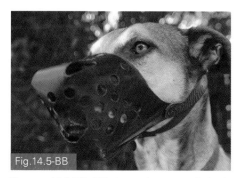

Fig.14.5-BB

Figures 14.5-BB: This is another type of plastic basket muzzle.

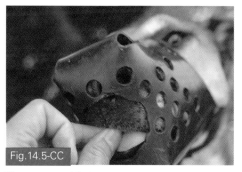

Fig.14.5-CC

Figures 14.5-CC: A hole can easily be made in the front of the muzzle. The dog can get food treats through the hole but cannot bite.

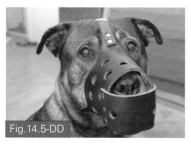

Fig.14.5-DD

Fig.14.5-DD: Leather basket muzzles are designed to stay securely on the dog. They strap around the back of the neck and also over the forehead.

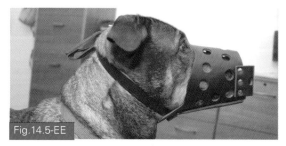

Fig.14.5-EE

Fig.14.5-EE: Because they require a metal buckle, the leather basket muzzles take slightly longer to put on the dog, but they stay on more securely. Dogs can be left in their cages with this or other basket muzzles because they can open their mouths and breathe as well as drink water.

14.5.4 Air muzzle restraint (www.Softpaws.com).

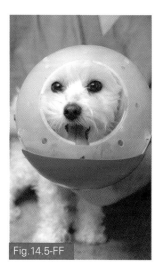

Fig.14.5-FF

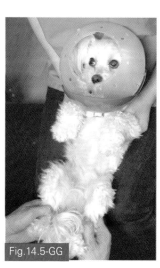

Fig.14.5-GG

Fig.14.5-FF: Air muzzles work on some dogs (and cats) who won't accept other muzzles without counterconditioning. An air muzzle also has an attachment that converts it to a nebulizing chamber.

Fig.14.5-GG: This muzzle works nicely when restraining dogs on their backs. The dog shown here did not resist placement of the air muzzle at all.

14.5.5 Putting on the muzzle.

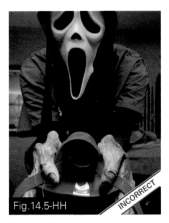 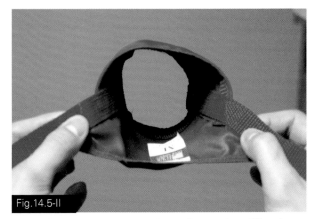

Fig.14.5-HH

Fig.14.5-II

Fig.14.5-HH, Incorrect: Placing a muzzle on a fearful or potentially resistant dog requires skill and practice. Fumbling can provide an opportunity for the dog to escape or become more anxious or aggressive. First, be aware that approaching from the front can look menacing. If you must approach from the front, avoid looming over the animal.

Fig.14.5-II, Step 1: Standing behind the dog with your outstretched arms holding the muzzle is less menacing, but requires more practice.

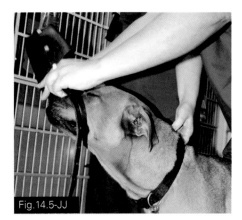 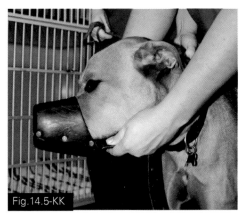

Fig.14.5-JJ

Fig.14.5-KK

Fig.14.5-JJ, Step 2: The muzzle should be placed in one smooth motion. One person should restrain the dog in a manner that prevents the dog from backing up and from moving her head around (e.g. by standing behind the dog and holding her head). In this photo, the dog is friendly and barely needs restraint. With one hand on each side of the muzzle, smoothly come from above to slip it on over the dog's nose.

Fig.14.5-KK, Step 3: The top of the muzzle opening should meet the top of the dog's nose first. Then pull the muzzle on all the way.

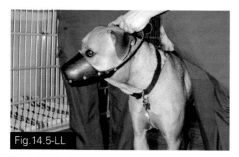

Fig.14.5-LL

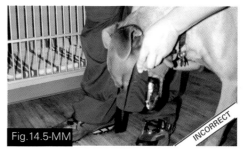

Fig.14.5-MM

Fig.14.5-LL, Step 4: Slide your hands down the straps and then tighten the straps behind the ears. The entire process should take 2 seconds or less.

Fig.14.5-MM, Incorrect: With the nylon muzzles, if the dog has her mouth open a little, you could end up putting a portion of the muzzle into the dog's mouth. Leather cone muzzles are generally easier to place than the nylon muzzles due to the rigidity of the leather.

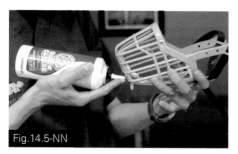

Fig.14.5-NN

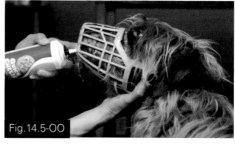

Fig.14.5-OO

Fig.14.5-NN: Many dogs will stick their heads into a muzzle on their own for goodies such as canned cheese paste, liver paste or semi-moist dog treats. If using a basket muzzle, just squirt the cheese on the muzzle.

Fig.14.5-OO: Let the dog stick her nose in. Then pull the muzzle away as the dog's finishing. Repeat. Once the dog readily puts her head in, fasten the muzzle behind her ears. The goal is to get the dog comfortable enough with the muzzle that she won't try to pull away when you fasten the straps, because you may only have one chance to get the muzzle on. Continue giving treats after the muzzle is on, as well.

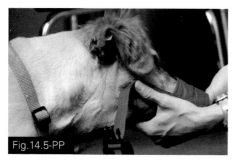

Fig.14.5-PP

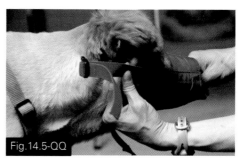

Fig.14.5-QQ

Fig.14.5-PP, Step 1: When placing the muzzle from the front, lure the dog with a treat to place her nose through the muzzle willingly. If food is not used, then you will most likely need a second person to restrain the dog so that she doesn't back away.

Fig.14.5-QQ, Step 2: Once the dog's nose is inserted, slide your free hand up the strap.

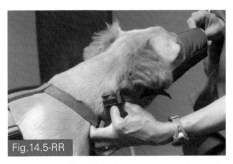
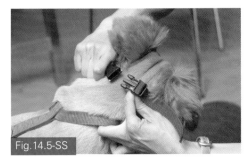

Fig.14.5-RR, Step 3: When you get as far as the collar, grab the collar so that the dog cannot back up.

Fig.14.5-SS, Step 4: Now fasten the muzzle straps.

The Gentle Leader can help when placing a muzzle. *(Video 10)*

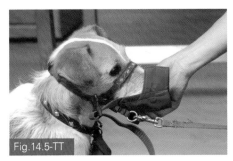
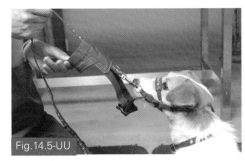

Fig.14.5-TT: In some cases, the muzzle can simply be placed over the Gentle Leader without needing to pull up the dog's head to close his mouth and direct the head in the right direction.

Fig.14.5-UU, Step 1: In other cases, you might need to put pressure on the Gentle Leader to get the muzzle on. Thread the leash through the muzzle, holding the muzzle upside down. If it's right-side-up, it's harder to get it over the nose.

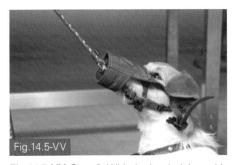
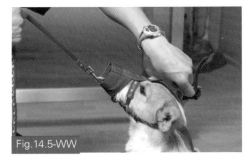

Fig.14.5-VV, Step 2: With the leash tight, guide the dog's head up. Then calmly lower the muzzle and place it over the dog's nose. If the dog struggles, get him under control by applying pressure to the Gentle Leader until he relaxes. Struggling should last less than 2-3 seconds. When the dog is relaxed, try again.

Fig.14.5-WW, Step 3: Once you've slipped the muzzle over the Gentle Leader, rotate it so that it is right side up. Keep pressure on the Gentle Leader. Then follow the procedure for placing a muzzle from the front.

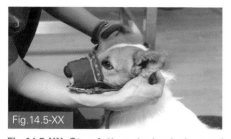

Fig.14.5-XX, Step 4: Keep the leash short and also hold the collar when fastening the muzzle.

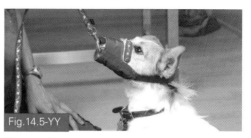

Fig.14.5-YY, Step 5: Once the muzzle is secured, the Gentle Leader will extend out the front of it.

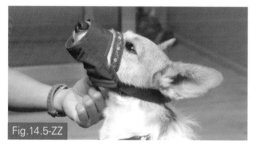

Fig.14.5-ZZ, Step 5 (variation): If you prefer, disconnect the leash and reconnect it from behind the muzzle. Only attempt this if you can do so safely.

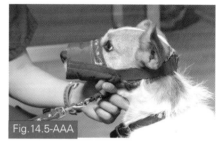

Fig.14.5-AAA: Now the Gentle Leader strap is in the correct configuration.

Muzzle problems. *(Video 11)*

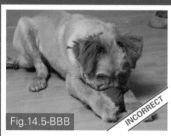

Fig.14.5-BBB, Incorrect: Never let the dog paw at her muzzle. She is likely to eventually get it off. Either distract (or countercondition) the dog, raise her collar or restrain her head while holding her leg. If the dog is also wearing a Gentle Leader, guide her head up high enough to prevent pawing at the muzzle. Then release the pressure when she relaxes and stops pawing.

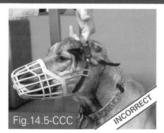

Fig.14.5-CCC, Incorrect: Never use the muzzle like a collar, or you will pull it off. Instead, be sure to hold the leash short enough so that you can control the dog's head and body. Better yet, use a Gentle Leader or Wonder Walker under the muzzle to gain better control of the head.

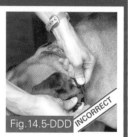

Fig.14.5-DDD, Incorrect: The snap from a basket muzzle can be difficult to fasten. Be sure you practice closing before using it on an aggressive dog.

If you can't easily get the muzzle on, ask the owner to do it. If the owner isn't able to get it on either, or if the dog resists at all, send the owner home to countercondition the dog to the muzzle. You can also try counterconditioning in the hospital. Often, it takes just 1 to 2 minutes if the dog isn't already aroused from repeated attempts at putting the muzzle on. Charge for the time it takes. This is an important behavioral service that's essential for the healthcare of some dogs.

If the animal has to stay at the hospital and needs to wear a muzzle continuously, a basket muzzle is best.

14.6 Practice Good Restraint Technique

Poor technique can cause the dog to go into escape mode. What starts as play for the dog can switch to aggression.

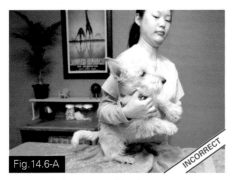

Fig.14.6-A, Incorrect: This dog is not being restrained well. The technician is unable to keep her from jumping and pawing.

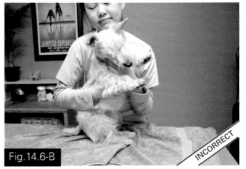

Fig.14.6-B, Incorrect: Now the dog is starting to get mouthy.

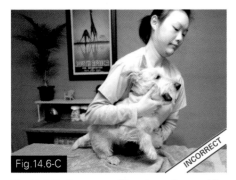

Fig.14.6-C, Incorrect: The dog tries to bite when the technician restrains her head.

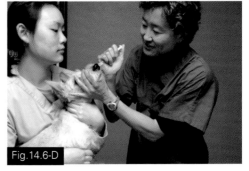

Fig.14.6-D, Correct: The technician released the dog and started over the correct way. Now she has a C hold on the dog's neck and is holding the leg above the elbow to prevent jumping. Now the dog is relaxed and does not try to struggle.

14.7 Use Minimal Restraint for Fearful Animals

Many fearful dogs do best with minimal restraint, meaning less surface area contact with your body. It's still essential to control the dog's body and keep it from moving in any direction, and to protect against injury, but try to do so without hugging the dog. Have as little physical contact with the dog as possible.

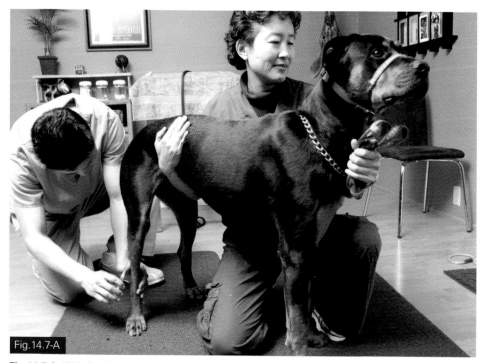

Fig.14.7-A

Fig.14.7-A: With fearful dogs, it's often easiest to draw blood from the rear leg. These dogs frequently become more anxious if a technician tries to restrain them by hugging them or using a large amount of body contact. This dog holds still with just a Gentle Leader and an arm under the abdomen. The dog has already received treats from the technician drawing blood, so she is only a little anxious about the technician being behind her.

Case 5: Mattie is afraid of all new people, including the veterinarian. *(Video 12)*
The last time Mattie had her blood drawn, the owner and a technician held her while she screamed and struggled, and a third technician drew the blood. An escape response like this can lead to aggression. Thus, a dog who had previously responded only by trying to escape could—due to mistakes made at just one visit—learn to exhibit aggression to defend herself. The dog enters the hospital fearful and then learns that her fear is justified. Not only does she fear veterinary staff, but now she might also fear unfamiliar people in general.

Prior to this visit, I have already worked with Mattie once at her regular veterinary hospital and once at her home. She's still extremely fearful and reactive, and today she's in a new location. She has allowed me to pet her while receiving treats and rubbed against my hand while I was petting. Now I want to take her blood. Both the technician who will be drawing blood today and I have given her at least 10 kibble-size treats today. She is still afraid of the technician.

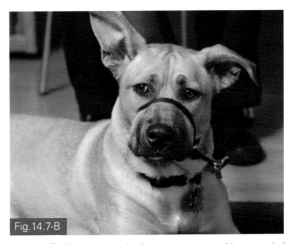

Fig.14.7-B

Fig.14.7-B: Mattie waits in the exam room with a worried look on her face.

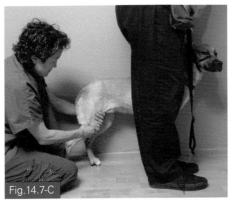

Fig.14.7-C

Fig.14.7-C: The owner has placed Mattie along the wall and is keeping her from moving forward by holding the Gentle Leader. By standing right next to her, the owner is also keeping Mattie from moving away from the wall, and I am in the back preventing her from backing up. She wants to sit, so I'm holding her in a stand with my left arm on her knee.

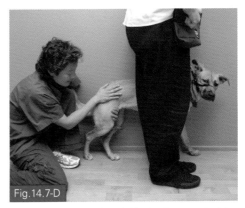

Fig.14.7-D

Fig.14.7-D: Mattie doesn't like it when a technician touches her below the hock, so I'm desensitizing her to the touch by giving her long strokes with my hand, starting at the hip and working down to the hock region. **When animals are sensitive to being touched, avoid patting the animal or touching her quickly and repeatedly. Each touch will cause the dog to startle. Instead, place your hand on the animal more proximally and keep it there until the dog relaxes.**

When animals are sensitive to being touched, avoid patting the animal or touching her quickly and repeatedly. Each touch will cause the dog to startle. Instead, place your hand on the animal more proximally and keep it there until the dog relaxes.

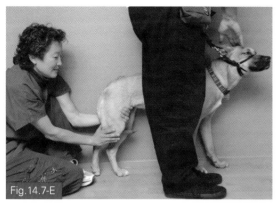

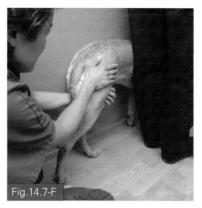

Fig.14.7-E: Now I'm moving my hand slowly down the leg in an even stroking gesture. You can stroke part way down the leg and then start over, or stroke all the way down the leg, depending on the dog's response. Note that the owner is petting the dog vigorously on the head to keep her distracted. The dog is responding well to petting.

Fig.14.7-F: For Mattie, stroking down the leg took over 5 seconds per stroke. But the whole process of desensitization took under 20 seconds.

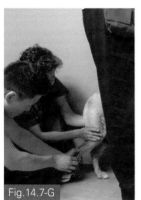

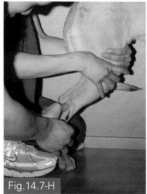

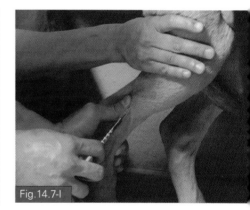

Fig.14.7-G, H: Now the technician, Jon, who has been right behind me all this time, can either repeat the stroking process or try to place his hand right where mine was so that he can draw blood. We ask Mattie's owner to pet her dog's head vigorously (since she enjoys being petted this way, at least at home) to distract her while the needle is inserted.

Fig.14.7-I: Mattie doesn't flinch, and we are able to collect blood easily and without a struggle. The owner could also give treats the entire time if she can coordinate holding the Gentle Leader in one hand, giving treats with the other and still keep the dog against the wall. Sometimes a technician can stand right behind the owner and take over restraint of the front end so that the owner can give the treats. Canned cheese, liver paste or peanut butter works well because this way fingers don't need to be near the dog's mouth.

Skill at performing the procedures is as important as skill in handling. When dealing with potentially difficult dogs, make sure you select the most skilled technician or veterinarian to perform the procedure as you may only have one chance.

14.8 Countercondition to Devices and Procedures

Many people refrain from using desensitization and counterconditioning techniques (referred to in much of this book simply as counterconditioning; see Chapter 4 for details), thinking they take too long. In actuality, over the course of several visits they end up saving time, manpower and lost work days due to bite-related injuries. In some cases, counterconditioning takes just minutes. These techniques improve the animal's overall demeanor and decrease stress at the hospital.

You may opt to charge for the time spent providing special behavioral care to fearful or aggressive dogs if doing so will allow you to provide this care.

Additionally, muzzles and chemical restraint are not adequate for many animals. Many dogs won't allow even their owners to place a muzzle on them. And with muzzles on, dogs can still struggle and cause injury. Another reason to countercondition to procedures is to make an extended hospital stay easier on the dog. During extended stays, wearing a nylon muzzle throughout the stay is not an option. Additionally, putting the muzzle on may be difficult. **Dogs should be routinely counterconditioned to muzzles, vaccines, toenail trims and other devices and procedures. Doing so is as important as completing pre-anesthetic blood work.** (Refer to the techniques in Chapter 18)

Also remember that any positive distractions (play, happy talk and other things that put the dog into a happy state) are a form of counterconditioning.

14.9 Understand Emergency Restraint Techniques for Injections

If an animal does not easily cooperate, we sometimes must use injectable chemical restraint. But if the dog is already aroused, the medications will not be as effective. Ideally, you should go to chemical restraint before the dog is highly aroused. Keeping the dog calm prior to injection is a good idea; try walking her in a more comfortable location for a few minutes. If the dog cannot be restrained easily for the injection, use the following techniques.

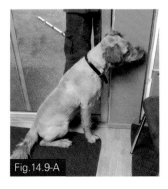
Fig.14.9-A

Fig.14.9-A, Method 1, Step 1: This technique can be performed in a very low-key manner. You're trying to get the dog to position herself the way you want her. First, inch the slip lead as high up on the neck as possible. Then walk through a doorway, keeping the leash taut but not pulling the dog yet. Close the door, but not all the way; leave about an inch-wide opening. Usually the dog will walk right up to the door. Pull the leash gently and keep it at that length to give the dog a chance to move parallel to the door on her own. Do not drag the dog's head to the door. The person giving the injection is still in the room with the dog, standing out of her personal space but near the back of her. Some dogs will easily position themselves parallel to the door.

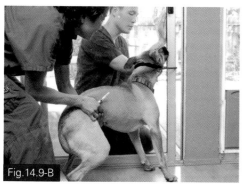
Fig.14.9-B

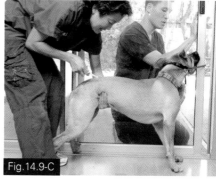
Fig.14.9-C

Fig.14.9-B, C, Method 1, Step 2: The person holding the lead should hold it level with the dog. Otherwise, pulling on the lead will cause the dog to jump up. The leash-holder can pull the dog's neck closer to the door if it isn't yet all the way up to the door. The technician giving the injection should simultaneously step toward the dog and quickly stabilize the dog's rear end against the wall with both hands and a leg, as the leash-holder pulls the lead tight. Then, while stabilizing with the leg, inject the dog with the chemical agent. The injection can be given IM in the back leg or SQ. The process should only take 2 seconds if the technicians have practiced and are skilled at the procedure. Technicians should practice this with non-aggressive dogs first so that they are aware of how performing this improperly can increase the dog's arousal.

> Technicians should practice this with non-aggressive dogs first so that they are aware of how performing this improperly can increase the dog's arousal.

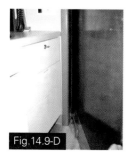
Fig.14.9-D

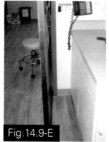
Fig.14.9-E

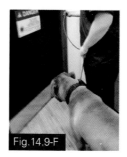
Fig.14.9-F

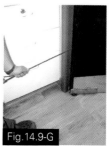
Fig.14.9-G

Fig.14.9-D, Method 2: In this method, you'll be confining the dog between a door and a wall. Start with a doorway that has at least 6 inches of room between the door and the wall that you will squeeze the dog against. The area shown here is appropriate.

Fig.14.9-E, Method 2: The space here is too narrow. You won't be able to squeeze the dog between the door and the wall (or drawers, in this case) because there is not enough room for the dog's head.

Fig.14.9-F, Method 2, Step 1: Once you've selected the door, thread the leash through the opening and pass it to the technician on the other side.

Fig.14.9-G, Method 2, Step 2: The technician on the other side should draw up slack in the leash without dragging the dog forward and wait for the injector's cue. The leash-holder must hold the leash at the level of the dog's neck or lower so that the dog cannot jump up. When the injector gives the cue, the leash-holder pulls the leash tight enough to pull the dog close to the front of the door (if she hasn't already positioned herself there).

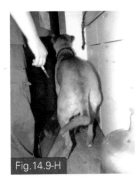

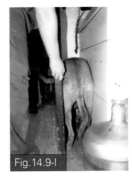

Fig.14.9-H, Method 2, Step 3: The injector, standing behind the dog, presses the door into the dog like a squeeze chute to hold the dog steady.

Fig.14.9-I, Method 2, Step 4: Immediately give the dog the injection before she has time to struggle much. The process should take just several seconds. If the dog struggles at all, it should be for no more than 2-3 seconds. Ideally, no struggling is involved.

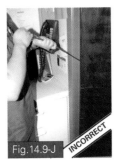

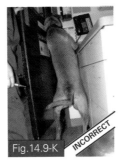

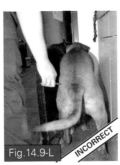

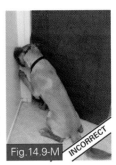

Fig.14.9-J, Method 2, Incorrect: The technician is pulling the leash up instead of keeping it level with the dog.

Fig.14.9-K, Method 2, Incorrect: Doing so causes the dog to jump up to escape the pressure.

Fig.14.9-L, Method 2, Incorrect: Here, the dog's paw prevents the door from closing. The technician can either secure the dog's back end with her leg or move the paw out of the way.

Fig.14.9-M, Method 2, Incorrect: Avoid pulling so tightly that the dog has nowhere to go with her head. Even friendly dogs will struggle when this is done.

14.10 Use Chemical Restraint if Needed

Chemical restraint should be used before the dog becomes anxious. Tranquilizers have more variable efficacy in animals who are highly aroused than in those who are not. If you predict that a dog will be difficult and are unsure of your abilities to perform the techniques described, using chemical restraint right away might be the best choice.

14.10.1 Use of oral medications prior to entering the hospital.

In general, oral anxiolytics and sedation are not that effective. Dogs might appear sedated, but when stimulated or aroused they can suddenly snap, lunge or bite quickly, as if they were not sedated. Ironically, these sedatives can lead to an increased likelihood of injury. If sedatives are used, the dog should be muzzled immediately, and the person placing the muzzle must do so in such a way that they can protect themself from being bitten.

Acepromazine should generally be avoided, especially when used as the sole agent rather than in combination with other drugs. It is not a true anxiolytic drug and patients still react to stimuli. It can also cause hypotension and bradycardia that could then preclude the use of other drugs.

Diazepam (Valium), a benzodiazepine, is a true anxiolytic. It can be given orally at up to 2.2 mg/kg in dogs. One caution with diazepam is that it can have a disinhibitory effect on some patients; for instance, if the animal is fear aggressive, she could become more so (Dyer 2008). It can also have a paradoxical hyperexcitable effect. Clients should administer a test dose a day or two before they need it, to determine the dog's reaction to the drug.

Alprazolam (Xanax), another benzodiazepine anxiolytic, can be administered orally at 0.1 mg/kg in dogs. Like diazepam, it can also have a disinhibitory effect.

Tiletamine/zolazepam (Telazol) (20 mg/kg powder [placed into a capsule]) or Telazol (20 mg/kg powder) combined with acepromazine (2 mg/kg) can be mixed in food for dogs who are extremely difficult. At these doses, both telazol alone, and in combination with acepromazine cause such extreme sedation that 50% or more of dogs sedated this way become laterally recumbent. In fact, these oral dosages were tested for the purpose of sedating dogs who were to be euthanized at a shelter. Thus, the long-term effects were not tested (Ramsay and Wetzel 1998).

14.10.2 Use of injectable agents.

In most cases, it's prudent to skip oral sedatives and go right to injectable agents due to the more predictable response of dogs to injectables. Owners should be warned of the risks of sedating an aggressive dog.

Medetomidine (Domitor) can be administered at 0.002 to 0.02 mg/kg (Moffat 2008), with or without an opioid such as **Torbugesic** at 0.1 to 0.4 mg/kg (Moffat 2008). **Acepromazine** can be added to this combination at a dose of 0.03-0.05 mg/kg if the medetomidine dose is halved (Moffat 2008).

References

Dyer, A. 2008. Oral sedation for difficult dogs. *Veterinary Anesthesia and Analgesia Support Group*, May 28, 2008 (accessedJune 28, 2008). Available online, URL: http://www.vasg.org/oral_sedation_for_difficult_dogs.htm.

Moffat, K. 2008. Addressing canine and feline aggression in the veterinary clinic. Veterinary Clinics of North America: Small Animal Practice 38 (5):983-1003.

Price, E.O. 2002. *Animal Domestication and Behavior*. New York: CABI Publishing.

Ramsay, E.C., and R.W. Wetzel. 1998. Comparison of five regimens for oral administration of medication to induce sedation in dogs prior to euthanasia. *Journal of the American Veterinary Medical Association* 213(2):240-42.

Tod, E., D. Brander, and N. Waran. 2005. Efficacy of dog appeasing pheromone in reducing stress and fear related behaviour in shelter dogs. *Applied Animal Behaviour Science* 93:295-308.

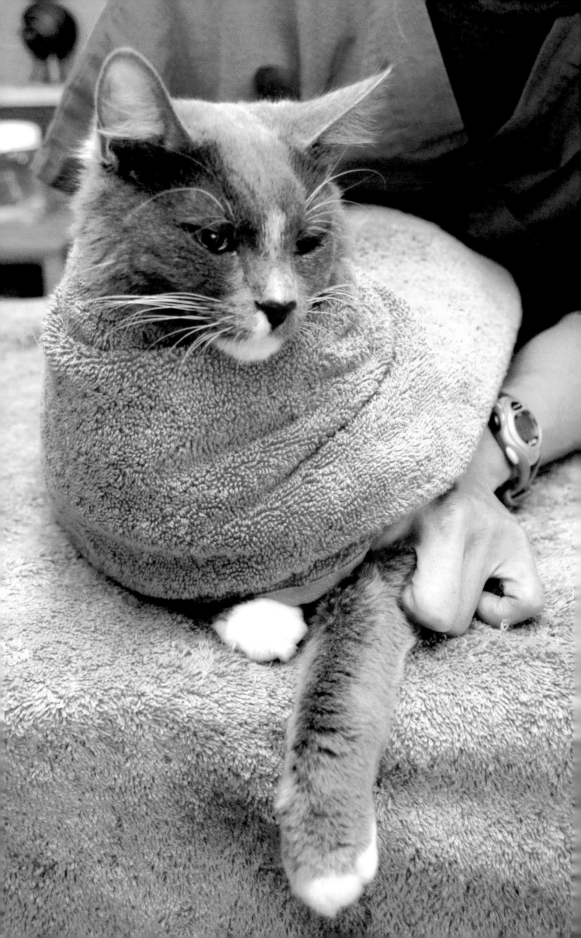

CHAPTER 15. RESTRAINT FOR STANDARD
Positions in Cats

Many veterinarians and technicians are comfortable handling dogs but insecure when it comes to cats. Cats can be more difficult to restrain for several reasons. In general, cats receive less socialization and handling than dogs and consequently are less accepting of restraint. Their evolutionary history as a prey species can also cause them to feel more vulnerable when restrained. Additionally, because they have sharp claws and are extremely dexterous, they can often pull free more easily than dogs and then bite or scratch.

While our initial response to struggling is probably to restrain the cat more firmly and hold him down while he's fighting, a better strategy is to find the position in which the cat feels most safe and comfortable so that he will cooperate. Toweling methods and distractions can be helpful.

In tests, 100% of people who only looked at the photos failed to imitate the photos correctly. Be sure to look at the photos, read the text, and when possible, watch the corresponding DVD clips.

15.1 Restraint While Standing

Many cats can be restrained and positioned in a manner similar to that used for dogs (see Chapter 12).

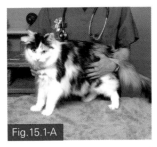

Fig.15.1-A

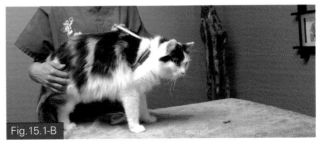

Fig.15.1-B

Fig.15.1-A: Place a C hold or U hold loosely around the neck. The other hand can be used to control the rear end. Keep your arm close to the cat's chest so that he cannot place his front feet on your arm.

Fig.15.1-B: For cats who squirm, try a leash harness (see section 15.8). It works well for some cats who are restless or want to explore because it allows them to move a little while requiring minimal contact on your part. The harness is fashioned from a 4-foot cotton British-style show slip lead made for dogs, but a standard hospital slip lead works too. Allow the cat several inches of slack on the leash so he can move a little, or hold the cat closer to you if necessary. Remove the harness from the cat if he shows any signs that he is not comfortable.

15.2 Positioning Cats Into a Sit

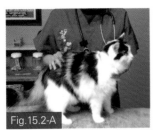

Fig.15.2-A

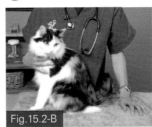

Fig.15.2-B

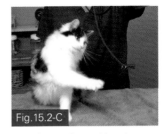

Fig.15.2-C

Fig.15.2-A: Most cats prefer to sit or lie down on the table, and exams can be performed in whatever position they choose. Sometimes having them sit can be more convenient for you and more comfortable and calming for the cat. To get the cat to sit, place one hand on the chest to keep the cat from moving forward. Place the other hand just above the base of the tail and gently push, while using the hand on the chest to shift the cat's front body up and back. If the cat does not sit with minor pressure, do not force him to sit. Just perform the procedure with him standing.

Fig.15.2-B: Once the cat is sitting, keep one hand lightly around the neck in a U hold and the other on the rear end, if needed. Many cats remain seated with just a hand around the neck.

Fig.15.2-C: Keep the cat relaxed and comfortable while waiting between procedures. You can even entertain him with toys or treats as long as you do not cause him to become overly aroused.

15.3 Positioning Cats Into a Down

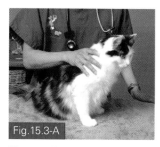
Fig.15.3-A

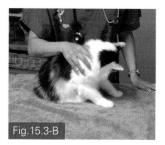
Fig.15.3-B

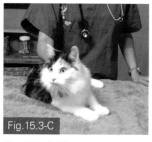
Fig.15.3-C

Fig.15.3-A: Many cats will lie down if you place gentle pressure over the shoulders.

Fig.15.3-B: Continue placing pressure until the cat lies down, as long as she is not becoming anxious or agitated. Alternatively, use the same technique as described for small dogs (see Chapter 12, Section 12.4).

Fig.15.3-C: Then just rest your hand lightly over the cat and be ready to scruff if needed.

15.4 Scruffing a Cat

While scruffing used to be the first technique recommended for restraint in cats, its use is now controversial among veterinary behaviorists. With some animals, scruffing appears to have a calming effect, while in others it may cause immobilization in which the cat barely tolerates the handling. A third groups of cats immediately becomes distressed. In general, scruffing should not be used automatically; rather, it should be applied on a case by case basis. *(Refer to Chapter 8, Video 2)*

Scruffing should not be used automatically in cats. Rather it should be used only when it will cause the animal to relax and allow restraint.

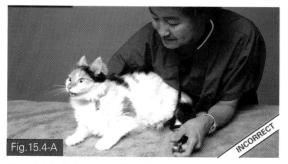
Fig.15.4-A — INCORRECT

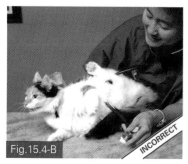
Fig.15.4-B — INCORRECT

Fig.15.4-A, B, Incorrect: Problems with scruffing: Many cats barely tolerate scruffing and others immediately become distressed. This cat quickly becomes difficult when scruffed. Once a cat becomes aroused like this, further examination and treatment may be impossible without chemical restraint or counterconditioning. This cat may need to go home and come back in another day. **Scruffing should not be used automatically in cats. Rather it should be used only when it will cause the animal to relax and allow restraint.**

Box 15-A: Two alternatives to scruffing.

Alternative 1: Restrain the cat similar to a dog.

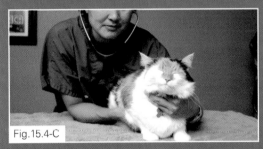

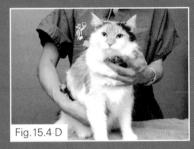

Fig.15.4-C

Fig.15.4 D

Fig.15.4-C, D, Alternative to scruffing 1: This cat remains relaxed when just held in place using restraint similar to that used for a small dog. If the cat is handled in a manner that keeps him calm and relaxed, he is more likely to cooperate for the procedure while needing only a minimal amount of restraint. Note that I have this cat's rear end against me and my arms along his side to support him. The hand in front can massage his chest, neck or head.

Alternative 2: Hold the head.

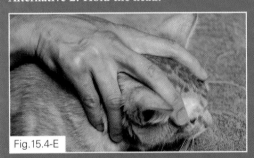

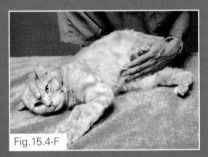

Fig.15.4-E

Fig.15.4-F

Fig.15.4-E, F, Alternative to scruffing 2: Some cats prefer having their head grasped rather than being scruffed, and will relax when handled this way. Only use this technique with cats who remain relaxed while you are using it. This hold can be used in any case where one might otherwise scruff the cat.

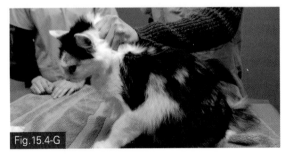

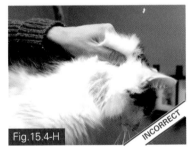

Fig.15.4-G

Fig.15.4-H

INCORRECT

Fig.15.4-G: When scruffing, grasp the scruff with your entire hand. Feel the skin firmly through all your fingers.

Fig.15.4-H, Incorrect: If you only grasp the scruff with your thumb and one or two fingers, the cat is more likely to get loose if he struggles.

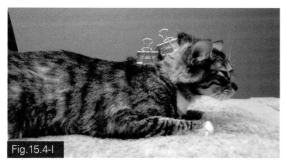
Fig.15.4-I

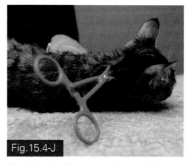
Fig.15.4-J

Fig.15.4-I, Mechanical scruffing: For cats who don't mind scruffing, mechanical clips can be useful (Pozza et al. 2008), for instance, during radiographs so that fewer handlers are needed. Although this technique has been shown to work well in colony cats, it's controversial among behaviorists regarding whether its success involves discomfort or incites a fear-based freeze response in at least some cats. More research should be performed.

Fig.15.4-J Mechanical scruffing: I prefer the Cat Scruffer Clamp (Campbell Pet Company, Brush Prairie, Washington). Avoid using this technique in cats who respond at all aversely to scruffing by hand or who are already aroused. Select cats carefully when using this technique.

15.5 Placing Cats Into Lateral Recumbency
There's no need for rough handling when getting a cat to lie on his side.

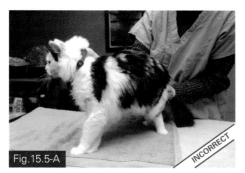
Fig.15.5-A INCORRECT

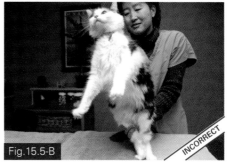
Fig.15.5-B INCORRECT

Fig.15.5-A, B, Incorrect: Technicians sometimes place cats into lateral recumbency in the manner depicted here, without considering whether other methods might be less stressful. Lifting up like a crane to place the cat on his side is unnecessary.

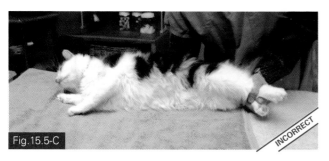
Fig.15.5-C INCORRECT

Fig.15.5-C, Incorrect: Avoid automatically stretching cats. Stretched positions are uncomfortable for the cat and can result in struggling.

15.5.1 From sternal to lateral recumbency

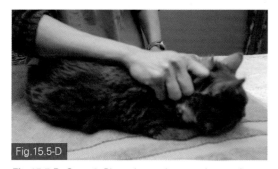

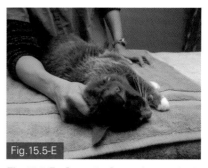

Fig.15.5-D, Step 1: Place the cat in sternal recumbency first, then roll him onto his side. Grasp the scruff and lay your arm flat across his back.

Fig.15.5-E, Step 2: Once the cat is in lateral recumbency, your arm will already be in position across the cat's back.

15.5.2 From standing to lateral recumbency

Method 1

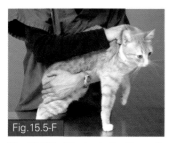

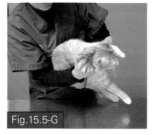

Fig.15.5-F, Method 1, Step 1: With one hand, grasp the scruff. Reach under the abdomen with the other hand and place it on the cat's upper thigh.

Fig.15.5-G, H, Method 1, Step 2: With your arms working in concert, rotate the cat into a lateral position.

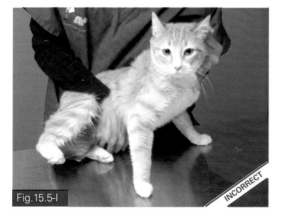

Fig.15.5-I, Method 1, Incorrect: If your arm is not placed correctly, you'll have problems positioning the cat. Here, the cat is able to plant his front leg due to poor positioning.

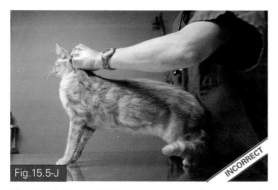

Fig.15.5-J, Method 1, Incorrect: In this photo, the technician's arm is not along the cat's back. This makes it harder to rotate the front of the cat's body. Her hand is also not supporting the cat's hip. Thus, she is relying on the rotation of the front half of the cat's body to rotate the back half.

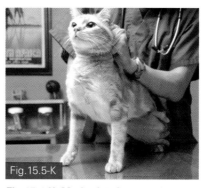

Fig.15.4-K, Method 1, Correct: Here, the hand is in the correct location on the hip.

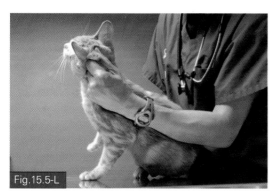

Fig.15.5-L, Method 1, Correct: Now the technician must rotate the front half of the body by rotating her wrist. This causes the cat's body to rotate over onto his side.

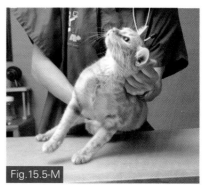

Fig.15.4-M, Method 1, Correct: This causes the leg to be pulled off the table.

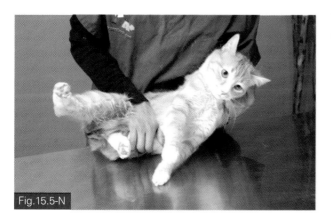

Fig.15.5-N, Method 1, Correct: And now the cat goes into lateral recumbency.

Method 2

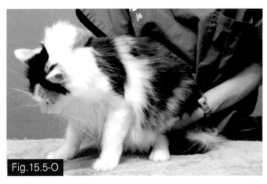

Fig.15.5-O

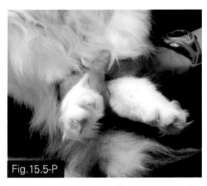

Fig.15.5-P

Fig.15.5-O, Method 2: In this variation, you control the rear end by gently grasping the hind legs in the hock region. The other hand is holding the scruff, with your arm along the cat's back.

Fig.15.5-P, Method 2, Step 1: The index finger should be placed between the legs.

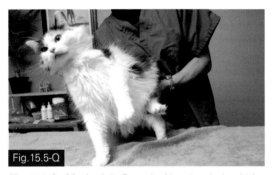

Fig.15.5-Q

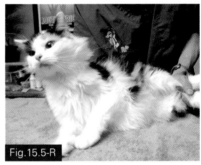

Fig.15.5-R

Fig.15.5-Q, Method 2, Step 2: Your hand should be placed as close to the hocks as possible when doing this. Then begin to rotate the cat.

Fig.15.5-R, Method 2, Step 3: The cat will lie down. Next rotate him onto his side.

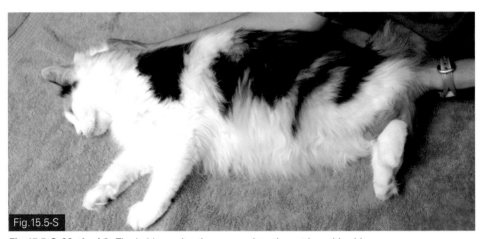

Fig.15.5-S

Fig.15.5-S, Method 2: The hold remains the same when the cat is on his side.

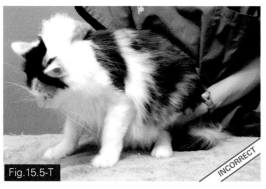

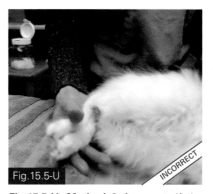

Fig.15.5-T, Method 2, Incorrect: If you only grasp one leg, the cat can plant the other hind leg on the table, making it difficult to get him on his side.

Fig.15.5-U, Method 2, Incorrect: If the legs are grasped in this manner, without a finger between them, the cat can easily pull a foot loose.

15.5.3 Correct handling once the cat is in lateral recumbency.

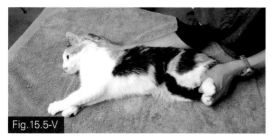

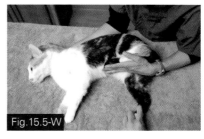

Fig.15.5-V: Grasp the rear legs, making sure that your index finger is between the two legs so that each leg is individually gripped. Again, avoid stretching the cat. Instead, if the cat struggles in this position, try a different position or a toweling method.

Fig.15.5-W: From lateral recumbency, the holder can place her hand perpendicular to the cat's hind leg to occlude the medial saphenous for a blood draw.

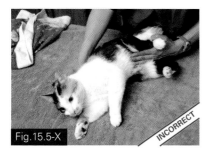

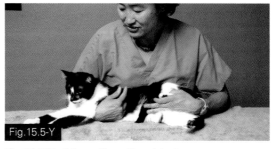

Fig.15.5-X, Incorrect: The technician's right arm is not supporting the cat's back. As a result, this hold is not secure. If the cat starts to struggle, he is likely to get free or become aroused trying.

Fig.15.5-Y, Alternative: Surprisingly, many cats can be restrained on their side without scruffing. This cat is very relaxed in this position (front end sternal) and he remained relaxed when we took blood from his medial saphenous vein (see Chapter 16, Section 16.6).

15.6 Placing Cats Onto Their Backs

This technique is similar to that used for small dogs (see Chapter 12, Section 12.7).

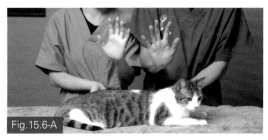

Fig.15.6-A

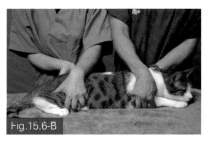

Fig.15.6-B

Fig.15.6-A: When placing cats onto their backs, many can be manipulated in a manner similar to the way dogs are handled. The handlers should position their hands so that they won't need to be repositioned once the cat is on his back. Their outside hands will grasp the legs of the cat that are closest to them. Their inside hands will reach over the cat to grasp his legs on the other side.

Fig.15.6-B: The technician in the front places her hands around the cat's elbows, while the person in the rear grasps the cat's knees.

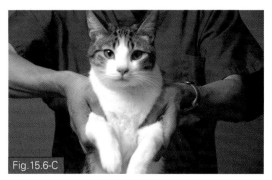

Fig.15.6-C

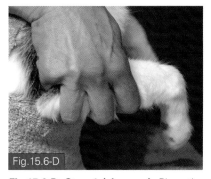

Fig.15.6-D

Fig.15.6-C, Step 1 (close-up): This photo shows the correct position of the front technician's hands, with one hand around each of the cat's elbows.

Fig.15.6-D, Step 1 (close-up): Place the pinky above the elbow and the other fingers below it.

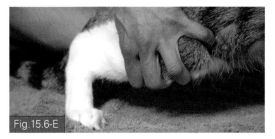

Fig.15.6-E

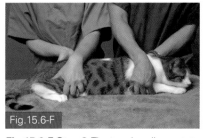

Fig.15.6-F

Fig.15.6-E, Step 1 (close-up): This photo shows the correct position of the rear handler's hands. She is grasping each leg around the knee, with the pinky above the knee and the rest of her fingers below it.

Fig.15.6-F, Step 2: The two handlers rotate the cat in a coordinated fashion, with the outside legs coming up and toward them.

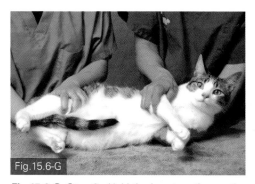

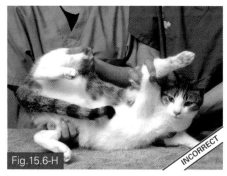

Fig.15.6-G, Step 3: Hold the legs together as the cat is rotated.

Fig.15.6-H, Step 3, Incorrect: Avoid splitting the cat's legs apart when you rotate him.

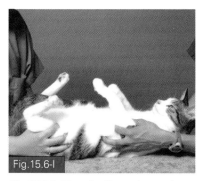

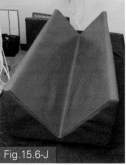

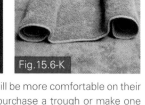

Fig.15.6-I, Step 4: Once the cat is on his back, the handlers' arms form a short trough to keep him balanced.

Fig.15.6-J, K: Many cats will be more comfortable on their back in a trough. You can purchase a trough or make one using a towel and rolling up the ends. The towel should sit rolled-side-down so that it does not unroll.

With trough

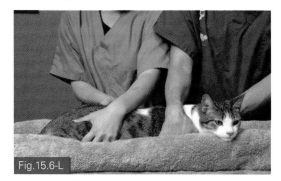

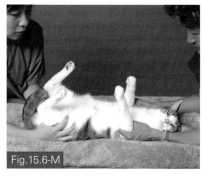

Fig.15.6-L, With trough, Step 1: Start with the cat in the trough and then rotate him onto his back using the method described above.

Fig.15.6-M, With trough, Step 2: The restraint remains the same.

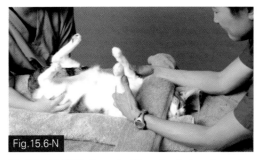

Fig.15.6-N, With trough, Step 3: A towel can be placed over the cat's neck to help prevent him from mouthing the technician's arms. If the cat struggles for more than 2-3 seconds, a different restraint should be tried. The goal is for the cat to remain relaxed.

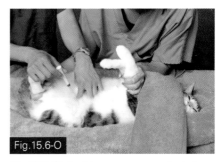

Fig.15.6-O: In this manner, one technician can hold the cat while a cystocentesis is performed. Be careful to keep the hind legs in a comfortable position.

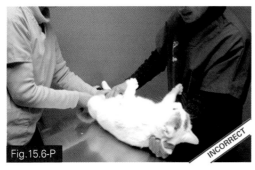

Fig.15.6-P, Incorrect: Some cats can be restrained better on their backs if they are scruffed. But holding a cat in this manner on the metal table is likely uncomfortable.

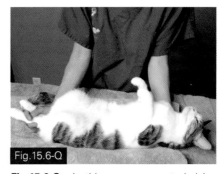

Fig.15.6-Q: In this manner, one technician can hold the cat while a cystocentesis is performed. Be careful to keep the hind legs in a comfortable position.

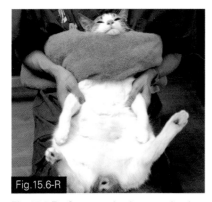

Fig.15.6-R: Cats can also be restrained on their backs in your lap.

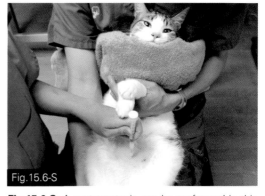

Fig.15.6-S: A cystocentesis can be performed in this position, although two technicians might be needed for restraint. As always, the goal is to keep the cat from struggling by keeping him as comfortable as possible.

15.7 Six Toweling Methods

Towels can make handling easier for many cats, especially those who are fearful. The wrap is not meant to be a straightjacket by which the cats can be held down screaming and hissing. Rather, the goal of a towel wrap is that the cat struggles less and remains calm. In general, the cat should struggle for less than 1-2 seconds and should not struggle repeatedly. If a cat is struggling for prolonged periods or repeatedly, then use a different method or chemical restraint. Switching to a more appropriate method before the cat becomes overly aroused means that you're more likely to be successful. Once the cat is highly aroused, even chemical restraint could become less effective.

Note that for some cats, first spraying the towel with Feliway (Ceva Animal Health, Lenexa, Kansas), a synthetic facial pheromone, may help.

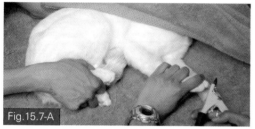 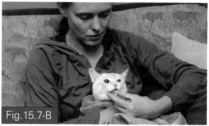

Fig.15.7-A: Sometimes just placing a towel over the cat's head so that he doesn't see his surroundings can calm the cat.

Fig.15.7-B: If you use these toweling techniques at the hospital, or if the owner will use them at home, have the owner make sure the cat develops a positive association with towels. Do this by giving the cat treats when he's sitting on or wrapped in a towel, or have petting sessions with the towel on him.

15.7.1 Method 1: The blanket wrap (head covered and clear access to rear end).

This method is especially useful to capture escaped cats or for getting difficult cats out of their cages. This method, and Method 2, involves covering the cat's head. The cat might feel less fearful with his eyes covered. *(Video 1) (Also refer to Chapter 10, Video 2)*

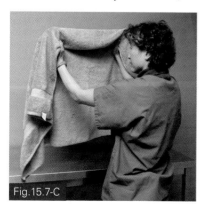

Fig.15.7-C, Method 1, Step 1: For cats who are fearful or difficult, remove them from the cage by placing a large towel, such as a thick 30 x 50-inch bath towel, over them. Hold your arms parallel with your hands several inches from the end of the towel. The end should be draped over your fingers. This is important, because you'll need to be able to wrap this portion of the towel over the front of the cat to cover his head, chest and feet.

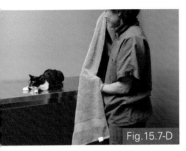
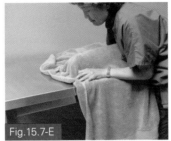
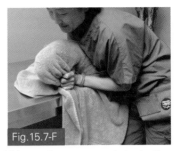

Fig.15.7-D

Fig.15.7-E

Fig.15.7-F

Fig.15.7-D, Method 1: If you're afraid the cat might bite, use two thick towels or one towel plus leather gloves. Use whichever provides you with better dexterity and ability to restrain the cat. Consider having a second person on hand with a towel or wearing gloves in case you need help.

Fig.15.7-E, Method 1, Step 2: In one smooth movement, place the towel over the cat.

Fig.15.7-F, Method 1, Step 3: Notice how the towel is wrapped over the cat's head and pushed under to include the head and feet. My arms are pulled together so that they're holding the towel snugly under the cat.

INCORRECT TOWELING EXAMPLES.

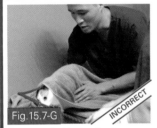
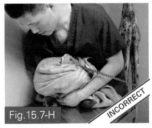
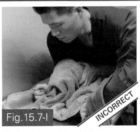

Fig.15.7-G   *INCORRECT*

Fig.15.7-H   *INCORRECT*

Fig.15.7-I   *INCORRECT*

Fig.15.7-G, Method 1, Incorrect: The towel is not wrapped over the cat's head and the sides are not pushed in snugly. Additionally, the technician is not using his body to block escape from the rear.

Fig.15.7-H, Method 1, Incorrect: The cat's head is covered but the towel is not wrapped snugly enough around the cat and the technician's arms have not formed a chute along the cat's sides.

Fig.15.7-I, Method 1, Incorrect: The towel is over the cat's head but is not tucked down over the front of the head and legs, and it's not pulled tightly under. The towel is also not tucked under the sides of the cat for control.

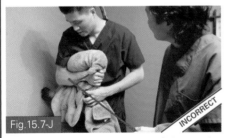
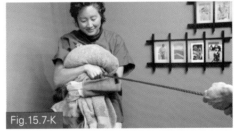

Fig.15.7-J   *INCORRECT*

Fig.15.7-K

Fig.15.7-J, Method 1, Incorrect: Only a portion of the cat is above the technician's arm. Thus the cat is not well contained in the towel.

Fig.15.7-K, Method 1, Correct: The entire cat is contained in the towel and held above the arms.

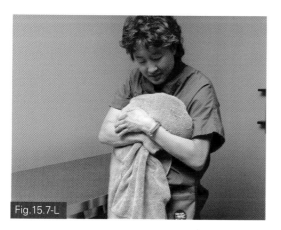

Fig.15.7-L

Fig.15.7-L, Method 1, Step 4: Now the cat can be repositioned so that you can finish wrapping him on the table or you can transport him to a different location. This is probably the most important wrap for cats who are difficult in their cage or carrier, so practice it until you can perform it skillfully. Unfortunately, there are many ways to perform it ineffectively.

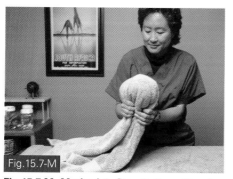

Fig.15.7-M

Fig.15.7-M, Method 1, Step 5: Reposition the cat so that all of the towel is on one side. Then lay the cat (that is, in the towel) on the table.

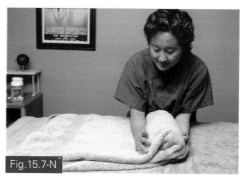

Fig.15.7-N

Fig.15.7-N, Method 1, Step 6: Tuck the towel in along the cat's body.

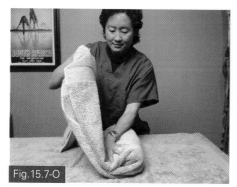

Fig.15.7-O

Fig.15.7-O, Method 1, Step 7: Then wrap the towel over the cat again.

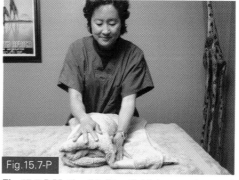

Fig.15.7-P

Fig.15.7-P, Method 1, Step 8: Make sure the towel is snug on the side, but avoid wrapping so tightly that the cat cannot breathe. Also, while the cat is wrapped always pay attention to his breathing.

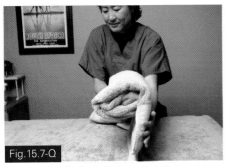

Fig.15.7-Q, Method 1, Step 9: Lift the cat so that the towel can wrap under him.

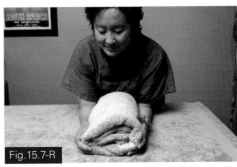

Fig.15.7-R, Method 1, Step 10: If there's more towel, wrap it around again.

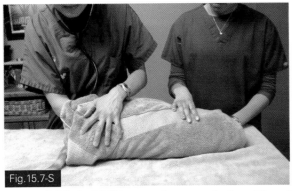

Fig.15.7-S, Method 1: This wrap allows examination of the cat from the chest to the rear end. For instance, you can loosen the back a little and then reach in with your arm and a stethoscope to listen to the heart, or you can palpate the abdomen.

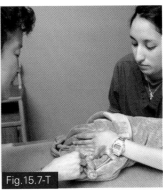

Fig.15.7-T, Method 1: Good access to the rear end allows medial saphenous venipuncture.

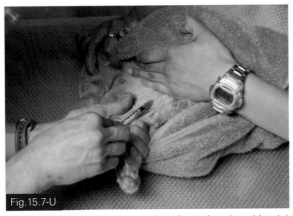

Fig.15.7-U, Method 1: The cat should remain calm with minimal struggling while you take blood.

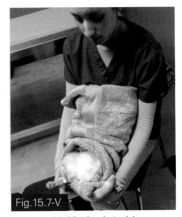

Fig.15.7-V, Method 1: Many cats will also allow cystocentesis when they are hidden in this wrap.

15.7.2 Method 2: The burrito wrap.

This is similar to the blanket wrap, but it begins with the cat lying on top of the towel. This and other wraps should be practiced first using a stuffed animal. *(Video 2)*

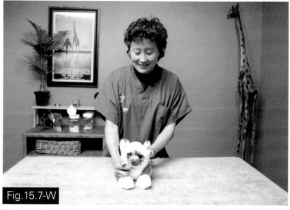

Fig.15.7-W

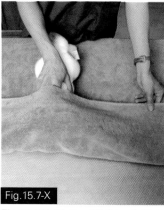

Fig.15.7-X

Fig.15.7-W, Method 2, Step 1: Place the cat (or your stuffed animal) on the towel far enough from the front so that the towel can be folded over his head. About 7 inches works well.

Fig.15.7-X, Method 2, Step 2: Hold the cat steady by placing a hand over the shoulders. Then fold the towel over his head.

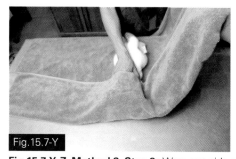

Fig.15.7-Y

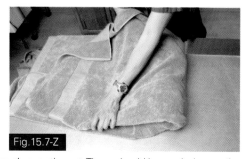

Fig.15.7-Z

Fig.15.7-Y, Z, Method 2, Step 3: Wrap one side snugly over the cat. There should be no slack once the towel is wrapped over the cat.

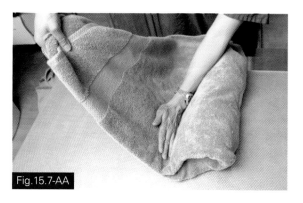

Fig.15.7-AA

Fig.15.7-AA, Method 2, Step 4: Wrap the towel back over the other side.

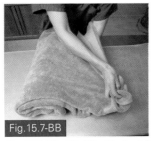
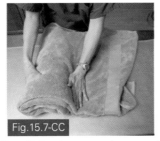
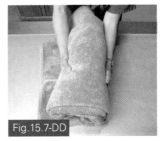

Fig.15.7-BB, CC, DD, Method 2, Step 5: Continue wrapping around and tucking in the towel.

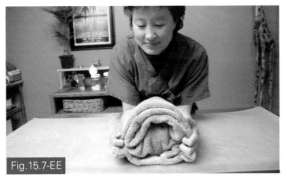

Fig.15.7-EE, Method 2, Final result: The wrap should be neat when it's all done. Check frequently to be sure the cat is comfortable and breathing easily.

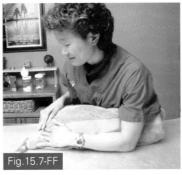

Fig.15.7-FF, Method 2: With this wrap and the previous one, one person can restrain a cat for examination of the rear end.

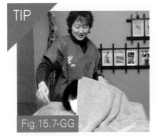
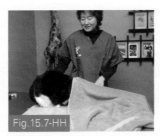
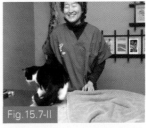

Fig.15.7-GG, HH, II, Tip: This cat doesn't like having his head covered. When I put the towel over his head, he immediately backs out. Some cats back out frantically. Once out, the cat calms down. A different toweling method where his head remains free might work for him. (See Methods 3 to 6.)

15.7.3 Method 3: The half burrito or reverse burrito wrap.

With this wrap, the cat's head remains free from the towel and the back end can be open or closed. Keep the back end open if you plan to examine the back half of the cat. Close it if the cat is likely to squirm out the back. This wrap is good for those cats who dislike having their heads covered but will remain calm in a towel with their heads out. These cats can easily be identified because they back out immediately when their head is covered by the towel. *(Video 3)*

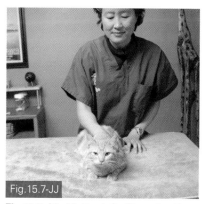

Fig.15.7-JJ, Method 3, Step 1: Start with the cat several inches from the front edge of the towel and about a foot from one side.

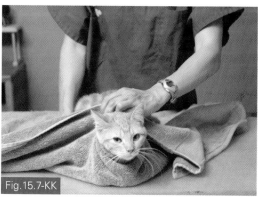

Fig.15.7-KK, Method 3, Step 2: Pull the front of the towel up around the cat's neck snugly so that he can't get his legs over the towel. Hold the towel ends together over the dorsal neck of the cat. Like the previous wrap, this one works best when the cat is lying down.

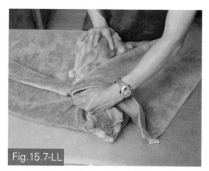

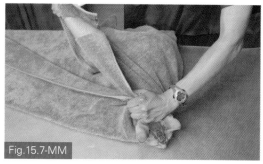

Fig.15.7-LL, MM, Method 3, Step 3: Hold the towel together with one hand. You might need to include the scruff in the hold to keep the cat in place if he tries to back out before you've wrapped him. With your free hand, wrap the towel over the cat.

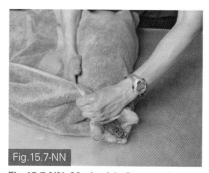

Fig.15.7-NN, Method 3, Step 4: Be sure to take up the slack on the side. There should be no room for the cat to squirm.

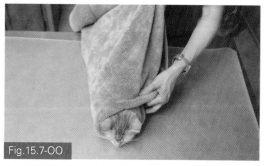

Fig.15.7-OO, Method 3, Step 5: Next, wrap the other side over snugly.

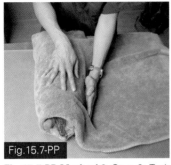
Fig.15.7-PP

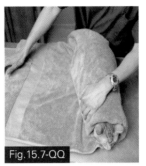
Fig.15.7-QQ

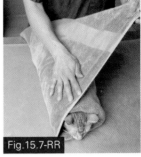
Fig.15.7-RR

Fig.15.7-PP, Method 3, Step 6: Tuck the towel in and then wrap it under the cat.

Fig.15.7-QQ, RR, Method 3, Step 7: Wrap the towel around the cat again.

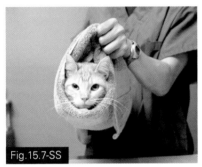
Fig.15.7-SS

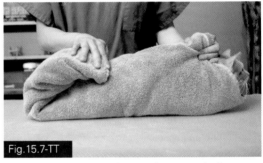
Fig.15.7-TT

Fig.15.7-SS, Method 3, Step 8: When the wrap is snug, you should be able to lift the cat by the towel and the cat should look comfortable.

Fig.15.7-TT, Method 3, Step 9: If the cat wiggles to get out the back, wrap the back of the towel up over the cat's hind end, or cover the rear with a second towel.

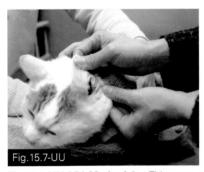
Fig.15.7-UU

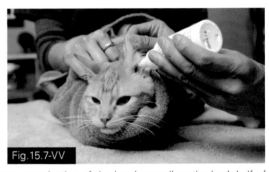
Fig.15.7-VV

Fig.15.7-UU, VV, Method 3: This wrap allows examination of the head as well as the back half of the body.

15.7.4 Method 4: The scarf wrap.

This wrap permits examination of the rear end, hind legs and abdomen, as well as the head. A variation also allows cephalic catheterization. *(Video 4)*

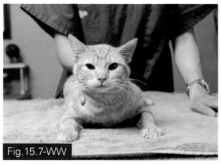

Fig.15.7-WW, Method 4, Step 1: Start with the cat several inches from the front edge of the towel and about a foot from one side.

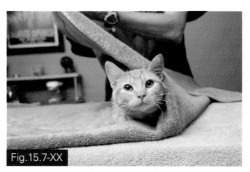

Fig.15.7-XX, Method 4, Step 2: Wrap the short side around the cat's neck snugly, like a scarf.

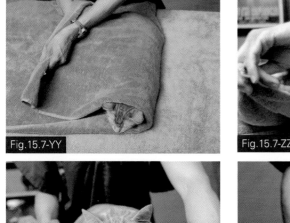

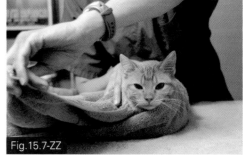

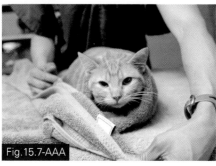

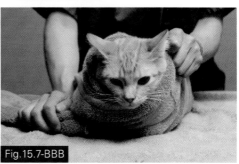

Fig.15.7-YY, ZZ, AAA, BBB, Method 4, Step 3: Pull the entire short side of the towel over the cat so that all of the cat is covered except his face. Then pull the front edge forward. This is the first "scarf" portion of the wrap, which will go under the cat's neck.

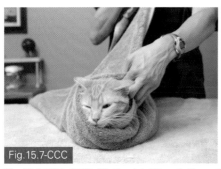

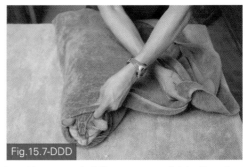

Fig.15.7-CCC, DDD, Method 4, Step 4: Once the towel is wrapped all the way around, take the other side and pull it over the cat. Make sure it's snug.

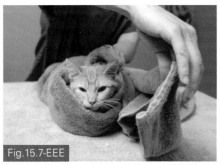

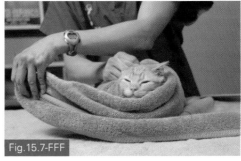

Fig.15.7-EEE, FFF, Method 4, Step 5: Now wrap this portion around the cat and under the neck like a scarf. Make sure it's snug.

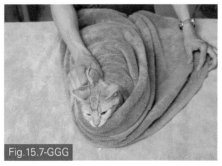

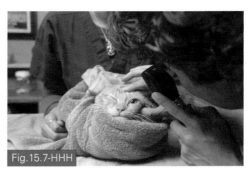

Fig.15.7-GGG, Method 4, Step 6: Keep the towel tight by scruffing the top of it. You can also make a trough with your arms on both sides of the towel.

Fig.15.7-HHH, Method 4: This wrap provides a lot of cushion around the cat's face.

Variation for the scarf wrap to allow access to a front leg (e.g., for catheterizing).

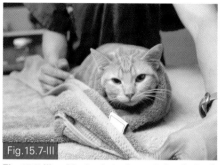

Fig.15.7-III, Method 4, Step 1 (variation): Once the first scarf portion of the wrap is done (Step 3 above) and you start to wrap the other side, leave the right leg out.

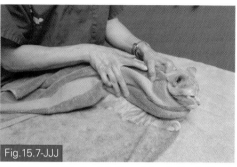

Fig.15.7-JJJ, Method 4, Step 1 (variation): Here's the view from the side.

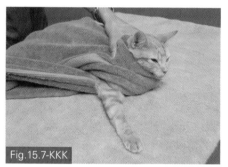

Fig.15.7-KKK, Method 4, Step 2 (variation): Gently pull the second half of the towel under the elbow.

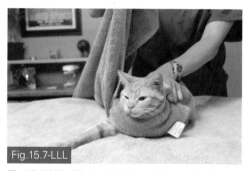

Fig.15.7-LLL, Method 4, Step 3 (variation): Then wrap the towel over the cat and around the front.

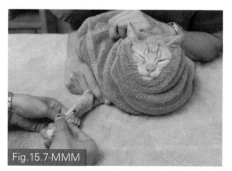

Fig.15.7-MMM, Method 4 (variation): Now the cat's front leg is free for venipuncture. This wrap can be used to examine the head, the back half of the body and one front leg.

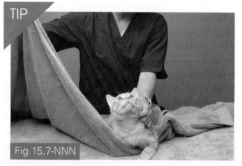

Fig.15.7-NNN, Tip: You can also start the scarf wrap with 1 front leg outside the wrap.

WHAT'S WRONG WITH THIS SCARF WRAP?

Example 1

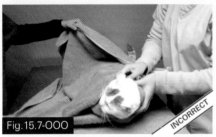

Fig.15.7-OOO

Fig.15.7-OOO, Example 1, Incorrect: This cat was wrapped but is still struggling. The wrap is too loose around the front half of the cat. Notice his legs extended under the towel; they should be folded against his body. The towel is also too loose around the back half.

Example 2

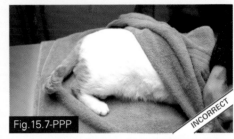

Fig.15.7-PPP

Fig.15.7-PPP, Example 2a, Incorrect: When wrapping the first side around the cat like a scarf, be sure to wrap the back half of the cat too, so that the pressure is even along the cat. Here, I failed to cover the cat's rear end.

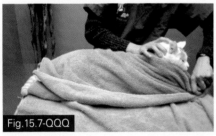

Fig.15.7-QQQ

Fig.15.7-QQQ, Example 2b, Correct: This time I covered the back end of the cat with the towel. It's not snug yet, but it will be when I wrap the other side over it.

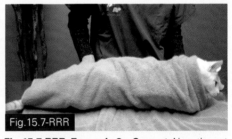

Fig.15.7-RRR

Fig.15.7-RRR, Example 2c, Correct: Now the cat is wrapped snugly. If he tries to back out, block his exit by placing your body behind him and your arms tight along both sides of him.

15.7.5 Method 5: The back wrap.

This wrap works well when you have to sneak the towel over the cat.

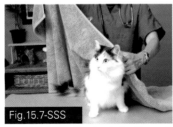

Fig.15.7-SSS

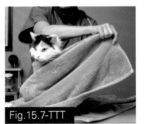

Fig.15.7-TTT

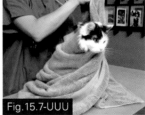

Fig.15.7-UUU

Fig.15.7-SSS, Method 5, Step 1: Hold the cat's scruff and the middle of the towel with one hand. The cat should be sitting.

Fig.15.7-TTT, UUU, Method 5, Step 2: Quickly wrap one side of the towel snugly around the cat.

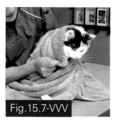 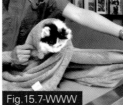 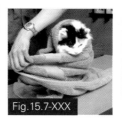 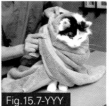

Fig.15.7-VVV to YYY, Method 5, Step 3: Hold that wrapped portion while you bring the other side of the towel around the front of the cat, making sure it's snug. For difficult or fearful cats, the wrapping of both sides can happen almost simultaneously.

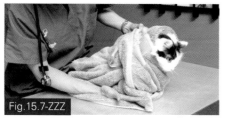 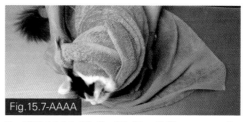

Fig.15.7-ZZZ, Method 5, Step 4: Now fold the towel under the cat from one side so that the towel is snug.

Fig.15.7-AAAA, Method 5, Step 5: Then repeat the process on the other side.

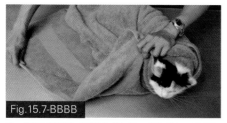 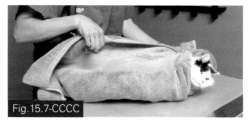

Fig.15.7-BBBB, CCCC, Method 5, Step 6: Wrap any remaining towel around the cat until the wrap is secure.

15.7.6 Method 6: The chin rest.

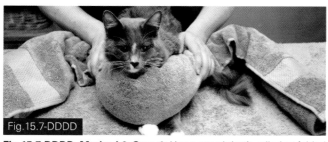 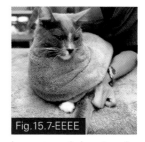

Fig.15.7-DDDD, Method 6, Step 1: Use a towel that's rolled or folded the long way and place it under the cat's chin but above the legs.

Fig.15.7-EEEE, Method 6, Step 2: Secure the cat by placing your arms like a trough along both sides of his body.

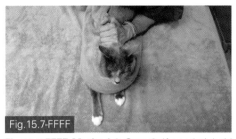

Fig.15.7-FFFF

Fig.15.7-FFFF, Method 6, Step 3: If needed, hold the towel securely by grasping the two sides just behind the neck. In essence, you are scruffing the towel rather than the cat. If the towel is folded instead of rolled, then it can also be used to cover the back half of the cat's body.

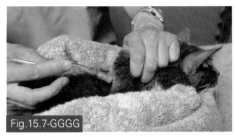

Fig.15.7-GGGG

Fig.15.7-GGGG, Method 6: This method can be used to help restrain cats for SQ fluids. Of course, cats can also be counterconditioned to accept SQ fluids and injections with little or no restraint.

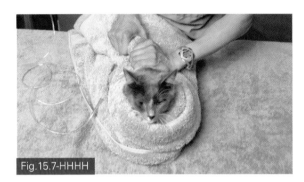

Fig.15.7-HHHH

Fig.15.7-HHHH, Method 6: Once the needle is inserted, the towel can be scruffed to keep the cat in place.

15.8 Minimal Restraint With a Leash Harness

Owners should be encouraged to bring squirmy cats in wearing a harness. (See Chapter 20 to learn how to countercondition cats to harnesses.) Harnesses are particularly useful for cats who are restless and don't like to be held or scruffed. We can also make a harness out of a leash for a cat to wear during an exam.

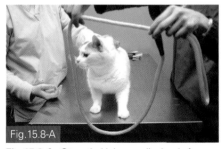

Fig.15.8-A

Fig.15.8-A, Step 1: Using a slip lead, form a loop that is much larger than the cat.

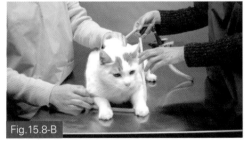

Fig.15.8-B

Fig.15.8-B, Step 2: Place the loop over the cat and pass his front legs through it so that the loop is right behind his armpits.

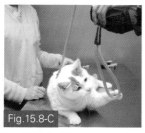
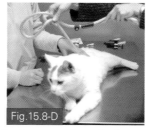
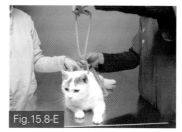

Fig.15.8-C: This cat was fearful a few seconds earlier but now wants to play with the leash. After engaging in play, the cat is calmer.

Fig.15.8-D, Step 3: Next, fold the remainder of the leash into another loop.

Fig.15.8-E, Step 4: Flip the loop so that the leash crosses itself in an X.

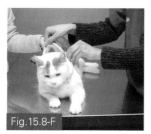
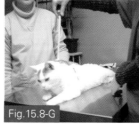
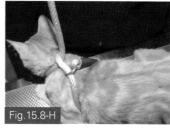

Fig.15.8-F, Step 5: Now flip the loop forward and over the cat's head.

Fig.15.8-G, Step 6: Holding onto the handle of the leash tightens the harness around the cat. Now you can let the energetic cat or the bolter move around without worrying that he will escape. As with dogs, keep the leash short so that the cat does not pace or move around frantically.

Fig.15.8-H: Do not leave cats tied up and unsupervised using this harness, because it can tighten around the neck if pulled in the wrong direction.

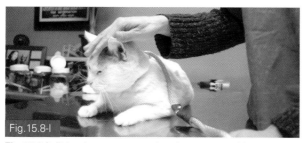
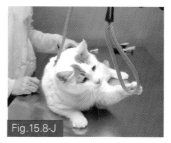

Fig.15.8-I: Take time to try to give the cat a positive experience. This cat enjoys being petted and scratched on the head.

Fig.15.8-J: And, as we saw earlier, he also enjoys playing with the leash.

References

Pozza, M.E., J.L. Stella, A. Chappuis-Gagnon, S.O. Wagner, and C.A.T. Buffington. 2008. Pinch-induced behavioral inhibition ('clipnosis') in domestic cats. *Journal of Feline Medicine and Surgery* 10:82-87.

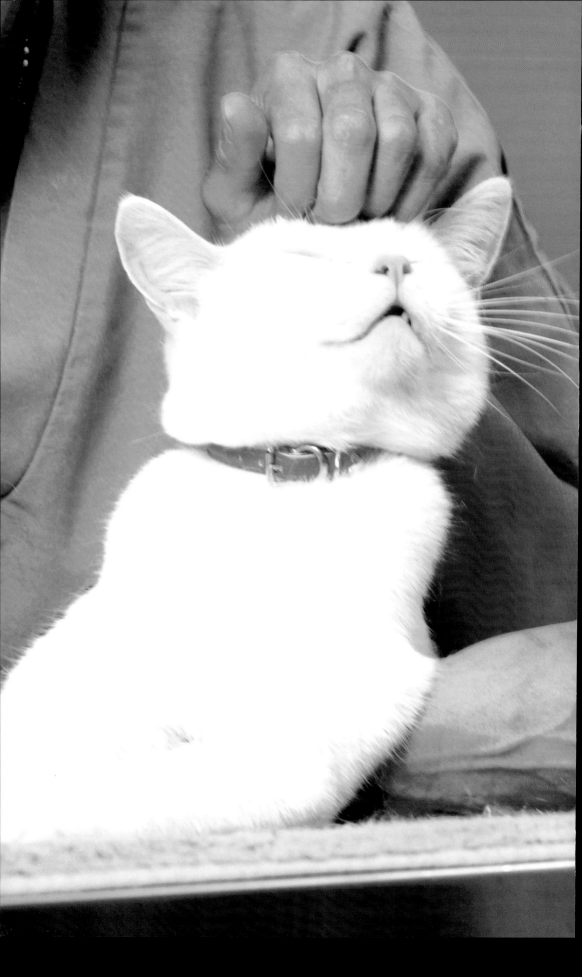

CHAPTER 16.
RESTRAINING
CATS
for Procedures

The technician carefully places the cat in sternal recumbency, grasps the cat's head with her left hand, and with the right hand stretches the cat's front legs down over the front edge of the table. As the veterinarian prepares to draw blood from the jugular vein, the cat struggles to get free. Unable to hold the cat, the technician lets go and the cat immediately starts to calm down. After letting the cat relax for a minute, they repeat the hold with the same results, except now the cat is hissing even after the struggle. "Let's try her on her back," suggests the veterinarian. Sounds like a good plan, except again, even before the veterinarian starts to insert the needle the cat struggles and hisses. "Too bad Gina's not here," says the technician. "She takes the difficult cats into a dark room and can take their blood by herself with hardly any restraint. It's like magic."

The reality here is that Gina is not getting blood in spite of using minimal restraint; she is able to take the blood because she is using minimal restraint. The standard restraint techniques that the technician and veterinarian are using are actually causing the cat to become aggressive. This chapter will demonstrate different techniques for restraining cats so that they feel comfortable and safe and consequently, they cooperate.

16.1 Eye, Ear and Mouth Exams

16.1.1 Restraining for eye exams.

Method 1

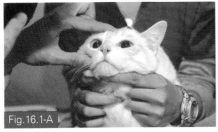

Fig.16.1-A

Fig.16.1-A, Method 1: Hold the cat's eye open with the thumb and index finger. A technician can help restrain the cat by gently holding the head in place.

Method 2

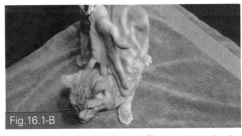

Fig.16.1-B

Fig.16.1-B, Method 2, Step 1: The head can also be restrained with just one hand. Start by placing your fourth and fifth fingers behind the skull to prevent the cat from moving her head backward.

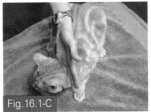

Fig.16.1-C

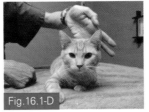

Fig.16.1-D

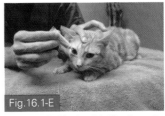

Fig.16.1-E

Fig.16.1-C, D, Method 2, Step 2: Slide your hand down so that the cat's neck sits against the webbing between your two fingers. While these fingers are behind the head, your thumb and index finger can be used to help examine the ears, eyes or mouth.

Fig.16.1-E, Method 2, Final result: Here, the index finger and thumb are being used to help hold the eyelids open.

Method 3

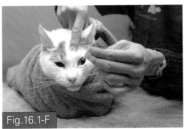

Fig.16.1-F

Fig.16.1-F, Method 3: A towel can be used to restrain a squirmy cat when only one person is available to treat the cat.

Box 16-A: Countercondition the cat to the towel.

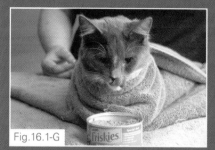

Fig.16.1-G

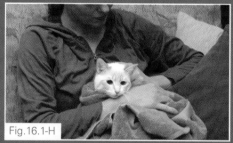

Fig.16.1-H

Fig.16.1-G: If the owners use a towel at home to help restrain the cat, then they should be instructed to also pair lying on the towel or being wrapped in it with positive experiences. For instance, they could bring the towel out and then open the cat's canned food. They should then place the food on the towel so that the cat has to lie on the towel to eat her meal. Or they can wrap the cat in the towel while she eats.

Fig.16.1-H: If the cat enjoys petting, she can lie on or be wrapped in the towel while on the owner's lap getting petted. Make sure that the cat is having a positive experience while she's in the towel. That is, if food is offered the cat should eat it, or else the food is not rewarding to her at that moment. If the cat is being stroked, she should show signs that she enjoys the stroking. She should not be trying to escape.

16.1.2 Restraining for ear exams.

Method 1

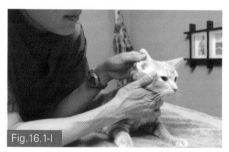

Fig.16.1-I

Fig.16.1-I, Method 1: The one-handed restraint described above can be used to examine the ears, too.

Method 2

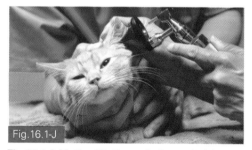

Fig.16.1-J

Fig.16.1-J, Method 2: Alternatively, a technician can gently tilt the head so that the ear closest to the veterinarian is facing upward. The technician must be sure to control the cat's body. Holds similar to those used with dogs can also be used with cats. However, less surface area contact generally works better with cats; dogs tend to require more contact.

Method 3

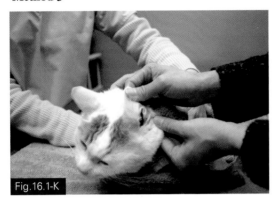

Fig.16.1-K, Method 3: If their ears are pruritic, cats will often claw or try to scratch them. A towel wrap—such as the scarf wrap or half-burrito wrap described in Chapter 15 (Section 15.7)—can be useful when you need to examine or clean the ears.

16.1.3 Restraining for mouth exams.

Method 1

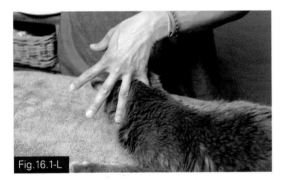

Fig.16.1-L, Method 1, Step 1: Place the fourth and fifth fingers behind the skull to keep the cat from moving her head backward. TIP: For cats that try to back up or squirm, have a technician place a hand on the cat's rear end.

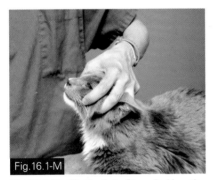

Fig.16.1-M, Method 1, Step 2: Use the thumb and forefinger on the proximal aspect of the zygomatic arch (cheek bones) to guide the mouth upward. Raising the cat's head usually causes her to open her mouth slightly.

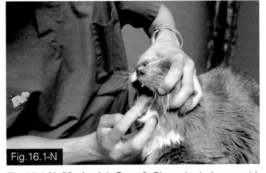

Fig.16.1-N, Method 1, Step 3: Place the index or middle finger of the free hand on the cat's mandible between the canines and pry the mouth open so that you can view the inside. Make sure that the lighting is good prior to doing this, as you might get only one chance to look in the mouth. Also, avoid pulling the jaw open too wide, or the cat will struggle.

Method 2

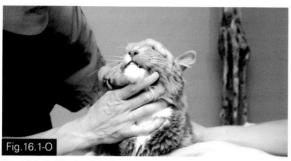

Fig.16.1-O

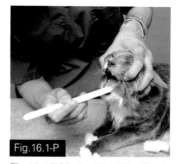

Fig.16.1-P

Fig.16.1-O, Method 1, Step 4: Be sure to release the cat's jaw before she starts to struggle. You might need to give the cat a break and reward her by scratching behind the ears (if the cat enjoys scratching at that moment). Or just let her rest and calm down before opening her mouth again.

Fig.16.1-P, Method 2: With difficult cats, try using a tongue depressor to open the mouth.

16.2 Oral Medications

16.2.1 Giving liquids.

Use the same head hold as when restraining for a mouth exam.

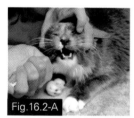

Fig.16.2-A

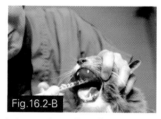

Fig.16.2-B

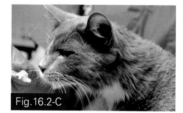

Fig.16.2-C

Fig.16.2-A, B: Open the mouth, insert the syringe from the side and squirt the liquid in. Because liquids are more likely than pills or capsules to enter the trachea, keep the head level. Do not tilt it backward, as is done when pilling. Alternatively, you can squirt the liquid onto the roof of the mouth if the cat's mouth is wide open.

Fig.16.2-C: Countercondition the cat to the syringe. If the cat is fearful of syringes, the owner could countercondition by regularly letting the cat eat treats such as canned food or tuna off the syringe. The owner might start the counterconditioning procedure by simply placing the syringe in or near the cat's food bowl during feeding time.

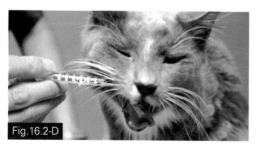

Fig.16.2-D

Fig.16.2-D: This cat needs no restraint to accept the tuna-laden syringe. The next step in counterconditioning is to restrain her head slightly and then present the tuna. This trains her to accept the head restraint.

16.2.2 Giving pills.

Use the same head hold as when restraining for a mouth exam.

Method 1

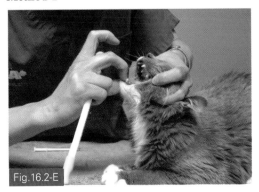

Fig.16.2-E

Fig.16.2-E, Method 1, Step 1: Prepare a syringe with water or a liquid that the cat likes, e.g., tuna juice or meat broth (with no onions or onion powder). The liquid will be used as a chaser to ensure that the pill or capsule does not get stuck in the esophagus, which could lead to esophagitis. (Note that in the research study [Westfall 2001] that revealed the benefits of a water chaser, 6 mL of water was administered per chaser). Next, place the pill in the pill gun. Tilt the cat's head back and open her mouth.

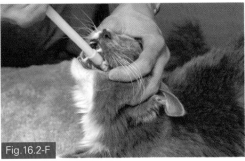

Fig.16.2-F

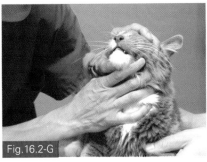

Fig.16.2-G

Fig.16.2-F, Method 1, Step 2: A small amount of meat baby food, canned cat food or other food the cat likes can be placed over the end of the pill gun to hide the pill, if needed. Insert the pill gun into the mouth and deposit the pill at the back of the cat's tongue.

Fig.16.2-G, Method 1, Step 3: Remove the pill gun and quickly close the mouth while continuing to tilt the head up. You can massage the throat to induce swallowing. Then follow up with the liquid chaser.

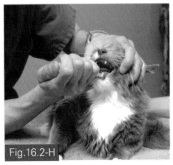

Fig.16.2-H

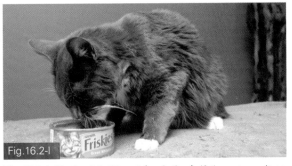

Fig.16.2-I

Fig.16.2-H, Method 1, Step 4: As with liquid medications, take care to leave the head level when giving the liquid chaser.

Fig.16.2-I, Method 1, Step 4 (variation): If the cat won't accept the liquid chaser (and requires counterconditioning to liquid administration), try feeding meat baby food, canned cat food or tuna juice from a bowl instead.

Fig.16.2-J , Method 1, Step 4 (variation): If she won't eat from a bowl either, then place Nutri-Cal on her paw or nose for her to lick off. Nutri-Cal may help lubricate the pill.

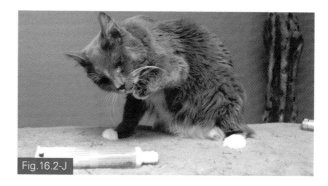

Method 2

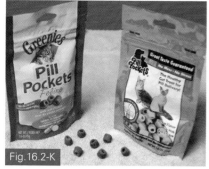

Fig.16.2-K, Method 2: Some cats will take pills hidden in Pill Pockets. These are semi-moist treats with a hole in them to place pills. Another option is to have the medications compounded into flavored liquids or pastes.

Method 3

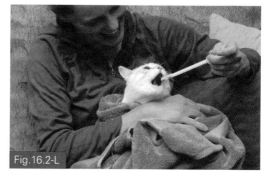

Fig.16.2-L, Method 3: Countercondition to pilling. Cats who are difficult to pill should be counterconditioned to the process. Here, the owner feeds her cat tuna using the pill gun. Difficulty pilling can lead to erosion of the owner-cat bond and non-compliance by the owner. Owners sometimes elect to euthanize their pets when they can't easily administer the medication the pet needs in order to cure or control a serious disease condition. Anything you can do to make medicating the cat pleasant for both owner and cat is important.

16.3 Subcutaneous Fluids and Injections

If a cat dislikes receiving fluids or shots, ask the owners if they would like their cat to have a less stressful and more enjoyable hospital visit. Also, inform them that many cats will need SQ fluids or injections to be administered at home at some time during their life. Ask if they would like to prepare now to make this process easy later. If the answer is yes to either question, send them home with a plan for conditioning their cat to injections. (See Chapters 18 and 20. You can download client handouts from the reader-only resources at www.nerdbook.com/lowstresshandling)

16.3.1 Giving subcutaneous (SQ) fluids.

Method 1

Method 2

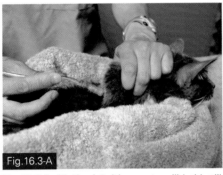

Fig.16.3-A

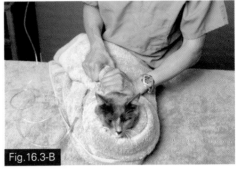

Fig.16.3-B

Fig.16.3-A, Method 1: Many cats will hold still with light scruffing. Tent the skin with the hand that's scruffing and inject the needle into the tented area.

Fig.16.3-B, Method 2: Towels can be used to help hold the cat in place. If the cat struggles a lot yet needs fluids frequently, the owner should prepare the cat by counterconditioning her at home to the feel of the needle and to the towel.

16.3.2 Giving SQ injections.

Method 1

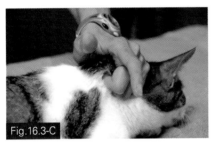

Fig.16.3-C

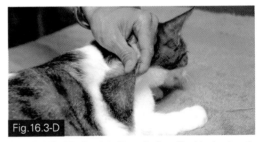

Fig.16.3-D

Fig.16.3-C, Method 1, Step 1: Use a small-gauge needle whenever possible. If the injection is to be given in the shoulder, neck or upper leg region, the cat can be scruffed.

Fig.16.3-D, Method 1, Step 2: Scruff with the fourth and fifth fingers while the thumb and index finger are used to tent the skin. For some cats, it's useful to desensitize them to the needle right before injection by tapping the area of injection several times. The cat should not respond to the tapping.

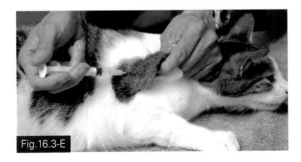

Fig.16.3-E

Fig.16.3-E, Method 1, Step 3: Inject the needle assertively and then inject the fluid. Slow placement of the needle is more likely to cause the cat to struggle.

Method 2

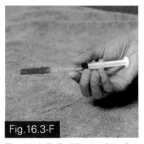

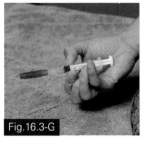

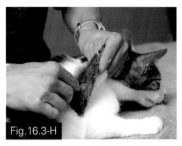

Fig.16.3-F, G, Method 2, Step 1: Another method of injecting the fluid is to hold the syringe so that the plunger sits in the heel of your hand. Fluid can be injected by pressing the palm of the hand on the syringe plunger.

Fig.16.3-H, Method 2, Step 2: When giving an injection this way, tell the client that you have done so, as they usually won't notice that the cat was actually injected.

16.4 Jugular Venipuncture *(Video 1)*

Method 1

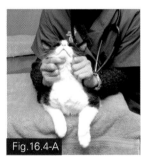

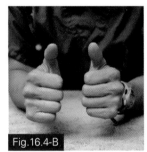

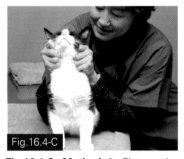

Fig.16.4-A, B, Method 1: If the cat is comfortable lying sternally, have her lie at the edge of the table. Elevate her head by placing a hand on either side of the neck and under the mandible. Fold your fingers under so that they do not block the jugular vein. The legs need not be restrained. If the cat is comfortable, she'll hold still. If she's going to strike out in an attempt to cause injury, she'll give ample warning; e.g., she'll first strike repeatedly but with low intensity or with claws not extended. If the cat jumps when poked with the needle or is tense when restrained in this position, change to a different venipuncture technique.

Fig.16.4-C, Method 1: Choose the position that's most comfortable for the cat. If she prefers to sit, let her sit. Even cats who are hissing can have blood drawn in this manner. If they struggle or claw, don't force them. Instead, try collecting blood from a different vein or position. Attempting to force a struggling, tense cat often results in scratch and bite injuries.

Method 2

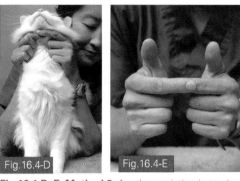

Fig.16.4-D

Fig.16.4-E

Method 3

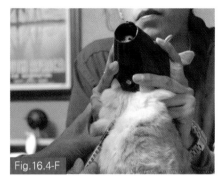

Fig.16.4-F

Fig.16.4-D, E, Method 2: Another variation is to place the index fingers across the mandible. With this method, if the cat struggles, the technician can hold on for 1-2 seconds before releasing the hold without getting bitten, which allows the person taking the blood to move away. Holding a struggling cat for a prolonged period can quickly result in injury to the technicians.

Fig.16.4-F, Method 3: A muzzle can be used if the cat is relaxed when wearing the muzzle. Some cats are more relaxed when they can't see. Others become distressed and struggle more. If the muzzled cat struggles, do not forcefully restrain her to take blood, or else you're likely to make the cat worse for the next procedure. Rather, change the handling technique.

Method 4

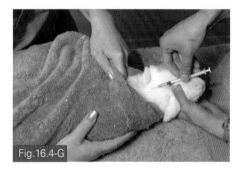

Fig.16.4-G

Fig.16.4-G, Method 4: Some cats tolerate being toweled in a reverse burrito (see Chapter 15, Section 15.7) and then lying on their sides or backs. Finding the position most comfortable for the cat is a trial-and-error process. Cats who struggle vigorously when one method is used are often very relaxed for others. Remember to note in the cat's file which positions worked and which didn't. The position shown in this photo is likely to work best in cats who like to lie on their backs in people's laps.

Box 16-B: Countercondition between procedures

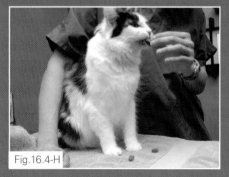

Fig.16.4-H

Fig.16.4-H: Countercondition between procedures. Technicians frequently spend time waiting for a second person or the veterinarian before a procedure can be performed. This provides the perfect opportunity to countercondition the cat. The cat shown here likes treats. Some cats will play with toys or leashes dangled in front of them. It only takes a little effort during this down time to see if the cat likes petting, treats or play. Just avoid food if the cat will need to be sedated or if it is otherwise contraindicated.

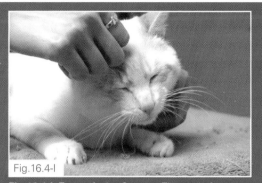

Fig.16.4-I

Fig.16.4-I, Example 1a, Correct: The goal of counter-conditioning between procedures is to help put the cat in a positive emotional state. If the cat likes being petted, scratch her head between procedures. Only do this if her body posture indicates that she likes it, or else you could be making her hospital experience worse. This cat is leaning into the technician's petting hand, obviously enjoying the attention.

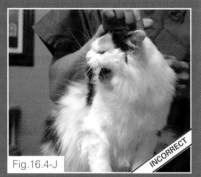

Fig.16.4-J   INCORRECT

Fig.16.4-J, Incorrect: This cat finds petting aversive at the moment. Other cats show more subtle signs or just tolerate the petting without really enjoying it. Only pet the cat if she's showing clear signs that she likes it.

Methods to avoid!!

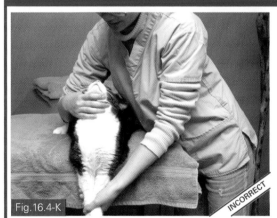

Fig.16.4-K   INCORRECT

Fig.16.4-K, Example 1, Incorrect: This method of restraint for jugular venipuncture is uncomfortable for many cats. The idea here is that holding the legs down will keep the cat from clawing. But this hold often increases the likelihood that the cat will struggle and bite or claw. Note that with this type of hold, the cat's body is not well supported. She can easily move her body sideways.

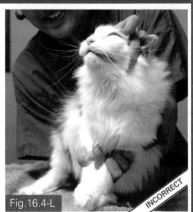

Fig.16.4-L   INCORRECT

Fig.16.4-L, Example 2, Incorrect: Restraining the head in this manner is also uncomfortable for the cat, and it provides poor support. There are no arms along the sides of the cat to act as railings so that the cat's body stays in position.

16.5 Cephalic Catheterization

Method 1

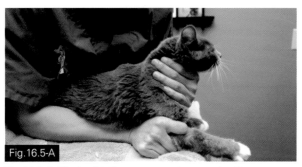

Fig.16.5-A

Fig.16.5-A, Method 1: Some cats can be restrained in a manner similar to that used for to dogs. Legs can be held in the same manner as for a dog (see Chapter 13, Section 13.5).

Method 2

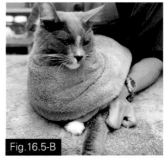

Fig.16.5-B

Fig.16.5-B, Method 2: This calm cat can be catheterized simply by placing a towel under her neck (refer to Chapter 15, Section 15.7) and extending her leg. If needed, the towel can be "scruffed" to hold the cat more securely.

Method 3

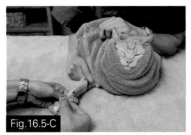

Fig.16.5-C

Fig.16.5-C, Method 3: Some cats are more relaxed with a more snugly fitting wrap, such as the scarf towel wrap (Chapter 15, Section 15.7).

Method 4

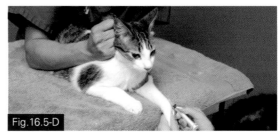

Fig.16.5-D

Fig.16.5-D, Method 4: Other cats are calmer when scruffed. But realize that if they try to bite, they can still reach the person placing the catheter. Thus, as with the other restraints, this method is best used with cats who remain calm in this hold.

Method 5

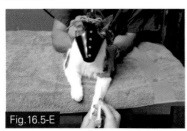

Fig.16.5-E

Fig.16.5-E, Method 5: A muzzle can be used if the cat does not react aversely to it.

Method 6

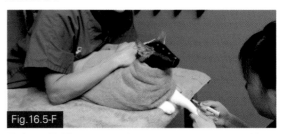

Fig.16.5-F

Fig.16.5-F, Method 6: Muzzling can also be combined with the chin rest toweling method. (See Chapter 15, Section 15.7.6.)

16.6 Medial Saphenous Venipuncture *(Video 2)*

Method 1

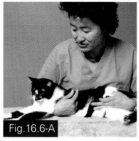
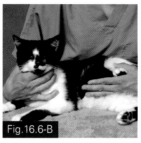
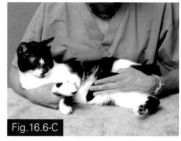

Fig.16.6-A, B, C, Method 1: Surprisingly, many cats will hold still for medial saphenous venipuncture without requiring head restraint if they are allowed to keep the front half of their body somewhat sternal (upright). The front end can be supported with your arm under the cat's armpit, with your hand in a C hold around the neck, or by holding their front legs with your index finger between the legs and as proximal (close to the body) as is comfortable for the cat. The ideal cat for this technique is one who remains relaxed in this position even when the venipuncture is being performed. The cat that's squirmy and trying to explore or play may not be the best candidate. When trying this technique, if you feel the cat tense up, switch to a different technique.

Method 2

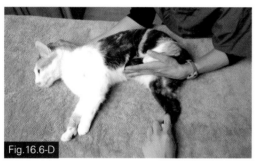
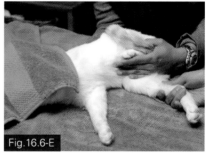

Fig.16.6-D, Method 2: With the cat in lateral recumbency, the restrainer should hold the cat's scruff firmly in her entire hand. Her arm supports the cat's back. The other hand should push the top hind leg up into the body and at the same time hold off the vein in the lower leg. Note that the cat is not stretched.

Fig.16.6-E, Method 2 (variation): Some cats are calmer if they have a towel covering their head so that they cannot see people, animals or objects that may scare them.

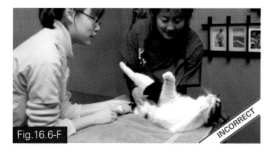

Fig.16.6-F, Method 2, Incorrect: If the cat struggles and tries to roll over, stretching won't help because you can't stretch the hind limbs to get blood. Sometimes vibrating the scruff can distract the cat. But if the cat repeatedly struggles or does so for more than a few seconds, change the technique.

Method 3

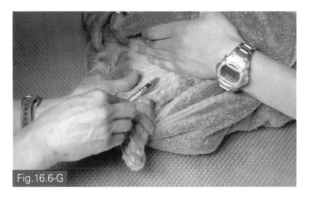

Fig.16.6-G

Fig.16.6-G, Method 3: Try one of the toweling methods described in Chapter 15 (Section 15.7) or use chemical restraint. Use a method where the cat remains relaxed. Struggling repeatedly for more than 1-2 seconds indicates that a different technique should be used or the procedure should be attempted in a quieter room.

16.7 Cystocentesis

Method 1

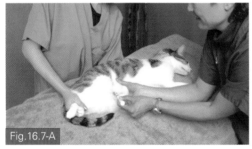

Fig.16.7-A

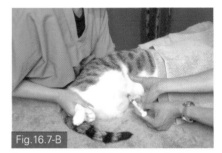

Fig.16.7-B

Fig.16.7-A, Method 1: A cystocentesis is typically performed with the cat on her back; however, many cats are uncomfortable with this restraint. Cats can instead be restrained on their sides for the procedure.

Fig.16.7-B, Method I (variation): Place a towel over the head of a fearful cat.

Method 2

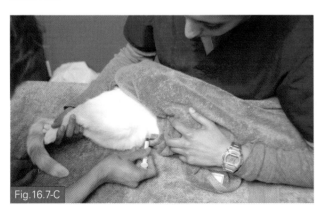

Fig.16.7-C

Fig.16.7-C, Method 2: Cats can also be wrapped in any of the wraps that leave the back half of the body open for examination (see Chapter 15, Section 15.7)

Method 3

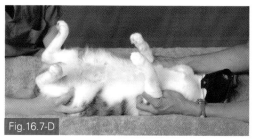

Fig.16.7-D

Fig.16.7-D, Method 3: If the cat is placed on her back on a table, either use a trough or be sure the cat is on a comfortable surface and is well balanced. A muzzle can also be used, if necessary.

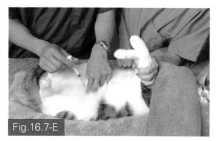

Fig.16.7-E

Fig.16.7-E, Method 3 (variation): Instead of a muzzle, you could try placing a folded towel across the cat's neck. The towel will not stay on, however, if she struggles for more than a second or 2.

Method 4

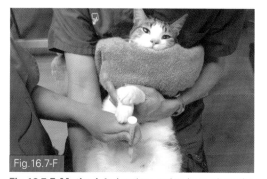

Fig.16.7-F

Fig.16.7-F, Method 4: Another option is to place the cat on her back in your lap.

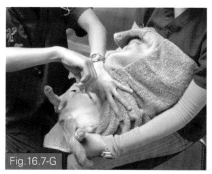

Fig.16.7-G

Fig.16.7-G, Method 4 (variation): A towel wrap such as the burrito or half-burrito wrap can also be used (see Chapter 15, Section 15.7).

16.8 Toenail Trims *(Refer to Chapter 18, Video 7)*

Perform nail trims in a position that keeps the cat comfortable. This means technicians should practice performing the procedure from many different angles. Toenail trims are an elective procedure that can make the cat much worse behaviorally if they are done without considering the cat's comfort level. A bad experience with a nail trim can teach the cat to be more fearful and aggressive at the hospital, thus making future care for important medical issues impossible. It can also make cats more fearful and aggressive around unfamiliar people and in response to small environmental changes. This anxiety can lead not only to aggression, but also to urinating or defecating outside the litter box.

If you see that the animal is nervous, point this out to the owner. Since toenail trims are not emergency procedures, take the time to show the owners how to counter-condition their cats to the procedure. Or show them how to trim nails on their own, so they can try when the cat is relaxed and sleeping at home. If the owner insists that you trim the nails, have them sign a consent form stating that they understand the procedure can cause the cat to become more fearful and aggressive for handling at home and in the hospital, and it can jeopardize the cat's ability to receive medical care in the future. Alternatively, you can require chemical restraint.

> Since toenail trims are not emergency procedures, take the time to show the owners how to countercondition their cats to the procedure. Or show them how to trim nails on their own, so they can try when the cat is relaxed and sleeping at home. If the owner insists that you trim the nails, have them sign a consent form stating that they understand the procedure can cause the cat to become more fearful and aggressive for handling at home and in the hospital, and it can jeopardize the cat's ability to receive medical care in the future.

Method 1

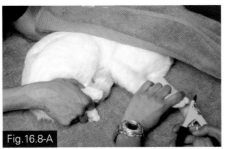

Fig.16.8-A

Fig.16.8-A, Method 1: A common restraint is to place the cat on her side. For a fearful cat, a towel can be placed over her head.

Method 2

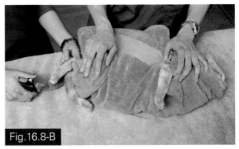

Fig.16.8-B

Fig.16.8-B, Method 2: Toweling in a scarf wrap (see Chapter 15, Section 15.7) allows access to 3 paws.

Method 3

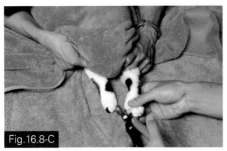

Fig.16.8-C

Fig.16.8-C, Method 3: Some fearful cats prefer lying sternally with their heads covered. The less manipulation needed, the better.

Method 4

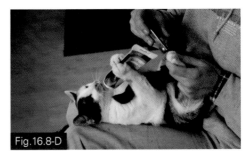

Fig.16.8-D

Fig.16.8-D, Method 4: Cats can be trained to lie on their backs for a toenail trim (see Chapter 20).

Method 5

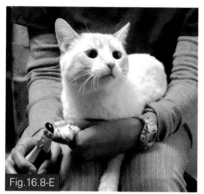

Fig.16.8-E

Fig.16.8-E, Method 5: Many cats object more to the restraint than the actual toenail trimming. See if you can find a position in which the cat is comfortable being held without restraint before moving on to other methods.

Method 6

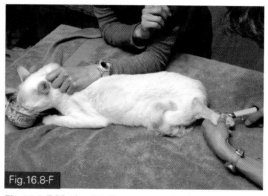

Fig.16.8-F

Fig.16.8-F, Method 6: Owners can also be taught to trim the nails themselves. Find a way to occupy the cat while they are doing so. This cat is eating her dinner while getting her rear toenails trimmed so she's developing a positive association.

References

Westfall, D.S., D.C. Twedt, P.F. Steyn, E.B. Oberhauser, and J.W. VanCleave. 2001. Evaluation of the passage of tablets and capsules through the esophagus in cats. *Journal of Veterinary Internal Medicine* 15:273.

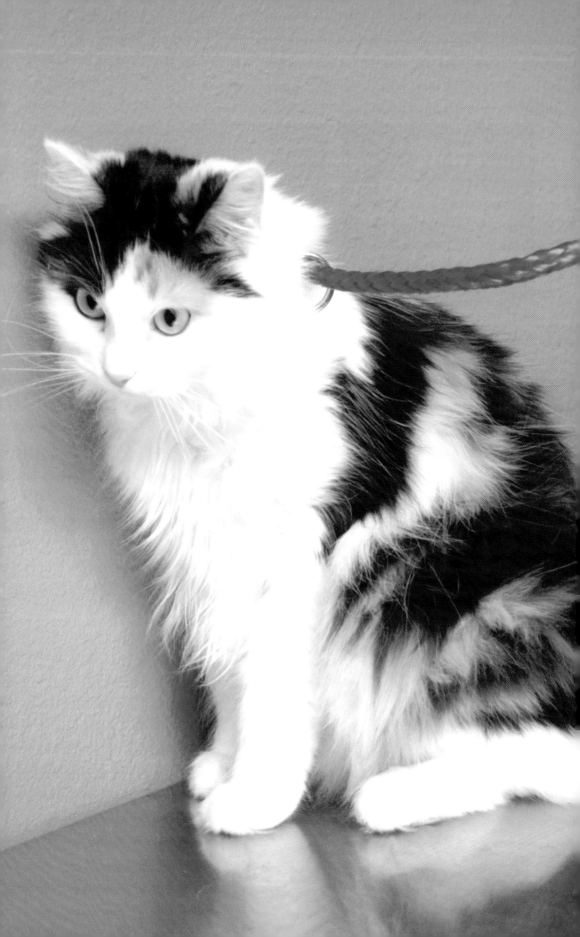

CHAPTER 17.
HANDLING
Difficult Cats

As with everything else, the handling of a difficult cat starts even before the cat comes in. The cat will be calmer if he's already been counterconditioned to the carrier and to car rides, and if he enters into a calm hospital environment. Regardless of how good your techniques are, some cats will require chemical restraint and others should receive—or their owners at least be offered the option of—a counterconditioning plan. As with dogs, fearful cats might be tolerant of handling on the initial visit but become worse with each subsequent visit. Thus, if a cat shows tendencies toward becoming difficult, the owner should be offered tips or plans to improve the cat's behavior—especially if he is likely to develop a disorder that will require management, such as diabetes. Many owners will choose to euthanize their cats for health problems rather than have to bring them in for unpleasant veterinary care.

17.1 Providing a Comfortable Environment

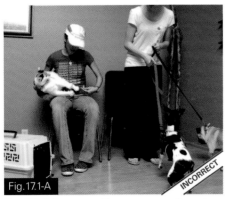

Fig.17.1-A

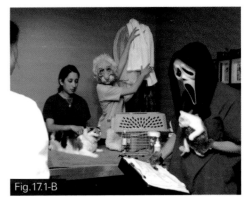

Fig.17.1-B

Fig.17.1-A, Incorrect: Keep cats away from dogs and other animals in the waiting area. Once a cat has one fearful experience, it sets the tone for the rest of his visit. It's best to have separate dog and cat areas in the waiting room and to have towels available for covering the cat carriers, because cats are often fearful of other cats, too. Also, move cats into an exam room as quickly as possible.

Fig.17.1-B: For animals who have not been socialized to all types of people and pets, seeing unfamiliar people and animals in a treatment room is like seeing monsters or aliens in a hospital emergency room.

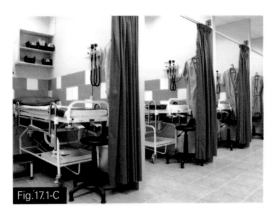

Fig.17.1-C

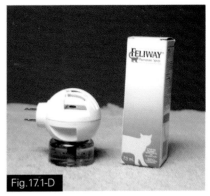

Fig.17.1-D

Fig.17.1-C: Human emergency hospitals are crowded but still provide some privacy with curtains. Fearful cats do better with privacy, too; they should be examined and have procedures performed in a quiet room such as an exam room. Visual barriers should be provided so that they don't have to see and hear people and animals whom they are afraid of.

Fig.17.1-D: Consider having the owner spray the cat's carrier or towel with Feliway (Ceva Animal Health, Lenexa, Kansas), a synthetic feline calming pheromone. The hospital can use Feliway, too, in diffusers in the rooms, on towels, or by spraying the cat cage 15 minutes before the cat enters (Griffith et al. 2000; Kronen et al. 2006; Landsberg 2006).

17.2 Removing Cats From Carriers

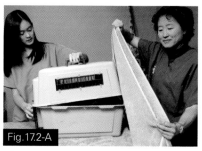
Fig.17.2-A

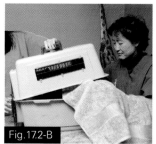
Fig.17.2-B

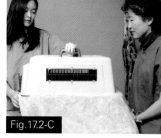
Fig.17.2-C

Fig.17.2-A, Step 1: Unscrew the screws from the carrier and lift the top while keeping the gate in place so that the cat does not dart out. One or two thick towels can be used, depending on how likely the cat is to try to bite or scratch.

Fig.17.2-B, C, Step 2: Elevate the rear portion of the top of the carrier so that the towel can slide in and cover the cat.

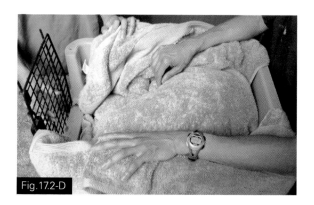
Fig.17.2-D

Fig.17.2-D, Step 3: Once the cat is covered, the top can be removed. Keep the gate in place until the cat's head is covered with the towel. Tuck the towel around the sides of the cat. Then lift the cat with the towel out of the carrier and onto a table (see Chapter 15, Section 15.7, Method 1).

17.3 Controlling Cats With Towels

Towels can often be used to help keep fearful cats calm. Some people use them to hold the cat still while he continues to struggle and scream, and even urinate and defecate. Cats who experience this type of treatment with or without a towel will be worse with each visit and might not be treatable in the near future. Usually, owned cats with repeated bad hospital experiences are more difficult to handle than feral cats. Always remember that the purpose of toweling is to keep the cat calm and prevent him from trying to struggle or escape. If this is not possible, then use chemical restraint. Refer to Chapter 15 for more information about toweling methods. *(Videos 1 and 2)*

Method 1

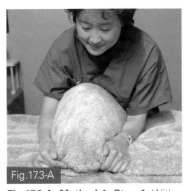
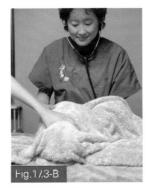
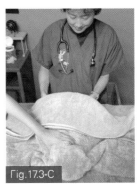

Fig.17.3-A, Method 1, Step 1: With a cat you've taken out of the carrier or cage using a towel, keep the towel on him once he's on the table. The towel covers the head, preventing the cat from bolting forward. Your arms on either side of the cat form a trough.

Fig.17.3-B, C, Method 1, Step 2: Often the cat can be examined from the back end with a technician just placing a hand on his neck to hold him in place. Now I can reach forward and auscultate the heart. I can also palpate the cat's abdomen and examine his rear end.

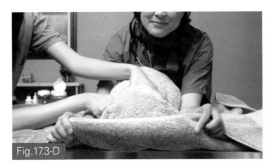
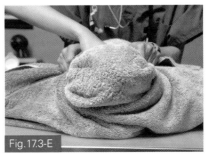

Fig.17.3-D, E, Method 1, Step 3: To examine the head, I use the lower towel in the first part of a half or reverse burrito wrap. The technician continues to put pressure on the cat's neck as I wrap the lower towel around it.

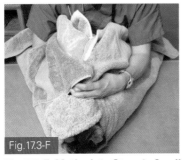
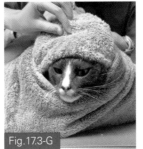
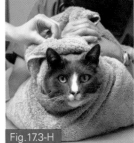

Fig.17.3-F, Method 1, Step 4: Scruff the lower (purple) towel to keep it tight around the cat.

Fig.17.3-G, H, Method 1, Step 5: Now the technician can pull the towels off the cat's head. Even with his head available for examination, he cannot escape out the front if I'm holding the towel firmly at the back of his neck.

With this wrap the cat's head can safely be examined

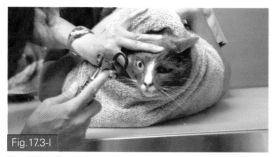

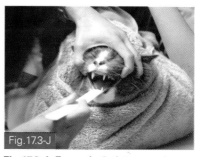

Fig.17.3-I, Example 1: The cat's eyes can be examined.

Fig.17.3-J, Example 2: A tongue depressor can be used to examine the mouth.

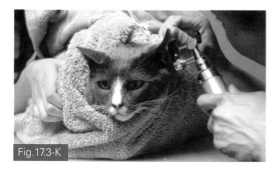

Fig.17.3-K, Example 3: If the cat is comfortable, the ears can also be examined. The technician is rotating the head slightly by pulling on one side of the towel.

Method 2

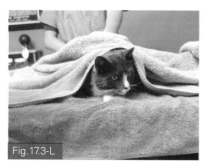

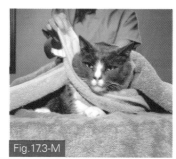

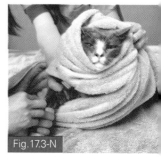

Fig.17.3-L, Method 2, Step 1: To place a catheter in the front leg, the towels must be adjusted. For an instant, there will be nothing in front of the cat. The technician still places pressure over the cat's neck to help prevent him from bolting.

Fig.17.3-M, Method 2, Step 2: Quickly wrap one end of the towel lying on the cat around the cat's neck. This is the first step of the scarf wrap.

Fig.17.3-N, Method 2, Step 3: Here the cat is in a completed scarf wrap. Now a catheter can be placed.

Method 3

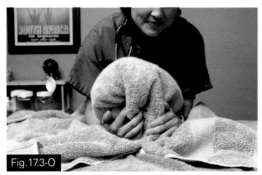

Fig.17.3-O

Fig.17.3-O, Method 3, Step 1: To perform a medial saphenous venipuncture or cystocentesis, the scarf wrap can be tucked over the rear end. However, in this case I'm using a blanket wrap instead.

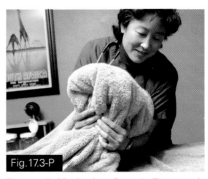

Fig.17.3-P

Fig.17.3-P, Method 3, Step 2: The towels are tucked over the top of the cat, and then he is laid on his side.

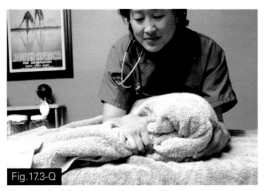

Fig.17.3-Q

Fig.17.3-Q, Method 3, Step 3: This particular cat is calm in the wrap, so the remainder of the towel does not need to be wrapped around him any further.

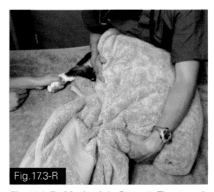

Fig.17.3-R

Fig.17.3-R, Method 3, Step 4: The towels can be bunched together to keep them snug, and the rear leg can be extended for medial saphenous venipuncture.

Method 4

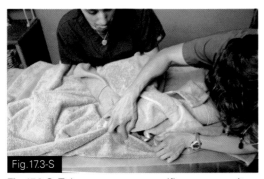

Fig.17.3-S

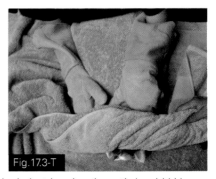

Fig.17.3-T

Fig.17.3-S, T: In many cases, specific wraps aren't required. Just keeping the cat's head hidden as much as possible works well. The technician can place pressure on the cat's shoulders and neck. If he is likely to bolt forward, the towel on the table can be wrapped around his chest and front legs.

Since the cat is calm the head can be examined

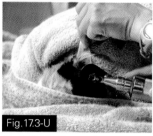

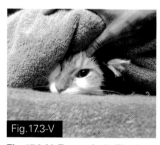

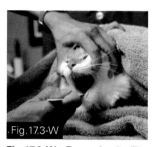

Fig.17.3-U, Example 1: Here, the towel is simply lifted to expose the ears while still covering the eyes.

Fig.17.3-V, Example 2: The lower towel can be moved out of the way to view the eyes.

Fig.17.3-W, Example 3: The mouth can be examined using a tongue depressor.

17.4 Using Muzzles Correctly

Using a muzzle does not give license to rough handling. The goal is to not only keep the handler safe, but also to keep the cat calm and prevent the cat from even attempting to bite. Several kinds of muzzles are available for use on cats. Use them if doing so keeps the cat calm. Use a different technique if the cat gets tense or agitated due to the muzzle.

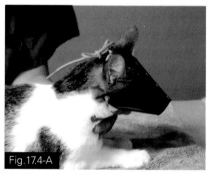

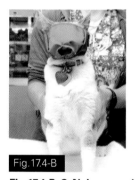

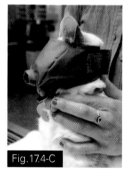

Fig.17.4-A, Cone Muzzle: The cone muzzle provides good protection from being bitten and is easy to put on safely while avoiding a bite.

Fig.17.4-B, C: Nylon muzzles aren't as easy to place as cone muzzles, and it can be difficult to see where the cat's mouth is. They can help calm the cat by covering the eyes.

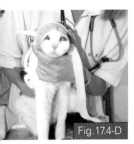
Fig.17.4-D

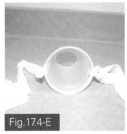
Fig.17.4-E

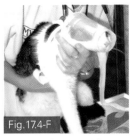
Fig.17.4-F

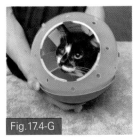
Fig.17.4-G

Fig.17.4-D, Makeshift muzzle: A muzzle can also be fashioned from a plastic or paper cup.

Fig.17.4-E, Makeshift muzzle, Step 1: Choose an appropriate size cup that will fit over the cat's head easily. Cut two holes, each near the rim on opposite sides. Use gauze wrap for the strap.

Fig.17.4-F, Makeshift muzzle, Step 2: The cup is easy to place over the cat's head, and it allows you to see where the mouth is. Tie the gauze wrap behind the cat's ears.

Fig.17.4-G, Air Muzzle: This muzzle works on some cats. It's especially helpful when combined with an attachment piece for use as a nebulizer.

17.5 Elizabethan Collars

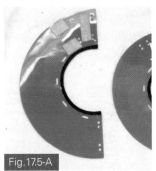
Fig.17.5-A

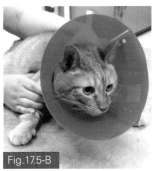
Fig.17.5-B

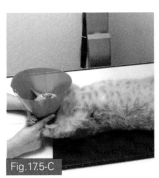
Fig.17.5-C

Fig.17.5-A, B, C: Elizabethan collars can also be used to protect the handlers. Use these collars if the particular cat allows you to easily place it. Velcro can be added to the collar so that it can be secured quickly. Some collars come with Velcro already applied. When wearing the collar, the cat can be restrained similar to the way a dog is, and all the rules that apply to restraint in these positions for dogs apply to cats too. (For example, in the photo above where the cat is on his back, most cats would be more comfortable if their legs were held together with their tibias parallel to the table, rather than stretched down onto the table. This would be indicated by how relaxed they are in the particular position.)

17.6 Capturing Escaped Cats

When cats escape, they can be captured using towels, nets or leashes. The use of a leash should be combined with the use of a towel; the blanket wrap (Chapter 15) is the most useful. Nets, if used, should be specifically designed for cats and small animals. The mesh must be small enough so that cats can't get their toes stuck in it and be injured.

17.6.1 Using the blanket wrap with a towel. *(Video 3)*

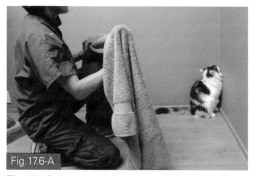

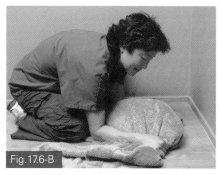

Fig.17.6-A: Use the blanket wrap described in Chapter 15 to capture cats in cages or corners.

Fig.17.6-B: You can use two towels or a towel plus gloves if you're concerned about being bitten. This technique requires practice.

17.6.2 Using the Snappy Snare in combination with a towel wrap.

This method works well for a cat planted at the back of his cage, and can also work for cats who have escaped and are hiding stationary under an object or high up. The Snappy Snare (available through Campbell Pet Company, Brush Prairie, Washington), an animal capturing device, helps move the cat forward so that he can be toweled and picked up. A slip lead can also be used, but the Snappy Snare is easier to remove and its loop is easily kept open.

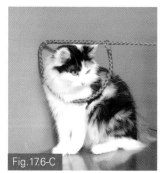

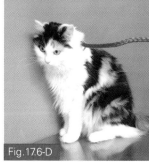

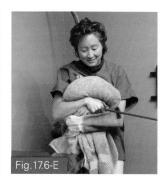

Fig.17.6-C, D: With the loop dangling, place the Snappy Snare over the cat's head and take up the slack by pulling the snare gently towards you. Then pull the cat into reach and place a towel over him.

Fig.17.6-E: Use the blanket wrap described in Chapter 15. (Section 15.7.1) Be sure to cover the cat immediately after capture, to help him calm down. This technique should be practiced prior to the emergency situation.

AVOID USING A SNAPPY SNARE LIKE THIS.

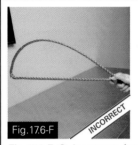

Fig. 17.6-F · INCORRECT

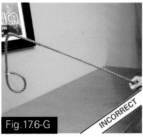

Fig. 17.6-G · INCORRECT

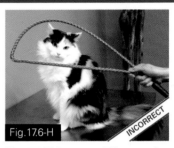

Fig. 17.6-H · INCORRECT

Fig. 17.6-F, G, Incorrect: Avoid using the Snappy Snare by pulling it open like a bow and then releasing it so that the loop suddenly gets small (snaps to a smaller size). When snapped without an animal in it, the loop immediately gets small. But this might not happen if snapped on a cat.

Fig. 17.6-H, Incorrect: When used on a cat, the snapping can scare him, or the metal ring—if it hits him—can sting. The sting is most likely to occur if the cat's neck sits along the flexed portion of the snare. Consider practicing first on a stuffed animal with the Snappy Snare.

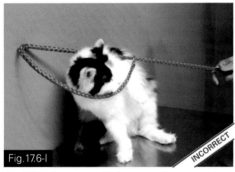

Fig. 17.6-I · INCORRECT

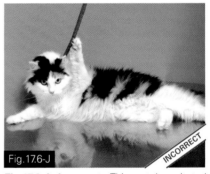

Fig. 17.6-J · INCORRECT

Fig. 17.6-I, Incorrect: If the snare is snapped on a cat, it tends to bounce off the cat and open up like so. So if you do use it you must be sure to start with the loop dangling loosely as depicted in **Fig. 17.6-C.**

Fig. 17.6-J, Incorrect: This cat is agitated from the snapping of the snare. If the cat bites the lead, it should be disinfected and may need to be disposed of, since thorough disinfecting can be difficult. The goal is to keep the cat from becoming so aroused or defensive that he bites the snare.

When to use a snappy snare.

This product is most appropriate for those cats who are huddled in the back of a cage or small space and are not easily reachable, but whom scruffing might make worse. Such cats could easily be toweled and then removed in a calm state. Avoid using this in cats that are attacking. These cats are better caught with a net or EZ Nabber because capture is faster and you are more likely to be able to calm them down faster.

17.6.3 Capturing with a net.

Net captures are primarily for capturing loose cats. Cats who hide under objects or in other small places can be gently encouraged to escape. Once they are out of hiding, they can be caught using the net.

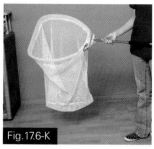
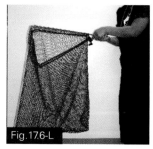
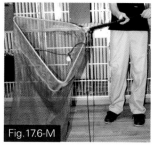

Fig.17.6-K

Fig.17.6-L

Fig.17.6-M

Fig.17.6-K, Versa-Net (Animal Capture Equipment, Inc., Bacliff, Texas, www.ace-cap.com): Commonly used in zoos, this lightweight, durable net has a flexible polycarbonate frame for maneuverability and to prevent accidental injury to the animal. The teardrop shape allows for the capture of animals in corners, against walls or running freely. The net is long enough that it can be flipped over the handle and squeezed down to immobilize the animal quickly. These nets come in many shapes and sizes, and can be custom designed based on your particular needs. *(Video 4)*

Fig.17.6-L, The Grab Bag (Campbell Pet Company, Bush Prairie, Washington): This triangular net is heavy and inflexible, but the short handle still makes it fairly easy to maneuver. The triangular shape makes it especially useful for capturing animals in corners or along walls. Once the animal is in the net, the metal frame can be slipped out and the drawstrings tightened. *(Video 5)*

Fig.17.6-M, The Extendable Capture Net (Campbell Pet Company): The amount of netting makes this heavy net bulky, too. The handle extends to 5 feet. Once the animal is captured, the drawstring can be pulled closed to prevent escape.

Netting technique: Practice netting before you have an emergency situation. A ball or other inanimate object can be used. If the cat is under furniture, encourage him to leave his spot and then net him or towel him in a corner. Don't try to grasp him with tongs that tighten around the neck, so that you have to drag him or lift him off the floor by his neck.

Exercise 1: Practice netting technique with a ball. Here, a Versa-Net is used.

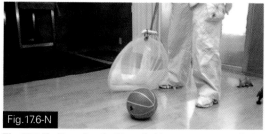
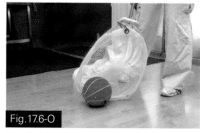

Fig.17.6-N

Fig.17.6-O

Fig.17.6-N, Exercise 1, Step 1: Have someone roll the ball toward the net that you're holding close to the floor.

Fig.17.6-O, Exercise 1, Step 2: As the ball gets close, scoop it up.

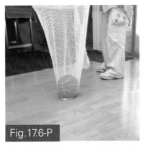

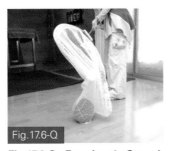

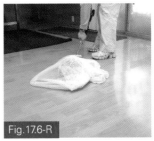

Fig.17.6-P, Exercise 1, Step 3: Immediately pull the net up around the ball.

Fig.17.6-Q, Exercise 1, Step 4: Twist the net on itself quickly; cats can climb out of nets in a split second.

Fig.17.6-R, Exercise 1, Step 5: Then lower the rim of the net over the ball to immobilize the ball.

Restraint once the animal is netted.

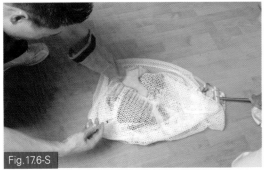

Fig.17.6-S: With a real cat captured securely in a net in the same way as the ball, it's at this point that you can inject a tranquilizer. Hold the cat down while you inject, because he might be able to wiggle a little in the net.

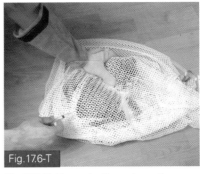

Fig.17.6-T: Use a leather glove, if necessary, to protect the restraining hand. It's important to complete the injection within a few seconds to reduce the arousal time.

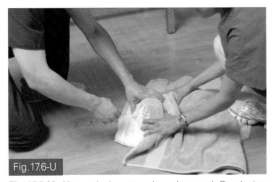

Fig.17.6-U: Alternatively, a towel can be used. By placing one foot on the handle or rim of the net, one technician can control the net and restrain the cat by placing pressure over the towel.

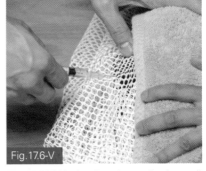

Fig.17.6-V: Notice that the netting is small enough that the cat cannot get his toes stuck, yet wide enough to easily inject through it.

Returning the cat to a cage or carrier.

Method 1

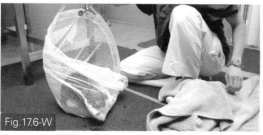

Fig.17.6-W, Method 1, Step 1: If you only need to get the cat back into a cage or carrier, raise the net and place a towel over the cat and the net.

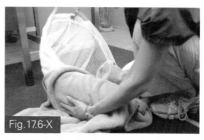

Fig.17.6-X, Method 1, Step 2: Carry the cat and net back to the carrier.

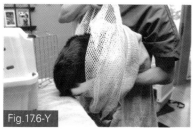

Fig.17.6-Y, Method 1, Step 3: Guide the cat into the carrier.

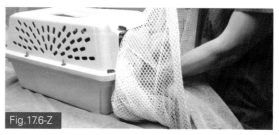

Fig.17.6-Z, Method 1, Step 4: Make sure he's all the way in before removing the net and towel and simultaneously closing the cage door.

Method 2

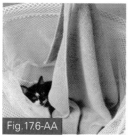

Fig.17.6-AA, Method 2, Step 1: Alternatively, drop a towel or two down into the net and onto the cat.

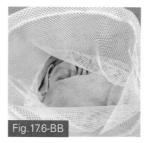

Fig.17.6-BB, Method 2, Step 2: Make sure the towel covers the cat.

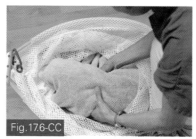

Fig.17.6-CC, Method 2, Step 3: Cover the cat's head and wrap the towel around his sides. Then lift him out and place him back in his cage, or perform the procedure or exam if the cat is calm enough.

17.6.4 Using an EZ Nabber to get cats out of cages.

Another type of net that can be useful is an EZ Nabber (Campbell Pet Company, Brush Prairie, Washington). This is most useful for getting cats out of their cages. Once captured, the net should be covered with a towel to decrease visual stimulation and thus decrease fear and arousal. The EZ Nabber can sometimes be used to capture cats out of corners, but it is not as versatile as the Versa-Net for this purpose. It's important to use the technique that can be performed the quickest and with the best skill, to keep the escaped animal from becoming even more agitated.

17.7 Equipment to Consider Avoiding

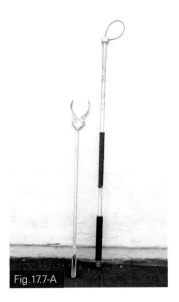

Fig.17.7-A

Fig.17.7-A: Avoid the rabies pole and the cat tongs. Rabies poles and cat tongs are often used without even considering one of the previously covered options. When cats are captured on such poles, lifted off the floor and then placed in a new location, they become extremely frightened and consequently, some can become extremely aroused and aggressive. This is not only a behavioral problem but a medical one too, especially in a shelter situation. When cats bite or scratch the pole, they can inoculate the pole with infectious organisms from their mouth. Also, the abrasions caused by the struggle can serve as portals through which infectious organisms embedded in the pole can infect these cats. Regular disinfection after this type of damage to the pole may not be adequate. In fact, in one case of necrotizing Staphylococccus canis outbreak affecting an animal shelter in California, the room affected was depopulated twice and the infections still came back. The source of reinfection was found to be a rabies pole that had been disinfected regularly, according to Kate Hurley, DVM, director of the shelter medicine program at University of California-Davis (Yin, in press).

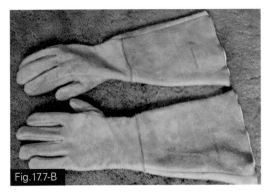

Fig.17.7-B

Fig.17.7-B: Limit the use of the leather gloves. Alone, leather gloves are usually insufficient because they don't prevent the cat from struggling or flailing. If used, they should be used in conjunction with one of the other techniques, such as toweling or netting, in which the animals' body is controlled and better supported. Another problem with leather gloves is that they cannot be easily disinfected.

17.8 Using Chemical Restraint

Chemical restraint should be used before the cat becomes highly aroused, or else a higher dose might be required and the drugs will have a more variable effect.

17.8.1 Mild restraint or sedation, such as for premedication or catheterization.

Acepromazine is most suitable for use in young and middle-aged healthy cats.

Combination	Acepromazine (IM or SQ)	Opioid (IM or SQ)
Acepromazine/oxymorphone	0.05 mg/kg	0.05 mg/kg oxymorphone
Acepromazine/butorphanol	0.05 mg/kg	0.2 mg/kg butorphanol
Acepromazine/buprenorphine	0.05 mg/kg	0.01 mg/kg buprenorphine

Midazolam is more suitable in older cats because it is less of a cardiovascular depressant.

Combination	Midazolam (IM or SQ)	Opioid (IM or SQ)
Midazolam/oxymorphone	0.2 mg/kg	0.05 mg/kg oxymorphone
Midazolam/butorphanol	0.2 mg/kg	0.2 mg/kg butorphanol
Midazolam/buprenorphine	0.2 mg/kg	0.01 mg/kg buprenorphine

Owners can also give alprazolam to cats orally before the pet comes in to the veterinary hospital. A test does should be given several days before the veterinary visit to ensure that the drug has the intended effect.

17.8.2 Mild restraint and skin analgesia.

Buprenorphine, a partial mu opioid agonist, can be administered at 20μ/kg oral, transmucosally (OTM) using a 1 mL TB syringe. When given OTM or IV, it has a peak effect at 90 minutes and this effect lasts up to 6 hours (Robertson et al. 2005). Cats given buprenorphine OTM in Robertson's study accepted the oral administration, did not salivate or vomit and were easy to handle after drug administration. They also showed signs of euphoria—increased purring, rubbing against handlers in the cage and kneading with their forepaws. All the cats ate food when it was offered. Buprenorphine might be indicated in cases where the cat is sensitive to injection, such as for venipuncture, or when a sensitive area of skin must be clipped.

17.8.3 Stronger restraint.

Combination	Dose
Ketamine (oral)	100-200 mg orally, sprayed into the mouth (avoid the eyes). This will cause transient excessive drooling. Only use this for cats whom you cannot inject.
Telazol (tiletamine/zolazepam) (IM)	2.0-3.0 mg/kg. Telazol can be associated with prolonged recovery time, especially on repeated dosing.
Ketamine/midazolam (IM)	Ketamine: 3.0-10.0 mg/kg Midazolam: 2.0 mg/kg
Ketamine/acepromazine (IM)	Ketamine: 3.0-10.0 mg/kg Acepromazine: 0.1 mg/kg
Medetomidine (Domitor) (IM)	Medetomidine: 0.01-0.02 mg/kg. In general, use this only in young, healthy cats.

Difficult cats can also be anesthetized through box induction. This should occur before they have become aroused or aggressive.

17.9 Keeping Owners Informed

If special techniques are needed because the cat is aggressive or fearful, a note regarding which handling techniques were successful should be placed in the records and only the most skilled staff should perform treatments or procedures. Additionally just as you would talk to an owner about a health issue discovered as an incidental finding, the behavioral issue should also be brought to the owner's attention and treatment offered. The owner should be told that the cat is likely to become increasingly difficult to treat, to the point where eventually he may no longer be able to receive medical attention. Clients should be given the options of applying simple counterconditioning protocols that they can do at home (see Chapter 20 and visit the readers-only resources at www.nerdbook.com/lowstresshandling for client handouts as well as client consent form), scheduling a technician behavior modification session, or seeing a veterinary behaviorist or veterinarian with a special interest in behavior.

> A note regarding which handling techniques were successful should be placed in the records and only the most skilled staff should perform treatments or procedures. Additionally owners should be informed of the situation and behavioral treatment offered.

References

Bednarski, R.M. 2007. "Dogs and Cats." In *Lumb & Jones Veterinary Anesthesia and Analgesia, 4th ed.*, edited by W. J. Tranquilli, J. C. Thurmon, and K. A. Grimm. Ames, Iowa: Blackwell Publishing. Pp. 705-16.

Griffith, C.A., E.S. Steigerwald, and C.A.T. Buffington. 2000. Effects of a synthetic facial pheromone on behavior of cats. *Journal of the American Veterinary Medical Association* 217:1154-56.

Kronen, P.W., J.W. Ludders, H.N. Erb, P.F. Moon, R.D. Gleed, and S. Koski. 2006. A synthetic fraction of feline facial pheromones calms but does not reduce struggling in cats before venous catheterization. *Veterinary Anaesthesia and Analgesia* 33:258-65.

Landsberg, G. 2006. "Why practitioners should feel comfortable with pheromones—The evidence to support pheromone use." Presented at *Small Animal and Exotics: Proceedings of the North American Veterinary Conference*. Orlando, Florida, January 7, 2006.

Robertson, S.A., B.D.X. Lascelles, P.M. Taylor, and J.W. Sear. 2005. PK-PD modeling of buprenorphine in cats: Intravenous and oral transmucosal administration. *Journal of Veterinary Pharmacology and Therapeutics* 28:453-460.

Yin, S. (In press). Necrotizing streptococcal infection. *Veterinary Forum*

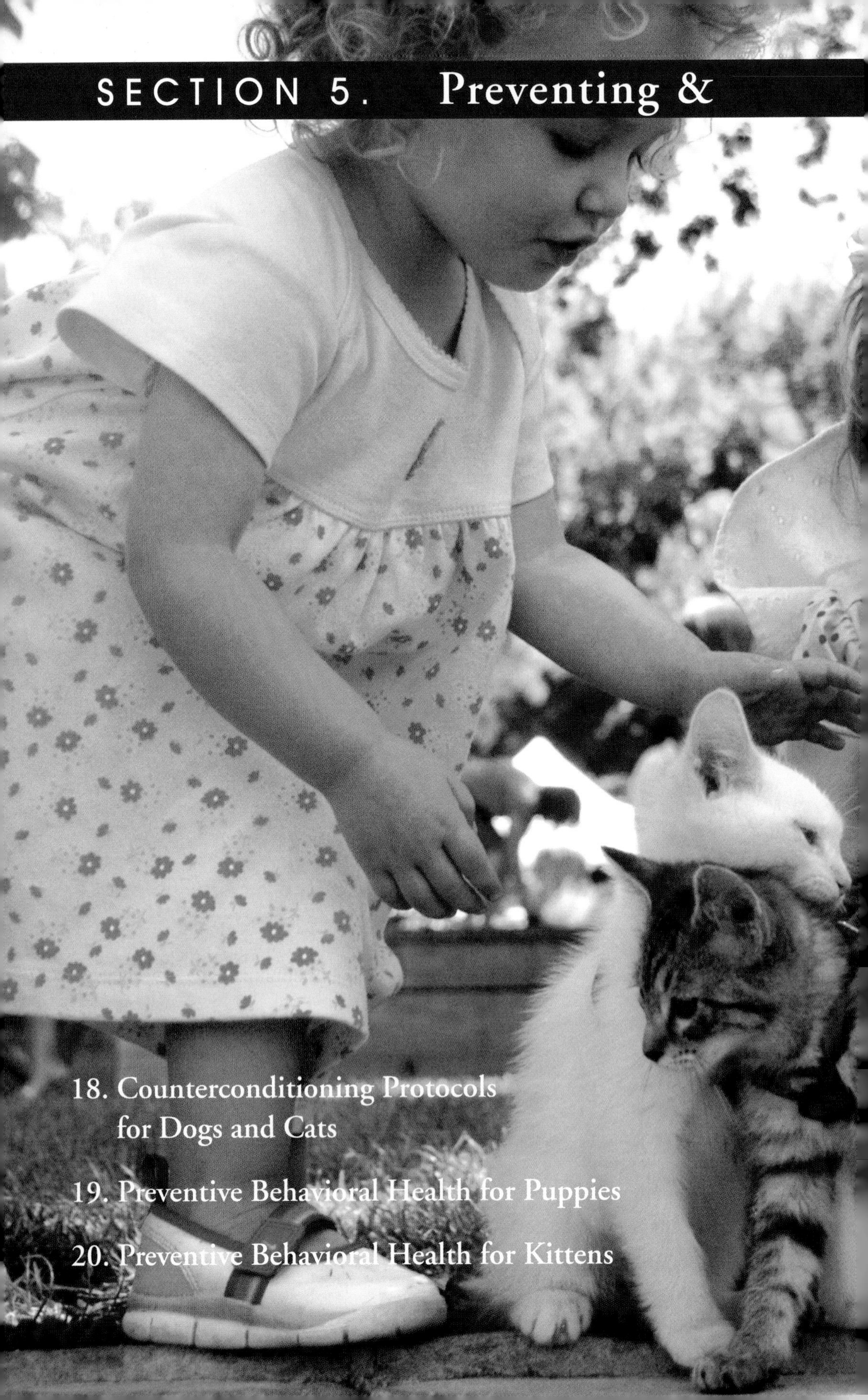

SECTION 5. Preventing &

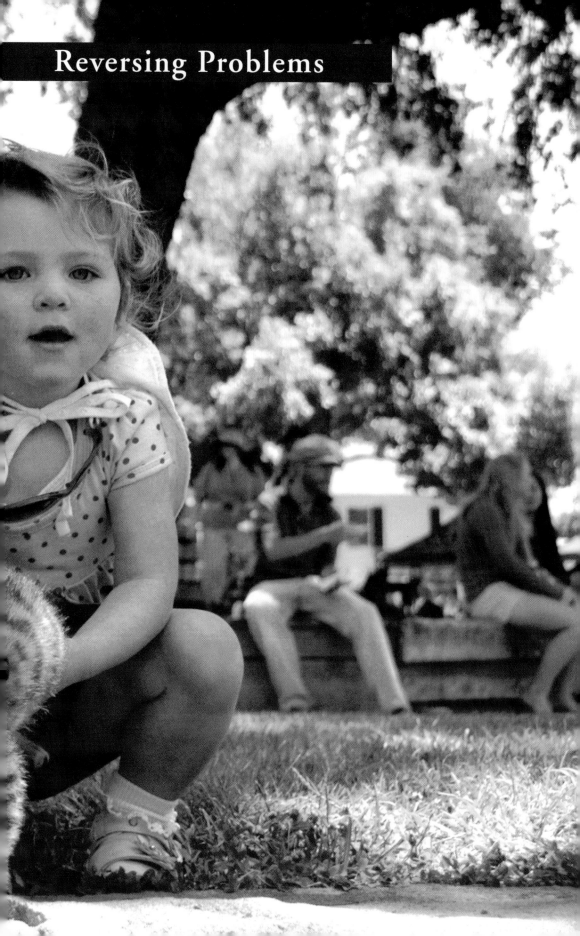

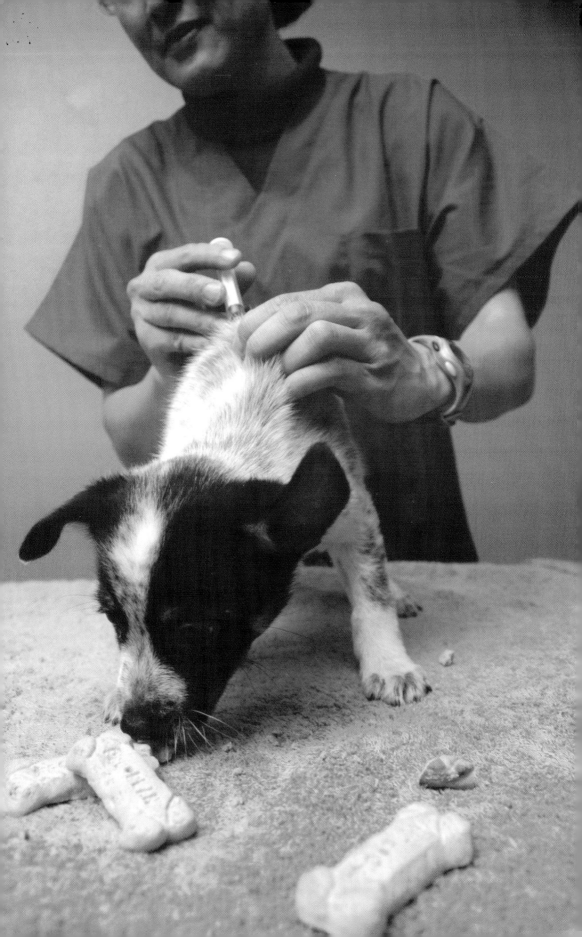

CHAPTER 18. COUNTER-CONDITIONING PROTOCOLS
for Dogs and Cats

"Technician to room 1," you hear over the intercom. A technician disappears into the exam room. A minute later you hear screaming. "Aeehaahehhaahhe." It stops for a moment, then starts and then stops. Several minutes later you hear the intercom again, "Technician to room 1," and a second technician enters the exam room. "Aeehaaehhaa" the screams pierce through the entire hospital. After several seconds, the exam door opens and out comes a veterinarian carrying a Dachshund pawing at her muzzle. The entourage of hospital staff walk past the pharmacy area into the treatment room, where they are joined by yet another technician. Now there's one person to sit

on the dog's back end, one to sit on the front, and one to hold her legs out while the veterinarian trims her toenails. "Aeehaaheeaheh," the screams put everyone on edge until the procedure is finally over. The veterinarian removes the muzzle and reaches to comfort the Dachshund, but the once happy dog now only stares warily at the muzzle and the vet's hand. The entire ordeal has taken 10 to 15 minutes, three technicians, and one veterinarian. And in the process, it's raised the blood pressure of the entire staff, the patients and even the clients sitting in the waiting room.

Many veterinarians and technicians avoid desensitization and counterconditioning (DS and CC) because they think they don't have time. In reality, force often takes more time and manpower, and this extra effort is often not covered in the treatment fee. Desensitization and counterconditioning, on the other hand, can often be done with the help of the owner and may take as little as several minutes. Additionally, DS and CC will save time and manpower at future visits and can be offered as a valued service.

18.1 Veterinarian-Supervised Technician Behavior Modification Sessions

When handling problems are identified during an office visit, clients should be informed of the issues and offered appropriate solutions. Owners need not automatically be sent to one of the few veterinary or Ph.D. behaviorists in practice. Early on, the problems can be addressed in technician counterconditioning (CC) sessions. Even if the client seeks a consult with a veterinary behaviorist, a behavior modification program for training pets to be manageable in the hospital will still require the cooperation and help of the pet's regular veterinarian.

Hospitals can run several types of veterinarian-supervised technician behavior modification sessions, as described below. Pricing should be based partly on the cost of the technician's time.

18.1.1 Session type 1: Counterconditioning pets to the hospital, the technicians and the veterinarian.

Many pets are afraid of the hospital, the technicians, the noises and the veterinarian. In most cases with dogs, the diet can be altered so that the dog is food-motivated in the hospital, which helps CC to be successfully performed there. This involves tossing treats continuously to a dog who is extremely fearful and knowing how to approach the dog correctly. Once a dog is more comfortable, the technician can CC her to being touched (refer to Chapter 5, Videos 6 and 7, and Chapter 14, Videos 2 and 7). Sessions should last about 15 to 30 minutes.

To make sure the owner perceives the value of these sessions, rather than viewing them just as treat-tossing, the technician must explain what she's doing and why at all times. During the sessions, owners should also be taught to recognize signs of fear and anxiety in their pets (Chapter 1), why their pets act fearfully or aggressively to people (Chapter 1) and how to keep well-meaning people from greeting or approaching their dogs incorrectly, worsening the dogs' fears (Chapters 1 and 9). Remember that the goal is to get the animals into a happy state; thus, both food and play can be used. In fact, dogs and cats can be trained to perform tricks such as targeting (Chapter 20).

Cats can also be counterconditioned in the hospital, if properly prepared, or at least clients can learn what to do at home. The technician can counsel the owners about training the cat to enjoy her carrier and car rides and can discuss strategies to keep the cat calm. Video clips from the DVD accompanying this book can also be shown to owners.

18.1.2 Session type 2: Counterconditioning pets to specific handling situations.

Owners can be taught how to CC the pet to each handling problem the animal has. It's best to work on just one or two problems in each session. For pets who are too nervous to eat during the in-office CC session, owners can practice the timing of the techniques on a stuffed animal. Demonstrating and then having the owners perform the technique is vital so that they get the timing right, read the pet's body language correctly and expose the pet to the stimulus at the right level. Generally, if you do not have the owner physically practice techniques while you watch, they will perform them incorrectly or ineffectively. Usually such handling will start with classical counterconditioning and progress to operant counterconditioning (Chapters 3 and 4, respectively).

> Generally, if you do not have the owner physically practice techniques while you watch, they will perform them incorrectly or ineffectively.

18.1.3 Session type 3: Teaching pets to perform calm and focused behaviors.

With both cats and dogs, I usually start with an automatic sit. I then progress to targeting (touching an object with their nose). Both behaviors can be used as an alternate desirable behavior to replace undesirable ones.

If the technician determines that progress is happening too slowly or is unsure how to proceed, the pet can always be referred to a specialist.

> If the technician determines that progress is happening too slowly or is unsure how to proceed, the pet can always be referred to a specialist.

18.2 Counterconditioning Dogs to the Gentle Leader

Note that introducing cats to a harness is similar and is explained in Chapter 20.

18.2.1 Begin classically counter-conditioning the dog to the Gentle Leader (GL). *(Video 1)*

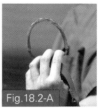 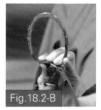

Fig.18.2-A, B, Step 1: Grasp the GL at the bottom of the nose loop in a manner that keeps it open.

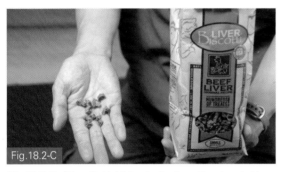

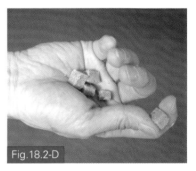

Fig.18.2-C, Step 2: Hold treats in the other hand. Have enough treats to occupy the dog for at least 3 seconds. One option is to use many small treats or kibble. Hold on to each treat so that the dog has to chew or lick it for a second or 2 before he takes it and so that you can dispense the treat in a controlled manner. For the tiny liver biscotti pictured above, if used with a large dog you can hold them as pictured here instead of presenting them individually.

Fig.18.2-D, Step 2: By holding the treats in the manner shown here, you can immediately follow one treat with another by rolling treats from the palm of your hand to your thumb and index finger. These are Natural Balance semi-moist food rolls cut into bite-size treats.

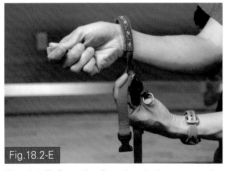

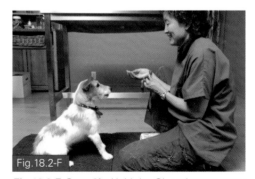

Fig.18.2-E, Step 3a: Start by placing your entire hand through the GL while holding the treats.

Fig.18.2-F, Step 3b: Hold the GL and treats away from the dog so that he does not try to jump on or nose you to get the treats.

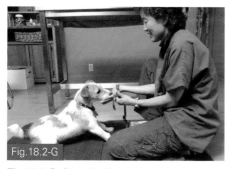 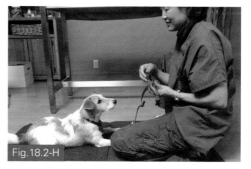

Fig.18.2-G, Step 3c: Then place the treats close to the dog's nose but far enough forward so that he has to reach to get them. He should immediately reach forward to eat them. It's important that he move forward to get them so that you can tell that it's his choice to come closer. If he looks wary of the GL, remove your hand and start again but this time with the GL farther up your arm.

Fig.18.2-H, Step 3d: Once he's finished the treat, immediately retract your hand and the GL so that he starts to understand that he loses the opportunity to receive treats when the GL is not close by. When the dog immediately takes treats in this manner 5 times in a row, continue to the next step.

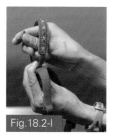 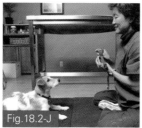 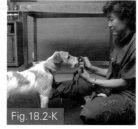 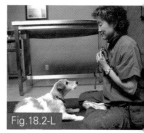

Fig.18.2-I, Step 4a: Extend the treat a shorter distance through the GL.

Fig.18.2-J, Step 4b: Again, start by holding the treat and GL out of the dog's reach so that you control his access to the treats.

Fig.18.2-K, Step 4c: Then place both within reach and let the dog move forward to eat the treat. Do not try to push the GL onto the dog's nose; just hold it steady.

Fig.18.2-L, Step 4d: As the dog finishes the treats, move the GL out of reach so that you're in control of the situation. When the dog takes treats without hesitation 5 or more times in a row, move on to the next step.

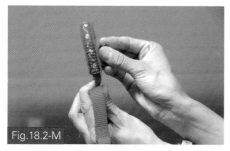 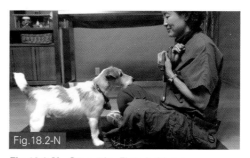

Fig.18.2-M, Step 5a: Now hold the treat right in the loop of the GL.

Fig.18.2-N, Step 5b: First hold the treats and GL away from the dog so that he must stand calmly.

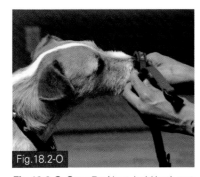

Fig.18.2-O, Step 5c: Next, hold both out so that the dog leans forward through the GL loop to eat the treats.

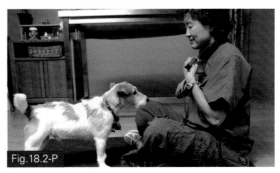

Fig.18.2-P, Step 5d: Retract your hand and the GL as the dog is finishing the last treat, so that he doesn't have the chance to pull his head away. Never let him do that; always move the GL and treats away before that can happen so you don't train the dog to pull his head away.

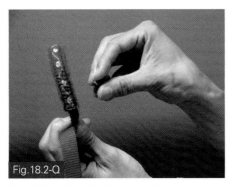

Fig.18.2-Q, Step 6a: Now hold the treat behind the loop so that the dog must stick his nose through it to get the food.

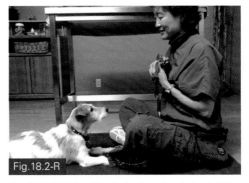

Fig.18.2-R, Step 6b: As before, begin by holding both the treat and the GL away from the dog.

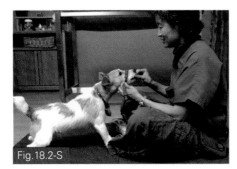

Fig.18.2-S, Step 6c: Then extend both toward him so that the dog pushes his nose through the loop to get the treat.

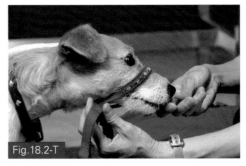

Fig.18.2-T, Step 6d: Be sure to hold the GL steady so that the dog can push his nose through. You want the dog to learn to shove his nose through against the pressure of the loop.

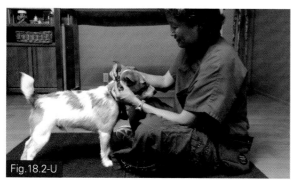

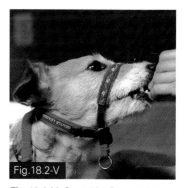

Fig.18.2-U, Step 7a: When the dog readily pushes his nose through several times in a row and looks completely comfortable doing so, snap the GL closed behind his ears. For dogs who have a history of hating the GL, you should keep repeating Step 6 until he's been putting his head in comfortably for at least several consecutive sessions. Or, for safety purposes, work on the operant counterconditioning steps in the next section prior to putting the GL on.

Fig.18.2-V, Step 7b: Give additional treats to keep him distracted and to continue building a positive association. Take off the GL before the dog is irritated or distracted by it.

18.2.2 Switch from classical to operant counterconditioning.

Perform these additional steps with dogs who already have an aversion to things being placed around their muzzle. These steps will ensure that they enjoy wearing the GL.

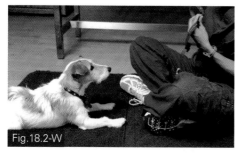

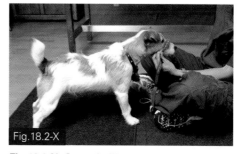

Fig.18.2-W, Step 1a: Once the dog is comfortable having you put on the GL with treats present, wean him off the treats by first switching to operant counterconditioning. As always, hold the GL away from the dog at first.

Fig.18.2-X, Step 1b: Then present the GL without treats. If the dog is ready for this step, he'll immediately stick his nose through the loop. This indicates his understanding of the association between the GL and treats.

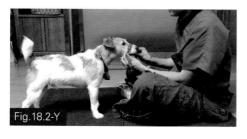

Fig.18.2-Y, Step 1c: Once he shoves his nose through, immediately reward him with treats. Then remove the GL and repeat.

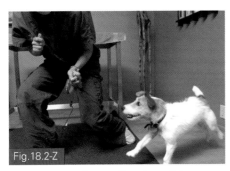 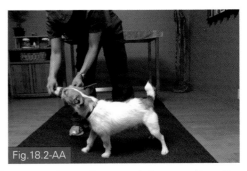

Fig.18.2-Z, AA, Step 2: Turn the training process into a game by running several steps away from the dog with the GL in your hand and then placing it within reach of the dog. The dog should rush after you to push his nose into the loop. When he does, reward him with treats. When he consistently runs after the GL and sticks his nose in, then you can put the GL on.

18.2.3 Potential problems

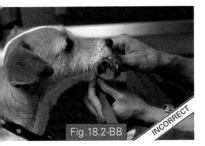 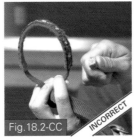 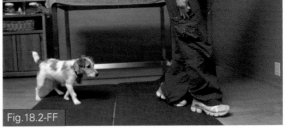

Fig.18.2-BB, Example 1a, Incorrect: The dog has shoved his nose over the GL and pushed it aside to get the treat.

Fig.18.2-CC, Example 1b, Incorrect: This occurred because the treat was placed too far to the side.

Fig.18.2-DD, Example 1c, Correct: Be sure to place the treat in the center and hold the GL steady so that the dog can get his muzzle through the loop.

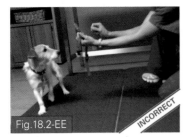 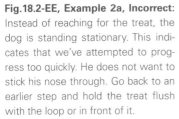

Fig.18.2-EE, Example 2a, Incorrect: Instead of reaching for the treat, the dog is standing stationary. This indicates that we've attempted to progress too quickly. He does not want to stick his nose through. Go back to an earlier step and hold the treat flush with the loop or in front of it.

Fig.18.2-FF, Example 2b, Correct: If you make the mistake of trying too much too soon, remove the GL and treats, and next time present the treats in such a way that the dog doesn't need to extend his nose through the loop as far. Additionally, you can walk away so that it's clear to the dog that he loses the opportunity to earn treats. You can even have a play session before starting the training session again to get him into a happy emotional state.

18.3 Counterconditioning Dogs and Cats to a Muzzle *(Video 2)*

The same method described here can be used with cats.

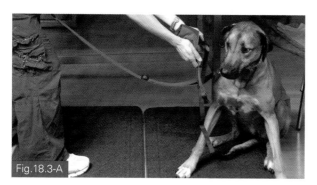

Fig.18.3-A: If a dog responds to a muzzle by pulling her head away, she should be trained to associate the muzzle with good things before muzzling becomes essential.

18.3.1 Begin classically counterconditioning the dog to the muzzle.

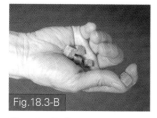
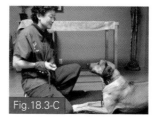
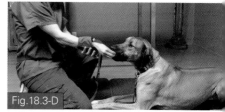

Fig.18.3-B, Step 1a: Start by holding multiple treats in one hand. By holding treats in this manner, they can be delivered consecutively while the dog's nose is through the muzzle.

Fig.18.3-C, Step 1b: Place your hand through the muzzle and away from the dog. The dog should be paying attention to you because you've already given treats and she knows you have more.

Fig.18.3-D, Step 1c: Put your hand forward and let the dog reach out her head to your hand. You should not push your hand and treat into her mouth, because dogs who dislike the muzzle may consider this a threat. It's essential that the dog reach forward to get the treat. Give her several treats continuously so that her nose is always on your hand.

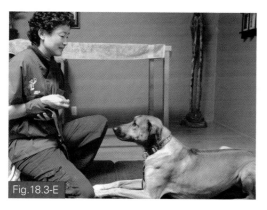

Fig.18.3-E, Step 1d: When she's finished with the treats, remove your hand and the muzzle before she has a chance to move her head away. You want it to be clear that you are taking the muzzle away from her rather than giving her the chance to move away from it. Disappearance of the muzzle equals disappearance of the treats. Repeat this step until she immediately reaches for and eats the treats 5-10 times in a row. Then repeat with a higher stimulus level; in other words, with the muzzle placed farther down on your hand.

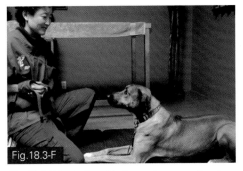

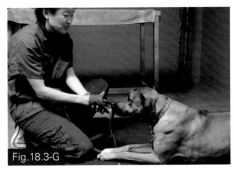

Fig.18.3-F, Step 2a: This time, place your hand so it protrudes halfway through the muzzle. Start by holding the muzzle out of reach. Note that if you can't fit your hand through the muzzle, just place the first two fingers through, use long treats such as jerky or pupperoni treats or use canned food on a spoon.

Fig.18.3-G, Step 2b: Present the muzzle and let her reach forward to grab the string of treats. She should be eating without hesitation. Note that here she's leaning forward as I bring the muzzle up to her. If the dog isn't leaning forward, pull the muzzle back to your body and repeat the process with your hand extended farther through the muzzle.

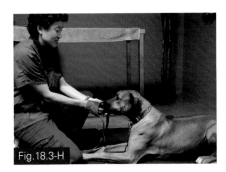

Fig.18.3-H, Step 2c: Now this dog readily takes the treat with my hand extended only slightly through the muzzle. Keep her eating for 3-10 seconds and then remove your hand and the muzzle and repeat the step. In general, stay at each step for 5-10 food trials (presentations of the string of treats). When she's successful 5-10 consecutive times, increase your expectations slightly. When moving to the next step, if the dog's response ever indicates that she does not want to immediately take treats, go back a step and repeat.

Box 18-A: Potential problem.

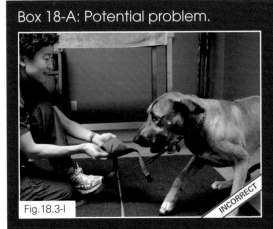

Fig.18.3-I, Incorrect: Avoid pushing the muzzle forward if the dog doesn't immediately reach for the treats. And don't try to slip the muzzle on farther once the dog is eating the treats. Trying to progress too quickly can cause the dog to be scared and move away (i.e., the stimulus level is too high). This will set the process back a few steps, because now she will be less trusting of you. Always stay below the dog's stimulus threshold—the point at which she will react aversely.

Box 18-B: Tips for counterconditioning to muzzles

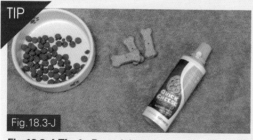

Fig.18.3-J

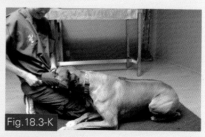

Fig.18.3-K

Fig.18.3-J, Tip 1: For training, you can use either the dog's meal or treats.

Fig.18.3-K, Tip 2: The dog should always reach forward to get the treat, as in this photo. She should look as if she doesn't even notice that a muzzle is present. Your goal should always be that the dog shows no adverse response—no withdrawal or hesitation to eat. She should act as though there is no scary stimulus present. If she hesitates, that means the stimulus level is too high and you need to back down to a previous step or somehow lower the stimulus level (e.g., by moving the muzzle farther back on your hand).

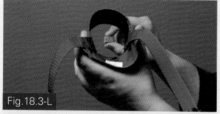

Fig.18.3-L

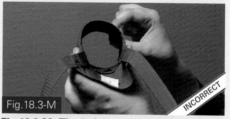

Fig.18.3-M

Fig.18.3-L, Tip 3, Correct: Where I hold the treat in relation to the muzzle determines where the dog's head is. Take care to hold the treat in the center so that she sticks her nose through the muzzle to get it.

Fig.18.3-M, Tip 3, Incorrect: In this case, the treat is too far from the center. The dog must reach around the outside of the muzzle to get it.

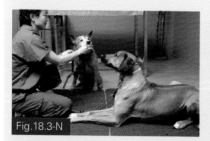

Fig.18.3-N

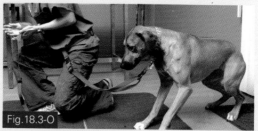

Fig.18.3-O

Fig.18.3-N, Tip 4: If the dog appears unmotivated or is not paying attention, try increasing the value of the food by feeding treats to another dog in front of the one you're training. Or, walk away so she knows she's losing the opportunity to get the food. Then try again.

Fig.18.3-O, Tip 5: Walk away or move to a different part of the room with each trial or each new step. If the dog is motivated by the treats, she should follow you.

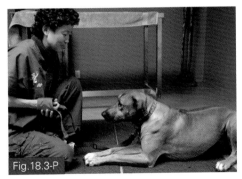

Fig.18.3-P, Step 3a: This time, place your hand so it barely protrudes through the muzzle. Start by holding the muzzle out of reach.

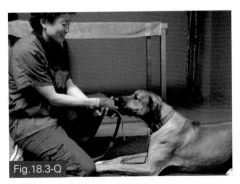

Fig.18.3-Q, Step 3b: Again, she should immediately reach for and take the treats when you present the muzzle.

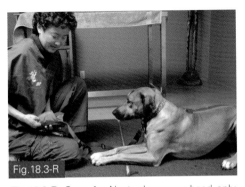

Fig.18.3-R, Step 4a: Next, place your hand only partway through the muzzle so that the dog has to stick her nose through a portion of the muzzle to get the treat.

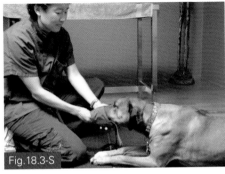

Fig.18.3-S, Step 4b: Remember to give treats continuously so that she does not have a chance to move her head away. If there's a gap in treats, she's likely to move.

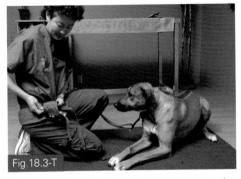

Fig.18.3-T, Step 5a: Next, place the treat at the far end of the muzzle so that she has to stick her nose all the way through it.

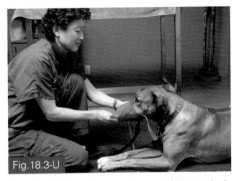

Fig.18.3-U, Step 5b: The dog should assertively push her head into the muzzle (even jam it in) to get the treat.

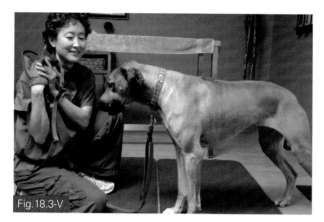

Fig.18.3-V: At this stage, when I remove the treats and muzzle, this dog gets up to follow my hand and try to grab more treats. This is a good sign; however, I still want the process to be under my control, so I'll move both the treats and muzzle far enough away that she understands she can't get them. When she's waiting patiently again, I will re-present the muzzle.

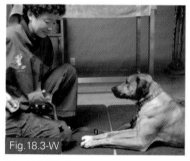

Fig.18.3-W, Step 6a: Now I can hold the treats far outside the muzzle and know that the dog will stick her nose in to get them.

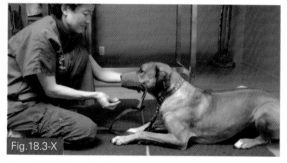

Fig.18.3-X, Step 6b: She understands that putting her nose into the muzzle predicts that she will get treats. I'm still showing her the treat first, but later I'll just show her the muzzle and then give her the treat afterwards. In this way, we move from classical conditioning (association of the treat with the muzzle) to operant conditioning (rewarding a desired behavior with the treat).

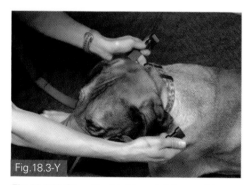

Fig.18.3-Y, Step 7a: At this point I can slide my hands down the straps and snap the muzzle on.

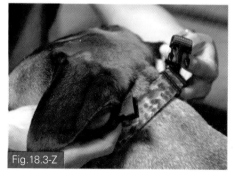

Fig.18.3-Z, Step 7b: Simultaneously grasp the collar with one hand so that the dog has no opportunity to back out.

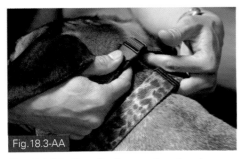

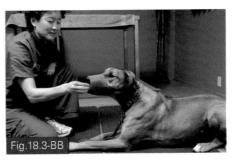

Fig.18.3-AA, Step 7c: Be sure there's only room for one finger under the muzzle strap.

Fig.18.3-BB, Step 7d: Once the muzzle is on, continue giving the dog treats to distract her.

18.3.2 Switching to operant counterconditioning. Dogs who have shown a strong aversion to the muzzle should go through this stage before the muzzle is put on.

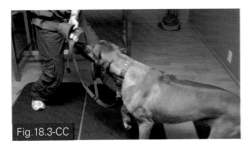

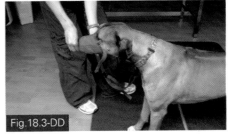

Fig.18.3-CC, Step 1: Now this dog likes the muzzle and I can make this process into a game. Here, I run backward with the muzzle and she chases after it to insert her nose into it.

Fig.18.3-DD, Step 2: Once her nose is inserted, I reward her with a treat. Repeat this procedure to reinforce the behavior and to strengthen the positive association with the muzzle.

Box 18-C: Placing the muzzle while simultaneously giving treats.
In some cases it's safer to place the muzzle while simultaneously giving treats. It's best to do this in a way that prevents the dog from backing out of the muzzle.

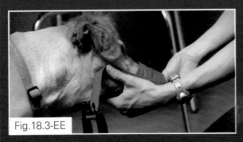

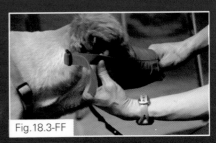

Fig.18.3-EE, Step 1: First be sure that the dog's nose is all the way through the muzzle.

Fig.18.3-FF, Step 2: Then guide one hand up the strap.

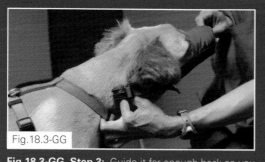

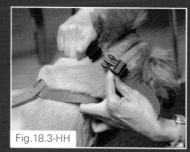

Fig.18.3-GG, Step 3: Guide it far enough back so you can grasp the dog's harness or collar. Once you have done so, the dog cannot back out of the muzzle.

Fig.18.3-HH, Step 4: Then use both hands to snap the muzzle on.

18.4 Counterconditioning Dogs and Cats to Toothbrushing

The steps shown below can be used with both dogs and cats.

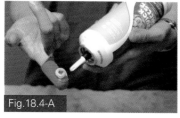

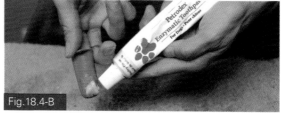

Fig.18.4-A, Step 1a: Place something tasty, such as canned cheese or Kong Stuff'N liver or peanut butter paste (The Kong Company, Golden, Colorado) onto a pet toothbrush.

Fig.18.4-B, Step 1b: Or use a tasty pet toothpaste. The toothpaste should be formulated just for pets. It has enzymes that degrade the bacteria on the teeth and is safe for pets to swallow. Regular toothpaste for humans is not meant to be swallowed and could cause an upset stomach.

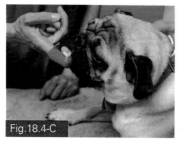

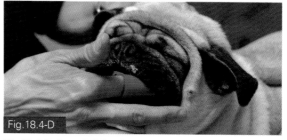

Fig.18.4-C, Step 2: Hold the toothpaste-smeared toothbrush to the dog's mouth to let him lick off the treat. If he likes it, you can reload and then move on to brushing his teeth.

Fig.18.4-D, Step 3: With the treat or toothpaste on the brush, insert the brush just inside his lips so that you can brush the outside of his teeth. Be careful not to insert your finger between his upper and lower tooth and accidentally get bitten. If done correctly, dogs (and cats) should look forward to their daily brushings.

18.5 Counterconditioning Cats to Pilling *(Video 3)*

To see this procedure for dogs, refer to Chapter 13 (Section 13.3).

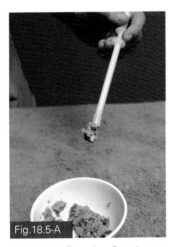

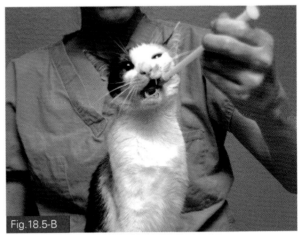

Fig.18.5-A, Step 1a: Start by putting treats (or wet food) in the pill gun and letting the cat eat from it.

Fig.18.5-B, Step 1b: When the cat consistently looks at the pill gun as if she is expecting a treat, continue to the next step.

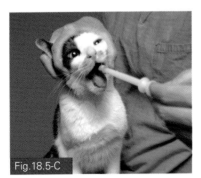

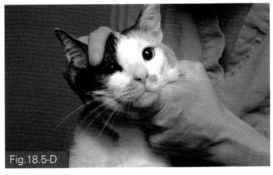

Fig.18.5-C, Step 2: Physically hold the cat's head up so she learns that restraint in this manner predicts a treat is coming. Place the pill gun in her mouth and deposit the treat or canned food.

Fig.18.5-D, Step 3: Immediately close the mouth and control the head. Repeat the process until it's clear she has a positive association with the restraint and pill gun. When you use an actual pill, open the mouth, place the pill in, close the mouth and immediately follow with a treat. The pill can be covered in canned food or baby food if needed.

18.6 Counterconditioning Dogs and Cats to Grooming.

Note that the process is the same whether you're brushing the pet or trimming the hair with clippers.

18.6.1 Start with classical counterconditioning

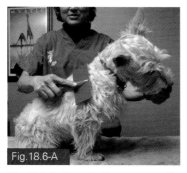

Fig.18.6-A, Step 1: Groom a specific location or at a specific level of pressure, with the dog's mouth physically on your hand eating treats the entire time. Feed enough kibble or treats to last about 5 seconds at first.

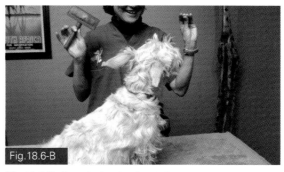

Fig.18.6-B, Step 2: As the dog is finishing the last treat (or kibble), remove both the brush and the treat hand so that it's clear that both the treats and the grooming are no longer accessible. Repeat this procedure until the dog is comfortable being groomed in this region of the body at this level of pressure at least 5 times in succession.

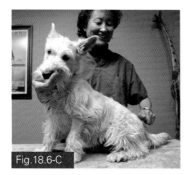

Fig.18.6-C, Step 3: Next, groom a different area starting with light pressure, or groom the same area with heavier pressure.

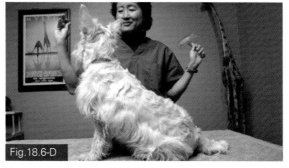

Fig.18.6-D, Step 4: Again, stop the treats and the grooming at the same time. In this manner, gradually increase the intensity or pressure of the grooming and slowly move to different areas of the body. You should be able to groom fairly vigorously as long as you never cross the dog's stimulus threshold.

18.6.2 Switch to operant counterconditioning

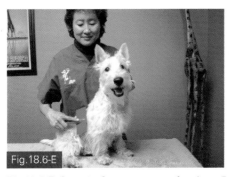

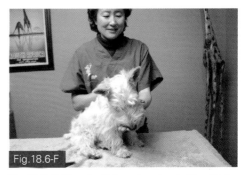

Fig.18.6-E, Step 1: Groom one area for about 5 seconds. Groom it for a short enough time period and at a light enough pressure that the dog never reacts aversely.

Fig.18.6-F, Step 2: When the dog holds still for grooming and shows no signs of struggling or aggression, reward her immediately with a treat. Repeat this 5 times in succession in the same location or with the same brush pressure; if she still remains calm, move on to a different area or a heavier brush pressure.

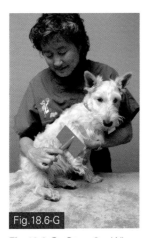

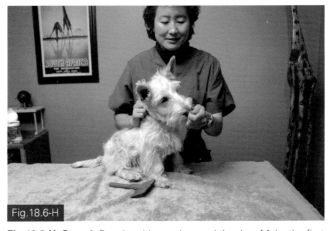

Fig.18.6-G, Step 3: When brushing in a new area or with heavier brush pressure, remember to always stay below the level that will cause the dog to react.

Fig.18.6-H, Step 4: Stop brushing and reward the dog. Make the first brush bouts short (5 seconds) so that the dog does not have much time to become irritated. This will also help her learn that sitting still for grooming leads to treats. If you have to put the brush down to give treats, then it's best to teach the dog (beforehand) that a marker word—such as "yes" spoken in a lively fashion—means a treat is coming. Do this by holding treats behind your back, saying "yes" and immediately delivering the treat to your dog. Repeat this 10-20 times per session. If you are good at delivering the treats suddenly and making your dog wait expectantly in between treats, she will quickly learn that "yes" predicts that a treat will come. It will come to signal her that she's performed a correct behavior and a treat is on the way. This will allow you a short delay between the correct behavior and the presentation of the food reward.

WHAT'S WRONG HERE?

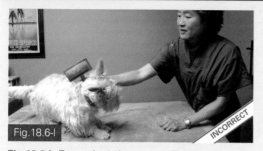

Fig.18.6-I

INCORRECT

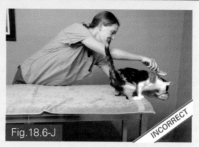

Fig.18.6-J

INCORRECT

Fig.18.6-I, Example 1, Incorrect: The dog is avoiding the brush here. Brushing in this way will sensitize the dog to grooming, worsening her behavior and setting back your training. If she reacts this way, either stop the session and try later—this time being more careful—or try going back to a lower-level brushing stimulus or higher-valued treats.

Fig.18.6-J, Example 2a, Incorrect: Holding the treat out too far can cause the pet to move all over the table and thus teach her to become unmanageable and wiggly while you groom.

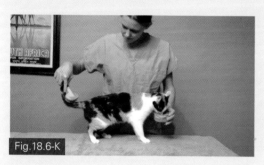

Fig.18.6-K

Fig.18.6-K, Example 2b, Correct: Now the technician holds the treats in a location that keeps the cat stationary.

18.6.3 Using the MannersMinder (Premier Pet, Midlothian, Virginia) to countercondition.

The MannersMinder, an automated treat dispenser, offers a convenient way to countercondition. Set the machine to release treats at a certain interval and then time the brushing to coincide with the dog or cat's snacking.

Classical counterconditioning with the MannersMinder. *(Video 4) (Also refer to Chapter 5, Video 4)*

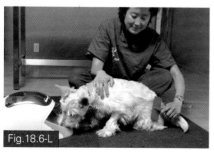

Fig.18.6-L

Fig.18.6-L, Step 1: Set the MannersMinder to "multi-treat" (to dispense 5 treats in succession) and set the treat rate to 10 or 15 seconds. The machine will dispense 5 treats every 10-15 seconds. Now set the ratio switch to "fixed" so that each session lasts 1 minute. Finally, press the "down-stay" button so that the treats will start dispensing as per your settings. Only brush when the dog's nose is physically in contact with the food bowl as she eats the treats out of it.

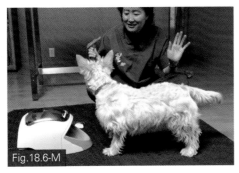

Fig.18.6-M, Step 2: Once the fifth treat has been released, stop brushing so that it's clear to the dog that brushing is associated with the treats. Be sure to stay under the level that irritates the dog.

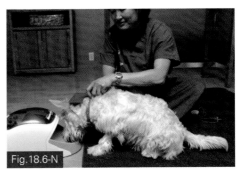

Fig.18.6-N, Step 3: Repeat the procedure at the same brush pressure or same spot on the dog 5 times in succession before moving to a different area of fur or increasing the brush pressure. That way, you're sure the dog understands the connection between brushing and food.

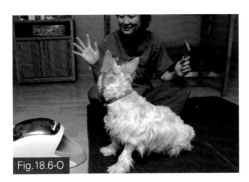

Fig.18.6-O: Always stop before the dog responds aversely. Note that the dog moving away from you could be an aversive reaction. You might want to place a hand on her to guide her or have her lie down so that she remains stationary.

Switch to operant counterconditioning with the MannersMinder.

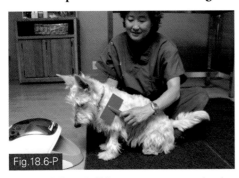

Fig.18.6-P, Step 1: When you can groom the dog anywhere on her body at the necessary level of pressure, switch to operant counterconditioning. Groom the dog for a short period (5 seconds). Ideally, because the dog knows she will get treats, she'll be paying more attention to the machine than to your grooming.

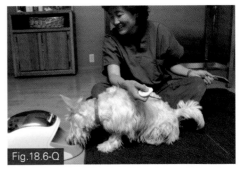

Fig.18.6-Q, Step 2: Stop grooming and dispense one or more treats from the MannersMinder. The advantage of giving treats by machine is that the dog will remain oriented toward the Manners-Minder between treats instead of moving to face you. Systematically increase the amount of time you brush prior to rewarding the dog.

An alternative method of using the MannersMinder is to set the machine to give a single treat every 3 seconds at a fixed rate. When doing this, at first brush only as the dog is eating a treat (e.g., her head is in the MannersMinder bowl). At the rate at which it's set, you'll get 20 opportunities to brush every minute. Then begin to brush more firmly as the dog eats. When the dog is non-reactive with this type of brushing, brush at more random intervals as treats are being dispensed. That is, do not time your brushing to occur only as the dog's head is in the bowl. When you can brush at the heaviest level of pressure necessary with treats coming every 3 seconds and the dog ignoring the grooming, increase the interval between treats. Intervals can be increased to 5, 7, 10, 15, 20, 25, 30, 45, 60 and 300 seconds. Thus you can systematically increase the intervals between treats, usually doing so within several 3-minute sessions.

18.7 Counterconditioning Dogs and Cats to Ear Handling

Many dogs and cats get ear infections or mites at some time in their lives and will require examination and medication. Taking just a few minutes a day for a week or so to countercondition a pet to ear handling can prevent problems down the road. Even pets who already have a bad association will soon learn to enjoy ear handling with good technique on your part. This protocol can be used with both dogs and cats.

18.7.1 Start with classical counterconditioning

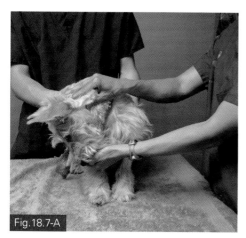

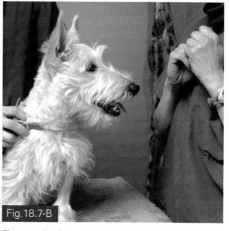

Fig.18.7-A, Step 1a: Rub the skin or fur near the ear vigorously while feeding treats. Feed the animal long enough so that you can rub the skin for 3-5 seconds. The dog's mouth should be physically on your hand eating treats the entire time. Make sure you start on an area that does not cause the dog to react to the handling.

Fig.18.7-B, Step 1b: As the dog finishes the treats, remove both the treat hand and the hand that's rubbing the dog.

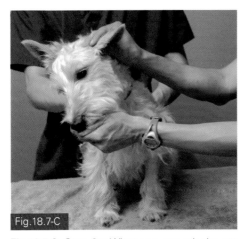

Fig.18.7-C

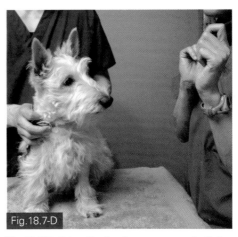

Fig.18.7-D

Fig.18.7-C, Step 2a: When you can rub the ear area in this manner several times in a row while the dog eats, begin to rub an area closer to the ear base, or rub the pinna instead. You might need to start with light pressure. Make sure the dog has begun eating the treat before you start rubbing the ear.

Fig.18.7-D, Step 2b: As always, remove both the treat hand and the rubbing hand before the dog is finished eating. When the dog is good at this step for several trials, move on to the next step. Systematically work your way into the ear and use more rigorous handling, but take care not to move along too quickly and elicit a bad reaction.

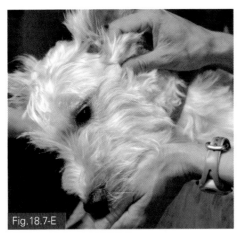

Fig.18.7-E

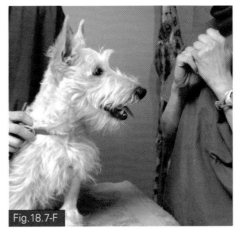

Fig.18.7-F

Fig.18.7-E, Step 3a: Get to the point where you can stick your finger in the ear while giving treats.

Fig.18.7-F, Step 3b: As the dog finishes the treat, stop handling. The dog should be focused on you with the expectation that she will get more treats.

18.7.2 Switch to operant counterconditioning.

The dog should now be accepting rigorous ear handling while receiving treats. Next, you'll use the treat as a reward for good behavior.

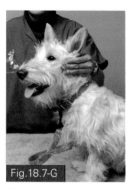 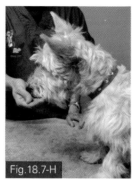 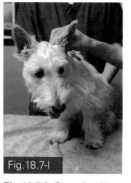 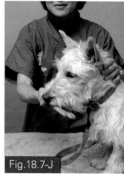

Fig.18.7-G | Fig.18.7-H | Fig.18.7-I | Fig.18.7-J

Fig.18.7-G, Step 1a: First rub around the ear. If you've counterconditioned well thus far, the dog should not react. Stop before she gets irritated.

Fig.18.7-H, Step 1b: Immediately after stopping, reward her for holding still and allowing you to handle her. You can use a marker word such as "yes" right as you stop handling the ear, if you've already trained it. That way, she knows exactly when she's done something good and what the reward is for. If you say "yes" just as you are finishing the rub, she'll understand that the reward is for holding still the entire time.

Fig.18.7-I, Step 2a: Now rub more vigorously but stay below the dog's threshold of tolerance.

Fig.18.7-J, Step 2b: Stop before she becomes irritated and reward her for holding still when you handle her.

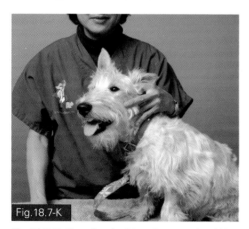 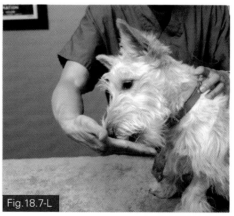

Fig.18.7-K | Fig.18.7-L

Fig.18.7-K, Step 3a: At this point, you should be able to stick a finger in the ear for several seconds prior to rewarding with treats.

Fig.18.7-L, Step 3b: Once you can rub any area for several seconds prior to giving a treat, increase the amount of time you can handle the ear before giving the treat. Eventually you might not need treats, and you can switch to praise or petting.

18.8 Counterconditioning Dogs and Cats to Injections *(Video 5)*

18.8.1 Countercondition to the syringe if necessary.

If the pet is already extremely fearful upon just seeing a syringe, then before counterconditioning to being injected, you'll need to train the dog or cat to accept the sight of a syringe.

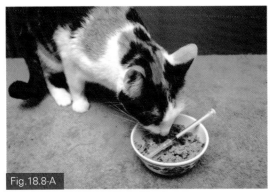

Fig.18.8-A

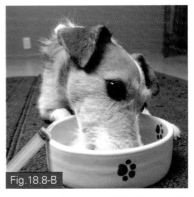

Fig.18.8-B

Fig.18.8-A, Step 1a: If the pet runs away as soon as she sees a syringe, start by placing one in or near her food. If she won't go near the food bowl with a syringe there, move it farther away from the bowl.

Fig.18.8-B, Step 1b: With dogs, make sure the syringe is a size that they will not eat. You can position it around the room with treats on it, or place it on or near the food bowl. Ideally, the pet should act as if he doesn't notice it.

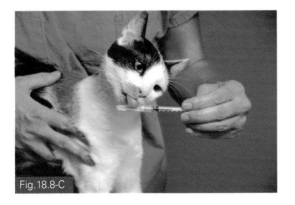

Fig.18.8-C

Fig.18.8-C, Step 2: Next, feed the cat or dog food off the syringe; use it like a spoon. When the pet sees you bring out the syringe, and looks as happy as she does when you're bringing out food, you know the counterconditioning was successful.

18.8.2 Classically countercondition to skin handling for subcutaneous injections.

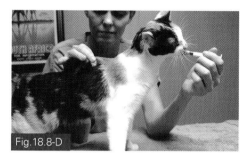

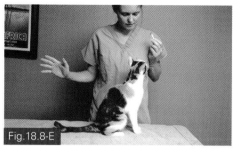

Fig.18.8-D, Step 1: Feed treats while handling the skin. Handle it firmly but gently enough so that the pet remains focused on the treats.

Fig.18.8-E, Step 2: After about 3-5 seconds of eating, remove the food and stop handling simultaneously. This way it's clear to the pet that having the skin handled is what gets her the treats.

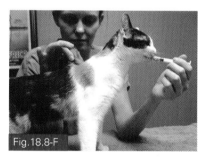

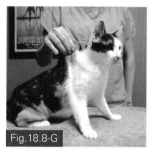

Fig.18.8-F, Step 3: Gradually get rougher—as rough as you'd need to be for an actual injection. But always stay under the pet's threshold of pain, because you want only a positive association.

Fig.18.8-G, H, Step 4: Eventually, you can change to operant counterconditioning. Handle the skin first, then give the treat. Use a marker word like "yes" or a clicker to mark good, calm behavior and signal that a treat is coming. (Remember, this marker must have been previously trained to be effective.)

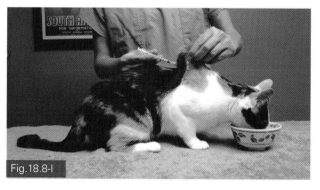

Fig.18.8-I, Step 5: Now get her used to having the skin not only handled but also jabbed with a capped needle. Do this while she's eating, or do it and when she holds still, say "yes" and feed immediately afterward.

18.9 Counterconditioning Cats to Being on Their Backs *(Video 6)*

This position is useful for performing a toenail trim.

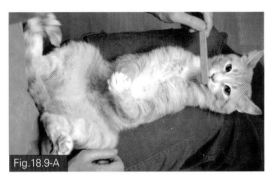 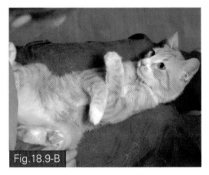

Fig.18.9-A, B: Place the cat on her back and immediately give treats. Gradually increase the interval between treats. If the cat tends to wiggle in between treats, stabilize her by holding her shoulder. Then reward her for remaining still for several seconds and gradually build up the time. Also refer to Chapter 20.

18.10 Counterconditioning Cats and Dogs to Toenail Trims *(Videos 7 and 8)*

The procedure below can be modified for use with dogs (see Chapter 19).

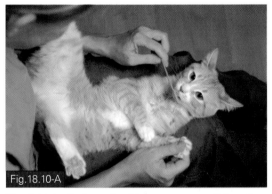 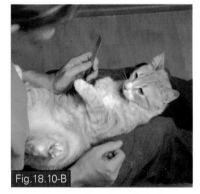

Fig.18.10-A, B, Step 1: First countercondition the pet to having her feet handled. Lay the cat on her back and touch her feet while feeding for several seconds. Then stop feeding and touching the feet simultaneously so that she learns that the food only appears when the feet are being handled. When the cat consistently holds still while you touch her feet, graduate to operant counterconditioning.

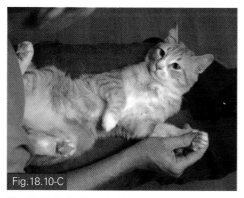
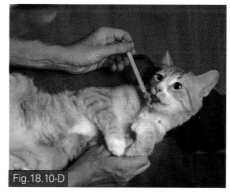

Fig.18.10-C, D, Step 2: Using operant counterconditioning, touch a paw for several seconds. If the cat holds still, reward with a treat. Always try to stop handling before the cat struggles, but systematically increase the handling time to a long enough period for you to be able to trim the nails. Once the cat lies calmly while you're touching her feet for about 10 seconds, you can go to the next step.

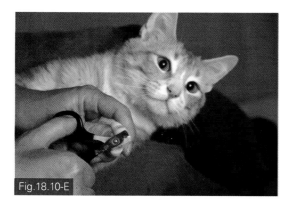
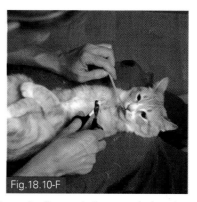

Fig.18.10-E, F, Step 3: Next, take the clippers out and trim a few nails. Stop and give treats before the cat has a chance to react aversely. Most kittens are not yet afraid of the nail trimmers, but if they are you may need to add a few steps, such as feeding treats in the presence of the nail trimmers, just touching the trimmers to the nail, trimming only one nail, and so on. Remember, the goal is to avoid any adverse reactions, so go as slowly as you need to.

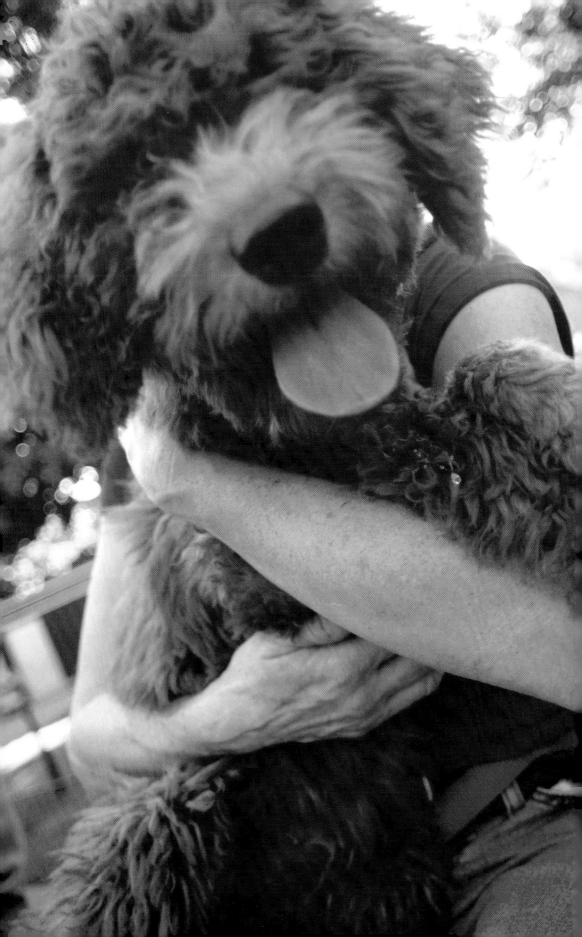

CHAPTER 19.
PREVENTIVE
BEHAVIORAL
HEALTH
for Puppies

The primary and most important time for puppy socialization is the first 3 months of life. During this time puppies should be exposed to as many new people, animals, stimuli and environments as can be achieved safely and without causing over-stimulation manifested as excessive fear, withdrawal or avoidance behavior. For this reason, the American Veterinary Society of Animal Behavior believes that it should be the standard of care for puppies to receive such socialization before they are fully vaccinated. (American Veterinary Society of Animal Behavior 2008)

We've all seen the puppy who hides in the corner when we enter the exam room, or the 8-week-old pup who squirms and growls when we try to examine him. These puppies clearly need socialization and handling to help them develop into behaviorally healthy dogs. But how about the adult dog who's friendly to his owner but aloof with everyone else because he's actually fearful? Or the dog who's great at home but intermittently barks and lunges at people, pets or passing bikes? These fear-related behaviors can drastically affect a dog's ability to go on walks and socialize with visitors. They can also deteriorate to actual biting and its sequelae. In most cases, these troublesome behaviors could have been prevented early with thorough socialization in puppyhood.

Since 28% of dogs (Salman et al. 2000) relinquished to shelters are relinquished due to behavior problems, puppy socialization can play an important role in keeping pets in people's homes. A study by Duxbury et al. (2003) found that participation in puppy socialization and training classes enhances the likelihood that puppies will remain in their first home. Consequently, early socialization can actually help save the puppy's life later on.

19.1 Early Socialization

In dogs, the prime time for socialization to people, pets and situations that dogs might come across later in life is between 3 and 12 weeks of age (Scott and Fuller 1965). During this period, puppies might startle easily but will recover more quickly and can more easily accept the new object, person, handling procedure or environment as safe. Early socialization helps puppies perceive unfamiliar people and environments as non-threatening, and it enables pets to easily assimilate new people and animals into their homes. It also helps them cope with potentially stressful events, such as schedule changes, the addition of new family members, a move to a new environment and rough handling or other fear-inducing events.

Continued periodic socialization through 6 to 8 months of age is probably important. Many dogs who are well socialized at 12 weeks will regress without such reinforcement—possibly due to a fear period or heightened sensitivity to fear that might occur around 4 to 6 months of age (Serpell and Jagoe 1995) or later.

19.2 Technician Preventive Behavior Health Sessions

Technicians can play a vital role in helping puppies develop into well-socialized dogs by offering puppy preventive behavioral health sessions. Such sessions should be offered to all clients with puppies. Individual behavioral health sessions last 20 to 30 minutes and focus on desensitization and counterconditioning to the handling procedures covered in this and previous chapters. Another important part of the session is teaching puppies one behavior—sit—that can be used as an alternate behavior to replace all kinds of unwanted behaviors.

In general, only 2 exercises should be taught per session so that the owner does not become overwhelmed. Have the owner bring the puppy to the session hungry. Each puppy should have 2 to 3 sessions, each about a week apart, so that the owner keeps up on the social-ization exercises during this sensitive period. Charge your normal fee for 20 to 30 minutes of technician time, or integrate individual sessions into your hospital's regular puppy package.

19.3 Puppy Preschool

All puppies between the ages of 7 and 16 weeks should be encouraged to attend puppy preschool in addition to or instead of the individual technician-run behavioral health sessions. Owners should be encouraged to start puppies in class as close to 7 or 8 weeks of age as possible. The advantage of a group class is that the puppies get to interact with other puppies and humans.

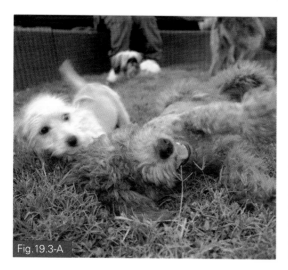
Fig.19.3-A

Fig.19.3-A: Because dogs need to be comfortable around other dogs in order to get along in high-density environments such as cities, it's extremely important that they learn how to interact appropri-ately with other puppies and adult dogs. Many dogs are interested in playing or in-teracting with other dogs but are socially inept or fearful. Their resulting improper behavior, such as greeting tensely or in an overly active manner, can be perceived by other dogs as a threat. These inexperi-enced dogs may also perceive other dogs that run up to them as a danger. Learning early how to interact properly with other puppies is imperative; puppies should perceive other puppies as fun and safe.

Technicians can run sessions consisting of approximately 4 hour-long classes in the hospital waiting room after hours, offered at weekly intervals. Classes should consist of handling exercises as well as time for play and appropriate socialization. It's often good to start with the handling exercises so that the puppies focus on the owners first and become accustomed to the area. The exercises can be performed on tables and countertops. Then some puppies can play while others continue different handling exercises. Prior to puppy play-time, owners should be taught how to recognize when play is becoming too arousing so that the puppies can be separated when necessary.

Puppy socialization is so important that the American Veterinary Society of Animal Behavior (AVSAB) considers it the standard of care that all puppies attend socialization class before their final vaccinations. Puppies should start preschool socialization classes as close to 7 or 8 weeks of age as possible. The younger they are, the more quickly they adapt to new people, animals, objects, handling and situations. They should have at least one vaccination and one deworming 7 to 10 days prior to the first class, and continue with their vaccinations throughout the sessions. Puppies who are coughing, sneezing, vomiting or have diarrhea should not come to class, but their owners can still attend.

Some activities that should take place during class are described below. Note: Most of the photos below showing grass were taken primarily during a class conducted on a soft, synthetic lawn (Heavenly Greens, San Jose, California) which could be disinfected if needed.

19.3.1 Make sure everyone has a chance to handle each puppy.

Play "pass the puppy" so that the puppies get used to associating other people with good things.

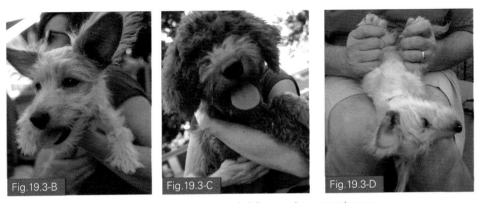

Fig.19.3-B, C, D: These class members take turns holding another person's puppy.

19.3.2 Countercondition to Gentle Leaders and muzzles.

Puppies should be counterconditioned to head collars such as the Gentle Leader in case they are needed at a later date. A study by Duxbury et al. (2003) found that the use of a head collar to redirect behaviors was associated with higher retention of puppies in their first homes.

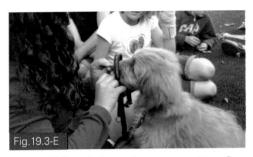

Fig.19.3-E, Step 1: To get the puppy used to a Gentle Leader (GL), place treats through the loop. When the pup sticks his nose through to get the treats, let him eat them.

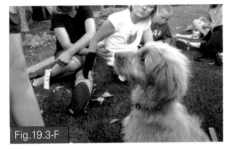

Fig.19.3-F, Step 2: When he's finished eating, remove the Gentle Leader before he pulls his head away. This way, you are in control of when he puts his nose through the loop.

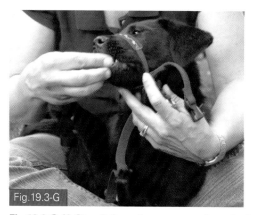

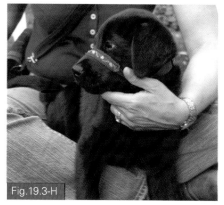

Fig.19.3-G, H, Step 3: Once the puppy consistently shoves his nose into the GL to get the treat, put the GL on and connect the straps behind the ears. Continue giving treats, and keep the puppy focused on the food and other exercises that he enjoys rather than allowing him to get distracted by the GL.

19.4 Handling

Countercondition puppies to handling and examination of different parts of their bodies. Offer treats while slowly and gently touching them all over, but work on one body part at a time. Avoid causing aversive reactions. Progress gradually until the puppy is comfortable with somewhat rough handling on various parts of his body.

19.4.1 General handling of body parts.

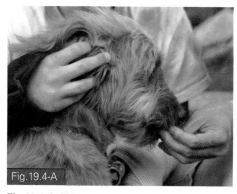

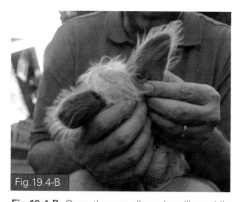

Fig.19.4-A: This puppy gets treats as his ears are examined and manipulated.

Fig.19.4-B: Once the pup allows handling while eating treats, work on handling without food and then reward him for calm behavior immediately afterward (i.e., switch from classical to operant counterconditioning).

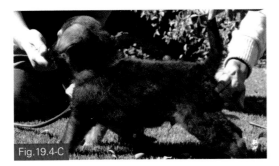

Fig.19.4-C: Here, the puppy is eating treats while his rear end is being examined.

19.4.2 Placing puppies on their backs in your lap. *(Video 1)*

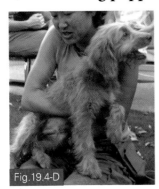
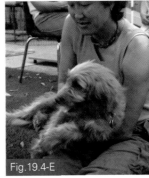
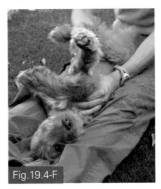

Fig.19.4-D, E, F: Owners should know how to properly restrain their puppies and place them on their backs so that the puppies are comfortable with the process. To move a pup of this size onto his left side, use your right hand to reach over the back and then behind the puppy's right foreleg to grasp the left leg above the elbow. Your left hand is on the dog's left hip. In one smooth motion, use both arms to rotate the dog onto his left side and then onto his back in your lap. Grasp each arm above the elbow to hold him there.

19.5 Pilling and Oral Examination

Use counterconditioning techniques to make handling the mouth pleasant for the puppy.

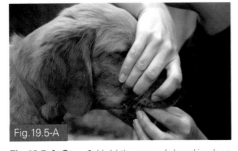
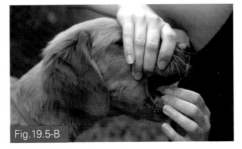

Fig.19.5-A, Step 1: Hold the puppy's head in place by placing your hand over his muzzle. Use your other hand on the incisors to open his mouth.

Fig.19.5-B, Step 2: Quickly place a treat in his mouth. The puppy should learn to associate getting treats with having his mouth pried open.

440

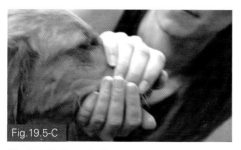

Fig.19.5-C, Step 3: Close the puppy's mouth before he has a chance to close it on his own or pull his head free. This puts you in control of the speed at which the mouth opens and closes.

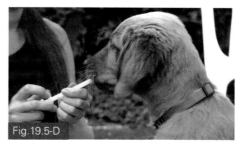

Fig.19.5-D, Step 4: Also feed treats using a pill gun so that he learns that this device predicts goodies.

19.6 Vaccinating

Use counterconditioning methods to teach puppies to accept vaccination procedures.

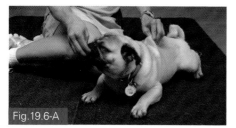

Fig.19.6-A, Step 1: Start by holding or pinching the dog's skin while feeding him a treat. The goal is to have him ignore the pinching and eat the entire time, so be sure you're not pinching hard enough to distract him from the treat.

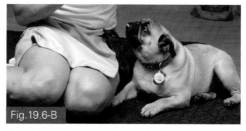

Fig.19.6-B, Step 2: When he's finished with the treat, pull away your feeding hand and pinching hand. Then repeat the procedure. The puppy should learn to associate skin handling with treats.

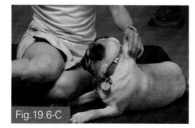

Fig.19.6-C, Step 3: When the pup stays calm no matter how rough you are or where you grasp the skin, you can either vaccinate him now or try some operant counterconditioning first. To continue training with the latter, grasp the skin for several seconds.

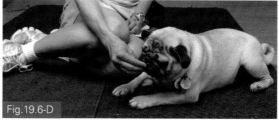

Fig.19.6-D, Step 4: Then release the skin and immediately follow with treats as long as he has remained still. This way, he learns that holding still while you grasp the skin leads to treats. Use a clicker or "yes" to mark the good behavior if the puppy is already familiar with this type of training. Refer to Chapter 18 (Section 18.8) for more details on counterconditioning to injections. *(See also Chapter 8, Video 5)*

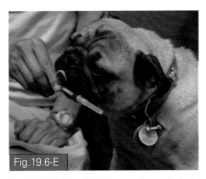

Fig.19.6-E

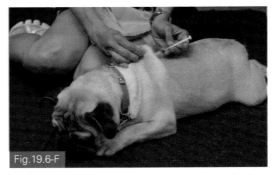

Fig.19.6-F

Fig.19.6-E, Step 5: If the pup is at all afraid of syringes, place food (try peanut butter or canned cheese) on the syringe and let him lick it off. When he consistently tries to lick the syringe as soon as he sees it, whether or not there's any food on it, you know he associates it with good things.

Fig.19.6-F, Step 6: Now place some treats on the floor for him to eat while you grasp his fur and poke his skin with the capped syringe. You can also distract him with food when giving actual vaccinations or other injections.

19.7 Grooming and Brushing Teeth

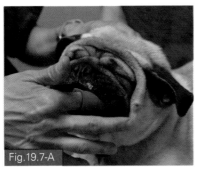

Fig.19.7-A

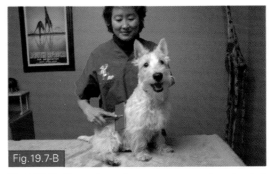

Fig.19.7-B

Fig.19.7-A Brushing teeth: With a treat or toothpaste on the brush, insert it just inside the puppy's lips so that you can brush the outside of his teeth. Be sure to avoid inserting your finger between his upper and lower teeth and accidentally getting bitten. If done the right way, the puppy should look forward to daily brushing. (See Chapter 18 for more details.)

Fig.19.7-B Grooming: Groom one area for about 5 seconds. Groom it for a short enough time period and at a low enough pressure that the puppy never reacts aversely. Gradually increase the pressure and length of time while providing treats and being sure to avoid adverse reactions. (See Chapter 18, Section 18.6 for more details.)

19.8 Toenail Trims

Toenail trims should not be a traumatic event. There's no need to forcefully hold down a puppy to keep him from struggling for this procedure. Use classical and operant counterconditioning techniques to help the puppy easily accept having his nails trimmed.

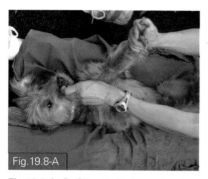
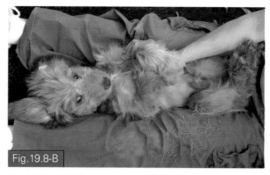

Fig.19.8-A, B, Step 1: First get the dog used to having his feet touched using classical counterconditioning. It might be easiest to place the puppy on his back on your lap. Handle his feet while giving treats. Then stop handling and stop giving treats simultaneously. Repeat.

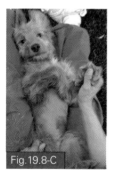
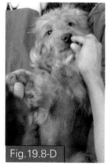
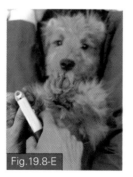
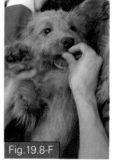

Fig.19.8-C, D, Step 2: Switching to operant counterconditioning, now handle the feet without giving treats. As soon as you stop touching the feet, reward the puppy for holding still.

Fig.19.8-E, F, Step 3: Add the toenail trimmers. Clip one or two nails and then reward for calm behavior before he struggles.

19.9 The Collar Grab

Puppies need to learn to calmly accept someone grabbing their collars or even their skin. People frequently get bitten when they suddenly grab their dogs to keep them from darting out the door or otherwise getting into trouble. One of the most common bite scenarios occurs during a dog fight when someone grabs one of the fighting dogs by the collar. When the aroused dog feels his collar being grabbed, he automatically turns and bites. We can decrease the chances of dogs being startled in this manner by desensitizing and counterconditioning puppies to collar grabs. Of course, all of these techniques work with adult dogs, too.

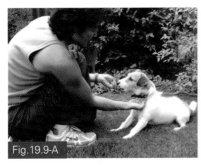

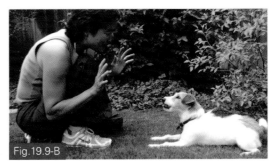

Fig.19.9-A, Step 1: Grasp the collar lightly while feeding the puppy a treat. The pup should ignore the hold on his collar and just focus on the treat.

Fig.19.9-B, Step 2: When he's finished with the treat, pull your feeding hand and the collar-holding hand away. Then repeat the procedure. Gradually grasp the collar more firmly until you can even drag the dog around a little with no adverse reaction while he's getting treats.

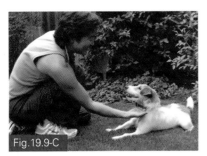

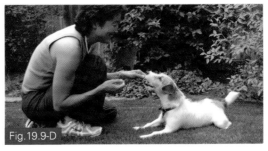

Fig.19.9-C, Step 3: When the puppy remains calm no matter how rough your collar grabbing, progress to operant counterconditioning. Grasp the collar and jiggle it, but don't feed treats yet.

Fig.19.9-D, Step 4: Stop touching his collar and simultaneously reward the puppy with a treat. You can even grasp the collar and drag him toward the treat, letting go as he starts to eat.

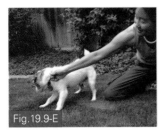

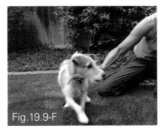

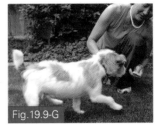

Fig.19.9-E, F, G: The goal is to be able to grab the puppy's collar or leash when he's focused on something else and pull him toward you and a treat that he can eat. He should think that grabbing and pulling on his collar equals a yummy treat for him. When he does he will actively run in the direction you're pulling in order to get to the expected reward.

19.10 The Automatic Sit

Puppies are distracted by many things throughout the day. It's essential that they learn to focus on their owners to offer a calm sit. That way, family members will have a positive method for getting their puppy's attention.

19.10.1 The basic exercise

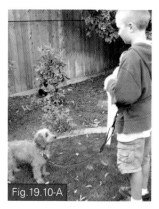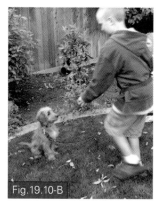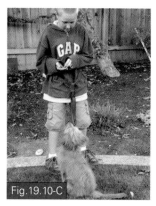

Fig.19.10-A, B, C: Start with a hungry puppy on leash while you stand stationary. When he sits, immediately reward him with a treat. Give additional rewards while he's still sitting to encourage him to remain in that position. Some people like to use food to lure the puppy into a sit. I find that usually a lure is not needed. Most puppies will eventually sit if the handler waits the puppy out. After the puppy gets lots of treats for sitting, sitting will quickly become a default behavior when he realizes other behaviors are not working to get him what he wants.

19.10.2 Suddenly settle and come when called

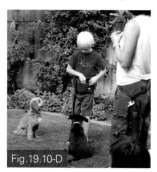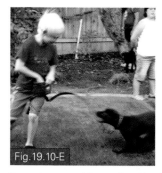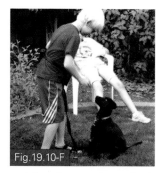

Fig.19.10-D, E, F: The automatic sit can be turned into a "suddenly settle" or "come when called." This exercise makes focusing on the owner more fun. This boy starts with his puppy sitting. Then he runs away from the pup quickly so that the puppy follows. When the boy stops, the puppy automatically sits in front of him and gets a treat. The puppy is learning that no matter how excited he is, he should have an "on/off" switch. When his handler stops, he stops too, and sits. This exercise can be converted to "come when called" just by saying "Rover, come!" right before you start running. The cue predicts that you will run away and that the puppy should run after you, stop and sit to get a treat.

19.10.3 Applying these exercises in distracting situations

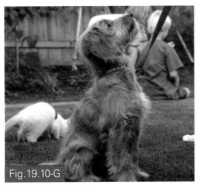 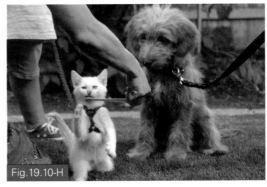

Fig.19.10-G, H: Similarly, puppies can get used to other pets and "distractions." This puppy is first focusing on his handler by performing sits, suddenly settle and come when called when near a kitten. Once he's calm, he is allowed to greet the kitten. In this manner he can learn to focus on his handler to be calm in many distracting, excitable situations.

19.11 Play Sessions *(Video 2)*

Puppies should also have play sessions with appropriately matched playmates. Sessions should be relatively short—several minutes at a time—and puppies should not be allowed to become overly aroused. It's important that they learn to play calmly rather than in an overly aroused manner. Two dogs can enjoy playing with each other in a highly aroused manner, but this type of play can escalate to aggression down the road. Aroused play can train puppies to greet and play inappropriately with other dogs. This in turn can cause fights and can cause fearful, shy or apprehensive dogs to become more fearful or apprehensive.

Interrupt play frequently and before it gets too excited. If the puppies are dragging leashes perform a "come when called" with leash assistance or perform a collar grab by pulling the puppies toward really tasty treats. After the puppies have focused on their handlers for several seconds, their additional reward is that they can play again.

> It's important that puppies learn to play calmly rather than in an overly aroused manner. Even if puppies enjoy playing in a highly aroused manner with each other, such play can escalate into aggression down the road. It can also train the puppies to greet and play inappropriately with other dogs.

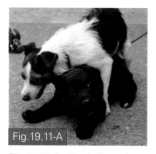
Fig.19.11-A

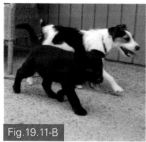
Fig.19.11-B

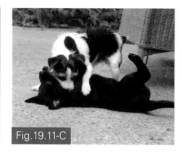
Fig.19.11-C

Fig.19.11-A: It's ok if puppies and dogs wrestle with each other in a manner where one is on top of the other as long as: 1) both dogs are relaxed, 2) the one on the bottom shows no signs of fear or stress (Refer to Chapter 1) and 3) the one on the bottom can easily get away at any instant if he wants and 4) once separated he wants to resume play with the same puppy.

Fig.19.11-B: The playmates should also frequently break off from play or slow play down for an instant by standing stationary or backing away for several seconds at a time. This puppy and adolescent have stopped play and are relaxedly walking side by side.

Fig.19.11-C: Puppies and adult dogs frequently mouth spar with each other. If the mouth contact is light (the puppy doing the mouthing is keeping his mouth open wide) and the puppy being mouthed remains relaxed and does not back away, then the sparring is acceptable. If one puppy starts to gnaw excitedly at, close the mouth or clamp down on the neck, then play should be stopped and his attention redirected, even if the other puppy does not object. If rough mouthy behavior is allowed the puppy will get practice using its teeth in an increasingly uninhibited manner that can lead to aggression in the future.

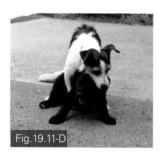
Fig.19.11-D

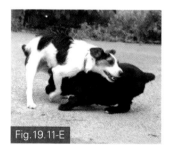
Fig.19.11-E

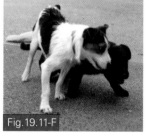
Fig.19.11-F

Fig.19.11-D: Separate puppies who try to mount other puppies. Just pull the mounting puppy off and direct his attention to a treat or perform a come when called and then keep him focused on you for several seconds before letting him resume play.

Fig.19.11-E, F: Overly aroused play can escalate to aggression. This Jack Russell Terrier, Homer, has been playing too roughly with the Labrador puppy and the puppy does not mind. He keeps coming back to play once the two are separated. But then Homer looks at the Labrador intensely the way he looks at a squeaking rat. He has to be separated before he bites the puppy.

References

American Veterinary Society of Animal Behavior. 2008. AVSAB *Position Statement on Puppy Socialization.* http://www.avsabonline.org/avsabonline/images/stories/Position_Statements/ puppy%20socialization.pdf (Accessed July 16, 2008).

Duxbury, M.M., J.A. Jackson, S.W. Line, R.K. Anderson. 2003. Evaluation of association between retention in the home and attendance at puppy socialization classes. *Journal of the American Veterinary Medical Association* 223:61-7.

Salman, M.D., J.C. New, P.H. Kass, and J.M. Scarlett. 2000. Behavioral reasons for relinquishment of dogs and cats to 12 shelters. *Journal of Applied Animal Welfare Science* 3 (2):93-106.

Serpell, J., and J.A. Jagoe. 1995. "Early experience and the development of behavior." In *The Domestic Dog: Its Evolution, Behaviour and Interactions With People*, ed. J. Serpell. Cambridge: Cambridge University Press. Pp. 80-102.

Scott J.P., and J.L. Fuller. 1965. *Genetics and the Social Behavior of the Dog*. Chicago: University of Chicago Press.

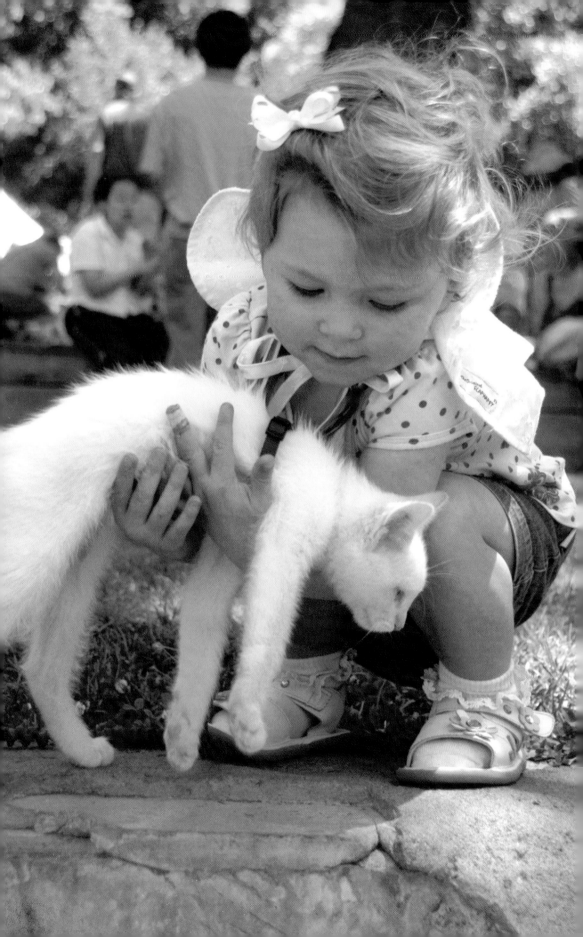

CHAPTER 20.
PREVENTIVE BEHAVIORAL HEALTH
for Kittens

Have you ever visited a home where the cats immediately ran away or hid when you entered? Or talked to a friend whose cat couldn't cope with the tiniest stressors? Perhaps a schedule change or an out-of-town visitor was enough to bring on anxiety-based urine spraying. Even worse, what if you want a new addition to your household—another cat, a dog, a boyfriend or a child—but your cat clearly doesn't? She hides, hisses, or even stalks the new arrival, and now you find potty presents around the house. Then there's the diabetic cat who needs regular injections but hates the treatments, is learning to hate her owners when they try to treat her, and has always hated the vet hospital.

These issues are difficult to deal with in adult cats, but they could have easily been prevented if these cats had received early socialization as kittens. Additionally, early socialization in kittens is relatively easy, especially when compared to similar socialization in puppies.

Early socialization can change the personality of a shy, aloof, even aggressive kitten to one who's outgoing, affectionate and adapts well to new people and environments. Such kittens can develop into cats who can go on walks just like dogs, come when called in the house even with distractions, and take environmental changes in stride rather than getting upset and urine marking.

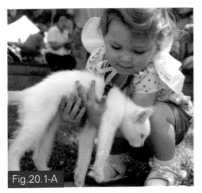
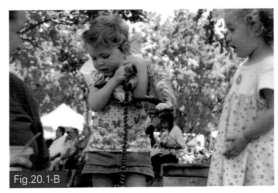

Fig.20.1-A, B: These well-socialized kittens didn't mind being picked up by unfamiliar children at the park. They remained relaxed and didn't struggle when lifted off the ground, even when carried improperly. This occurred during an outing to the local farmer's market, where the kittens were wearing leashes and harnesses.

20.1 Early Socialization

In cats, the prime time for socialization to people, pets and situations that cats might come across later in life is between 3 and 9 weeks of age (American Association of Feline Practitioners 2004). During this time, kittens might startle easily but they recover quickly and can accept new objects, people, handling procedures and environments as safe. Socialization must continue through adolescence to ensure that it is retained. The procedures and exercises are similar to those for puppies but, in my opinion, are much easier and less time consuming due in part to the kitten's size, relative independence and the expectations of them in a human household.

Although socializing kittens is relatively easy, it can have profound effects. Early socialization can completely change the personality of a shy, aloof, fear-aggressive kitten to a cat who is outgoing, affectionate and handles stress well. It can mean the difference between a cat who urine sprays when a new pet is introduced and one who takes new people, animals and environments in stride.

20.2 Technician Preventive Behavioral Health Sessions

Technicians can play a vital role in helping kittens develop into well-socialized cats by hosting kitten preventive behavioral health sessions. Such sessions should be offered to all clients with kittens. Individual behavioral health sessions last 20 to 30 minutes and focus on desensitizing and counterconditioning to the handling procedures covered in this and previous chapters. In addition, teaching kittens one behavior—sit—is important because it can be used as an alternate behavior to replace all kinds of unwanted behaviors.

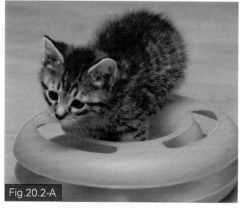

Fig.20.2-A

Fig.20.2-A: Kittens should start kitty kindergarten or structured socialization to unfamiliar pets, people and environments as close to 7-8 weeks of age as possible. The younger they are, the more quickly they adapt to the situation. In general, they should have at least one vaccination and deworming 7-10 days prior to the first class, and continue with their vaccinations throughout the sessions. Kittens who are coughing, sneezing, vomiting or have diarrhea should not come to class, but their owners can still attend.

Each kitten should have 2 to 3 sessions, each about a week apart so that the owner keeps up on the socialization exercises during this sensitive period. Teach only 2 exercises per session so that the owner is not overwhelmed. Have the owner bring the kitten in hungry. Charge your normal fee for 20 to 30 minutes of technician time, or integrate individual sessions into your hospital's regular kitten package.

20.3 Kitty Kindergarten

All kittens between 7 and 14 weeks of age should be encouraged to attend kitten kindergarten in addition to or instead of the individual technician-run behavioral health sessions. The advantage with a group class is that they get to interact with other kittens, humans and possibly other animals. Technicians can easily learn to run sessions of 2 or 3 classes, each lasting about an hour, in the hospital waiting room after hours. Kitty kindergartens are easier to run than puppy preschools because the inter-animal interactions and general movements of the kittens are easier to control—especially once the kittens are harness trained.

Spend the first 10 to 20 minutes of each session giving a short presentation on a topic such as the purpose of early socialization, litter box issues or handling problems. Kittens should be kept in their carriers during this portion of the session. When let out, immediately start with the handling exercises so that the kittens focus on the owners first and become accustomed to the area. The exercises can be performed on tables and countertops. Then some kittens can play while others continue different handling or training exercises. The kitty kindergarten should be set up and include activities as described below.

20.3.1 Provide plenty of toys evenly spaced throughout the room.

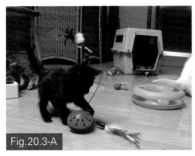 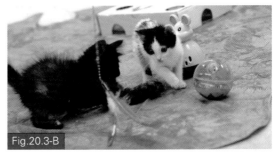

Fig.20.3-A, B: Toys help keep the kittens distracted from one another. This way, shy kittens are less likely to be bombarded by multiple kittens at once. **String-and-feather toys** are usually the most popular; have the owners dangle them for the kittens.

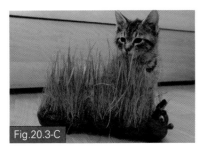 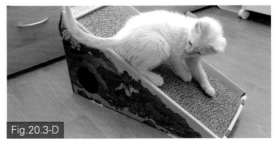

Fig.20.3-C: Kitty grass provides both an appropriate plant to play with and a hiding area.

Fig.20.3-D: Use disposable **scratching pads** or the replaceable cardboard type with a plastic frame that can be disinfected.

20.3.2 Introduce kittens to food puzzles.

Owners can make food puzzles or purchase them. Free-roaming cats spend several hours a day foraging for food. Food puzzles are a great way for kittens and adult cats to keep busy throughout the day. Cats can be fed their entire daily allotment of dry food using food puzzles.

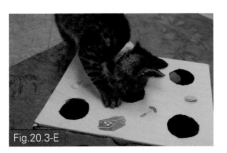

Fig.20.3-E: This homemade food puzzle is a cardboard box with holes cut on the top and sides. Cats can stick their paws in and bat the food out the sides. Similar boxes, such as the Peek A Prize Toy Box (SmartCat LLC, Cedarburg, Wisconsin), can be purchased.

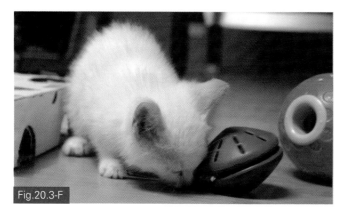

Fig.20.3-F: Other interactive toys include this Twist-n-Treat (Premier Pet, Midlothian, Virginia), a rubber toy that holds treats on the inside, and various balls that release kibble when they're rolled.

20.3.3 Offer hiding places and resting spots.

Kittens should have various hiding spots where they can play or escape from other kittens.

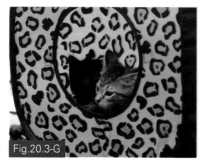

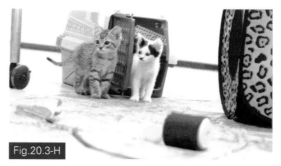

Fig.20.3-G: This is a nylon cube that folds up for easy storage. It is a kitty favorite.

Fig.20.3-H: Carriers also serve as good resting spots.

20.3.4 Don't forget litter boxes.

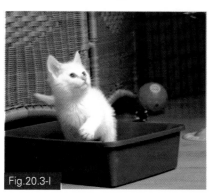

Fig.20.3-I: Include at least one litter box, and be sure that other kittens don't pounce on a kitten who is urinating or defecating in the box. We don't want the kitten to develop a litter box aversion after being pounced on while in the litter box.

20.3.5 Include other well-behaved, well-socialized species.

After the first class, you might opt to bring other well-socialized animals who are calm, healthy and fully vaccinated.

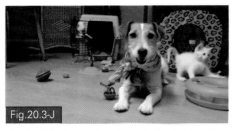 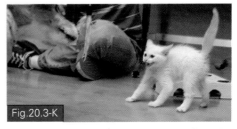

Fig.20.3-J: Jonesy has been trained to lie down calmly around kittens. Be sure to use a dog who moves slowly or who will remain in a down position so that the kittens can get used to him. Avoid pets who want to examine or play with the kittens, as this could scare them. Note that the kitten in the background is not even paying attention to the dog.

Fig.20.3-K: When this kitten comes face to face with the dog however, she is startled and fearful. Jonesy remains fairly stationary and doesn't move toward the kitten, so the kitten does not run away.

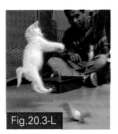 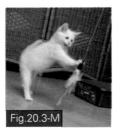 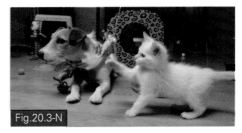

Fig.20.3-L, M: Instead, a class participant gets the kitten's attention with a toy, quickly engaging her in play. That is, the kitten's emotional state is quickly changed from fear to a happy state.

Fig.20.3-N: Now the kitten is comfortable with Jonesy even when she's right in front of him. When kittens are young they might hiss frequently at new things, but they recover quickly compared with adult cats. That is, they flee less often, flee a shorter distance, or return back to explore sooner than adult cats.

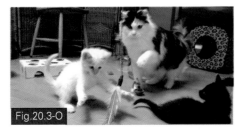 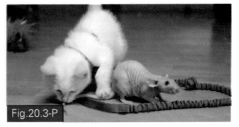

Fig.20.3-O: You can also introduce the kittens to friendly adult cats.

Fig.20.3-P: This kitten is greeting a pet rat. Notice she's on a leash. Overly rambunctious kittens and those who harass the others can play on leash. Use a leash any time you want to be able to control a kitten's movement. The Come With Me Kitty harness (Premier Pet, Midlothian, Virginia) fits well on cats of different sizes and has a bungee leash that allows cats to jump and play safely.

20.3.6 Provide good supervision.

Like children at a playground, kittens need to be supervised to ensure that they play appropriately.

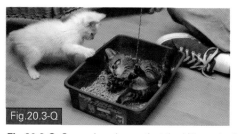 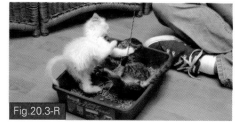

Fig.20.3-Q: Supervise play so that the kittens don't become overly aroused. They need to learn to calm down. Here, one kitten is engrossed in playing with the feather toy and another wants to join in. It's best to divert the incoming kitten's attention or temporarily remove the toy.

Fig.20.3-R: Otherwise, this can happen. The two kittens have begun to fight over the toy. Fighting can lead to bad relations with other cats.

20.4 Handling

All kittens should be taught to accept and enjoy handling. It's important to get them used to all the types of handling they might need throughout their lives. For this to occur, owners must first be taught effective ways to hold the kitten. Handlers must support the kitten well, or else she will try to escape. They must also hold the kitten in such a way that she cannot struggle and escape, or else she will learn to do just that.

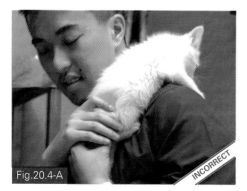 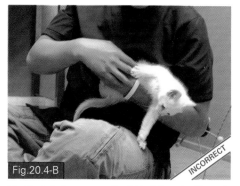

Fig.20.4-A, Incorrect: Avoid holding the kitten as if you're burping a baby. Don't allow front legs on your shoulder, or else the kitten is likely to climb up and escape over your shoulder, possibly leaving claw marks on your shoulder, neck and face.

Fig.20.4-B, Incorrect: Avoid holding the kitten in any way that allows her to struggle and escape. With every successful struggle and escape, her struggling is reinforced. We want her to learn to relax and accept handling.

20.4.1 Placing cats on their backs in your arms

This technique is similar to placing dogs on their backs. (see Chapter 12, Section 12.7, Method 4)

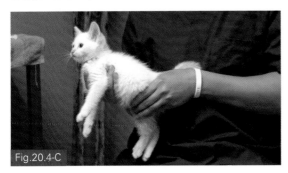

Fig.20.4-C

Fig.20.4-C: First hold the kitten by placing one hand under the chest so that your thumb is on the outside of one leg, your third finger is on the outside of the other leg, and your index finger sits between the legs. Then place the opposite hand on the kitten's hip.

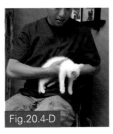
Fig.20.4-D

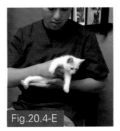
Fig.20.4-E

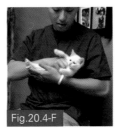
Fig.20.4-F

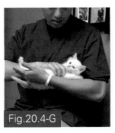
Fig.20.4-G

Fig.20.4-D to G: With both hands working in concert, rotate the kitten onto her back. Once she's on her back, countercondition her by giving food treats.

If the kitten doesn't like being held on her back, desensitize her (with or without counterconditioning with food).

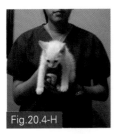
Fig.20.4-H

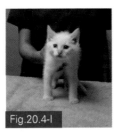
Fig.20.4-I

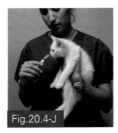
Fig.20.4-J

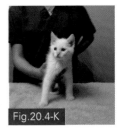
Fig.20.4-K

Fig.20.4-H, I, Step 1: If the kitten struggles when held on her back, even when given food, or if she's not hungry, go back and desensitize with or without counterconditioning. For example, starting with the kitten standing on a table, lift her off the table for a few seconds and then place her back into her comfortable standing position before she starts reacting to being held. Do this several times until the kitten is consistently relaxed when elevated off the table. Then repeat the procedure but hold the kitten elevated a little longer.

Fig.20.4-J, K, Step 2: Next, hold the kitten upright for a few seconds. If she'll take treats in this position, give her some so that she associates getting treats with being held. Place the kitten back onto the table before she starts to struggle. The goal is to always put the kitten back before any struggling occurs.

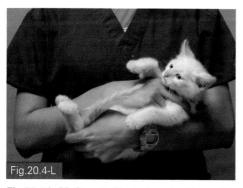
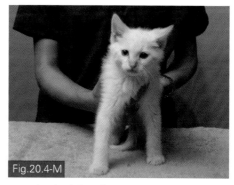

Fig.20.4-L, M, Step 3: Next, place the kitten all the way on her back for a few seconds. Again, put her back onto the table before she starts struggling. If she has been still, offer her treats once she's on the table, or give them while she's on her back. If she's not interested in treats, just make sure you quickly get her back onto the table in a comfortable position as her reward for being still.

20.4.2 Placing kittens on their backs in your lap. *(Video 1)*

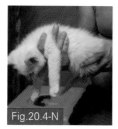
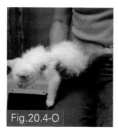
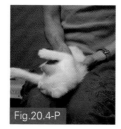
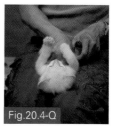

Fig.20.4-N to Q: A good position for a one-person toenail trim is to have the kitten lie on her back in your lap. With one hand, grasp the chest and control the front legs. With the other, support the rear end. In one smooth movement, rotate the cat onto her back in your lap. If you're supporting the kitten well, she should not be able to struggle.

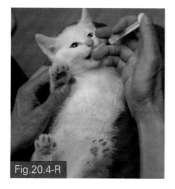
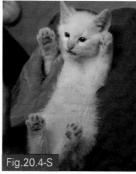

Fig.20.4-R, S: When she's on her back, if the kitten is likely to struggle, give treats. This kitten is getting tuna out of a syringe that has had its tip removed. Give a few bites, then remove the food syringe for several seconds. While the kitten is remaining still, give additional treats. Systematically increase the interval between treats. It might only take a minute for the kitten to learn to remain on her back.

20.4.3 Countercondition to being held in other positions. *(Video 2)*

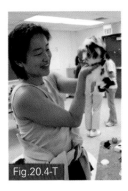
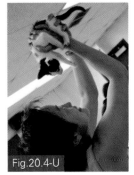

Fig.20.4-T, U: Hold the kitten in many different positions. Always do so for a shorter time period than she will tolerate. That is, put her down before she starts struggling. Avoid putting her down while she struggles, or you'll be rewarding her for struggling. If you must put her down when she's struggling, try again but this time hold her in a more readily tolerated position for a shorter time period, or countercondition with food.

20.4.4 Handle all body parts that might need to be examined.

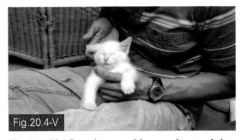
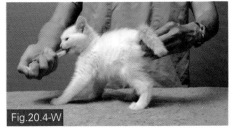

Fig.20.4-V: Practice touching and examining the ears. If the kitten likes having her ears rubbed, there's no need to use treats.

Fig.20.4-W: Countercondition to handling the rear end. Here, the handler is feeding canned food out of a syringe while rubbing the kitten's anal region.

20.5 Pilling and Oral Examination

This is easiest to do if the kitten has already been taught to sit. *(Refer to Chapter 18, Video 3)*

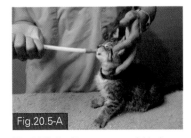
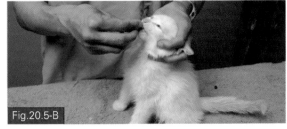

Fig.20.5-A: Kittens can quickly learn to associate pill guns with pleasant experiences if you feed them treats out of the pill gun. The handler can simultaneously put a hand behind the head as if to pill the kitten.

Fig.20.5-B: When the kitten is comfortable with having a hand behind her head, the handler can then start grasping the kitten's head as if for a pilling. By giving treats instead of a pill, the kitten will associate this hold with goodies. To countercondition to an oral exam, open the mouth, place a treat inside and then close the mouth.

20.6 Scruffing and Vaccinating
(Refer to Chapter 18, Video 5)

20.6.1 Countercondition to scruffing and skin pinching.

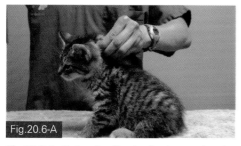 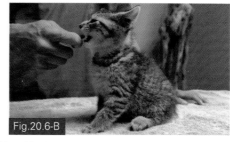

Fig.20.6-A, B: Practice first by firmly grasping the skin while feeding treats. Or grasp the skin and follow with a treat. Lightly pinch the skin in different locations around the body, including the back of the neck where you would scruff the kitten for restraint. The goal is to have the kitten never react to the grasping because you stop before it gets to be too much or you get the treat to her before she reacts. Work up to being able to handle the kitten rather roughly.

20.6.2 Countercondition to scruffing the kitten on her side, as you would for procedures such as blood draws.

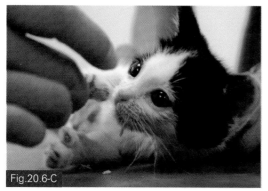 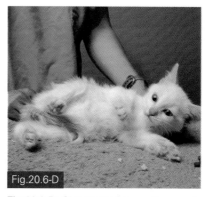

Fig.20.6-C: This kitten is being scruffed on her side. Many adult cats do not like being scruffed. But the kitten is not resisting; she's actually learning to associate scruffing with tuna. Note that the piece of tuna is large so that the kitten bites into only the tuna and not into the handler's finger. Kittens have difficulty distinguishing where the food ends and your finger begins.

Fig.20.6-D: Give treats frequently enough so that the kitten does not resist the handling. Systematically increase the interval between treats.

20.6.3 Countercondition to vaccination.

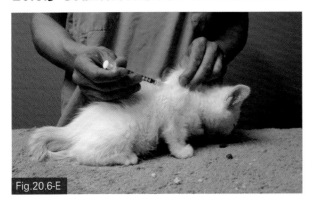

Fig.20.6-E

Fig.20.6-E: Once the kitten is used to having her skin grabbed roughly, countercondition to being vaccinated. The easiest way is to place food on the table. This kitten is eating kibble off the table while the handler is tenting the skin and jabbing the kitten with a capped syringe to mimic vaccination. The kitten should continue eating during the process. You might need to start by simply tapping lightly with the syringe instead of jabbing.

20.7 Grooming and Toenail Trims

20.7.1 Countercondition to being groomed.

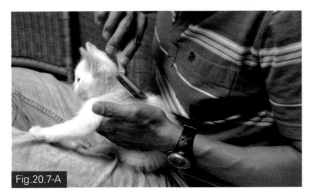

Fig.20.7-A

Fig.20.7-A: Practice brushing the kitten. If the kitten does not like being groomed, then pair brushing with treats.

20.7.2 Countercondition to nail trims. *(Refer to Chapter 18, Video 7)*

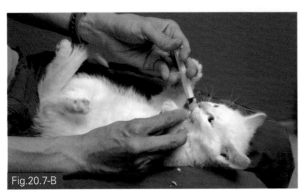

Fig.20.7-B

Fig.20.7-B, Step 1: First countercondition to having the feet handled. Lay the kitten on her back and touch the feet while feeding for several seconds. Then stop feeding and stop touching the feet simultaneously so that the kitten learns to associate foot handling with food. When she consistently holds still during the touching of her feet, graduate to operant counterconditioning.

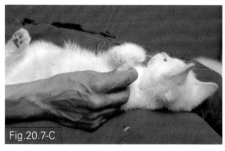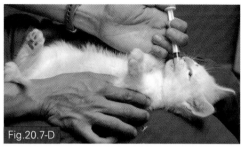

Fig.20.7-C

Fig.20.7-D

Fig.20.7-C, D, Step 2: Use operant counterconditioning by touching a paw for several seconds and then, if the kitten holds still, rewarding her with a treat. Always stop handling before the cat starts to struggle, but systematically increase the handling time to a period that's appropriate for a real nail trim.

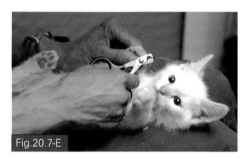

Fig.20.7-E

Fig.20.7-E, Step 3: Next, take the clippers out and trim a few nails. Stop and give treats before the kitten has a chance to react aversely. Most kittens are not yet afraid of the nail clippers, but if they are you'll need to add a few steps. For example, feed treats while you're simply holding the nail trimmers, then while you touch the trimmers to the nail, and then while trimming just one nail.

20.8 Wearing a Harness and Leash

Countercondition the kitten to wearing a harness and leash. Once they are used to being held in different positions, counterconditioning to a leash and harness is easy.

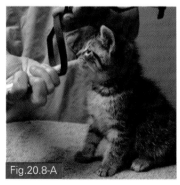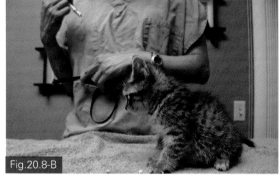

Fig.20.8-A

Fig.20.8-B

Fig.20.8-A, Step 1: First place food (canned cat food or tuna) in a syringe (without the needle) and place it through the harness so that the kitten is just near the harness.

Fig.20.8-B, Step 2: After several bites of food, remove both the food source and the harness simultaneously so that the kitten begins to associate the harness with receiving food. When the kitten performs this step with no adverse reaction several times in row, go to the next step.

™

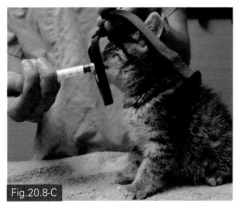

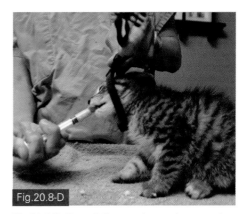

Fig.20.8-C, Step 3: Hold the food source so that the kitten has to hold her nose up to the harness. After several bites of food, simultaneously remove both the food source and the harness. When the kitten performs this step readily several times in row, progress to the next step.

Fig.20.8-D, Step 4: Repeat the previous step but this time hold the food so that the kitten must insert her head through the harness. Be sure to hold the harness in one position rather than move it around.

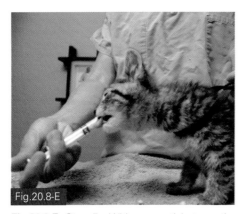

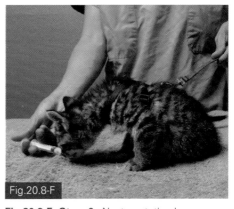

Fig.20.8-E, Step 5: With sequential steps, the kitten should soon be able to push her head and neck all the way through the harness so that her chest is pressing against it but with no sensitivity to the pressure. For this to occur, you must hold the harness stationary rather than letting it move with the kitten.

Fig.20.8-F, Step 6: Next, put the harness on completely and continue distracting the kitten with food. Now engage the kitten in other activities such as sit or targeting so that she does not focus on the harness and learns to associate it with positive experiences.

Realistically, kittens who already accept handling well can often skip many of the steps suggested for counterconditioning to the harness.

20.9 Going on Outings

Kittens should learn to be comfortable in new environments and with meeting new people.

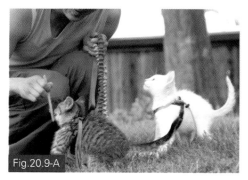 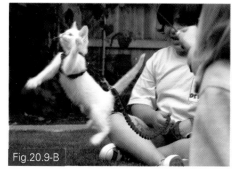

Fig.20.9-A, B: Once the kitten is counterconditioned to wearing a harness and leash, she can be taken on walks and can habituate to more environments, sounds and people. Now cats can learn to be as socialized, adaptable and outgoing as dogs. They can also be controlled better in situations around the house where running loose gets them in trouble. These kittens are wearing the Gentle Leader Come With Me Kitty (Premier Pet, Midlothian, Virginia) harness and bungee leash. These harnesses are especially effective because they adjust to fit the cat in a comfortable and secure manner. The bungee also allows kittens to explore without suddenly being jolted by the leash.

20.10 Teaching Behaviors

20.10.1 Teaching sit. *(Video 3)*

All kittens should learn to automatically sit quietly to receive treats, because this behavior can be used to prevent or fix many behavior problems. Kittens can be trained using their meals so that they get 10 to 30 food reinforcements for sitting during each session. They usually learn to sit within minutes, but to make sitting for treats and kibble a habit before they learn a less desirable behavior like clawing for treats, kittens should get lots of practice within a short time. Sitting for treats, no matter how excited they are to get the food, can be learned within days.

Kittens will learn to sit to solicit attention or food from their owners, instead of meowing, clawing or jumping on things. Sitting can be used as an alternative behavior to distract the kitten from undesirable behaviors such as scratching furniture, jumping on counters, climbing drapes or pestering another pet. Just get the cat's attention and ask for a sit, then reward her for it. Keep her involved long enough to make her forget about the previous unwanted behavior she was engaged in.

Cats are easier to train to sit than dogs because they naturally sit more frequently and remain seated longer. To train the sit, either just wait for the kitten to sit or lure her into position with food. For the latter technique, place the treat right up to the kitten's nose so that it's touching the nose, then raise it up and over the nose to make the kitten's weight shift onto her hind end, causing her to sit.

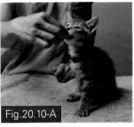
Fig.20.10-A

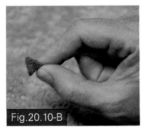
Fig.20.10-B

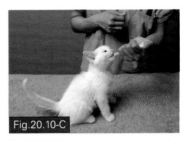
Fig.20.10-C

Fig.20.10-A, B: When using kibble to train, use a size that protrudes far enough from your fingers so that the kitten can distinguish between the kibble and your fingers. Kittens will often bite your fingers accidentally when trying to grasp food. Once the kitten is sitting, give 5 or more treats in a row to reward continued sitting. Then move away a few steps and repeat the exercise. The kitten should learn to follow you or walk up to you and sit quietly to get her treat.

Fig.20.10-C: You can also deliver the food through a syringe or pill gun, or put some on a spoon or tongue depressor. Each reward should last a few seconds or 1-2 bites. Then remove the delivery device for several seconds and give treats again if the kitten remains seated. This way you are rewarding continuous sitting.

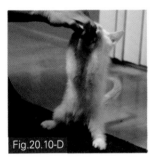
Fig.20.10-D

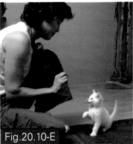
Fig.20.10-E

Fig.20.10-F

Fig.20.10-D: Avoid rewarding pawing or clawing behavior. If you do, you'll be teaching your cat to jump and claw you.

Fig.20.10-E, F: Instead, remove your hand quickly if the cat reaches with her paws (negative punishment). Now this kitty is sitting, but she still has one raised paw. Wait until all four feet are on the floor before rewarding.

What to do if kitty paws at the treat instead of sitting with all four feet on the floor. When kittens first learn sit, it's good to practice a lot (20 or more times for several days) so they quickly learn the behavior before they have a chance to learn to paw for the food. If your kitty is pawing, consider the following:

1. Sometimes kittens paw because they can't judge exactly where the food is, or they think they have to hold the food down to keep it from moving away. If this is the case, hold the food lower in spite of the pawing several times in a row and the kitten should stop pawing.

2. Alternatively, using canned food on a spoon or tongue depressor will stop the pawing because you will be able to deliver larger amounts of food that the kitten can easily see. Let her lick the food for up to 5 seconds and then remove it and use the rest for an another reward in several seconds.

3. Work on the scruffing exercise where you jiggle the scruff for a few seconds and then quickly follow with a treat. Only do this if it calms the kitten, allowing you to get the treat to her when her paws are on the floor. After several training sessions, you should not have to do this anymore.

4. Just drop the treat on the floor. To help the kitten understand when the treat is coming, train using a clicker; click and immediately drop the treat so that the kitten sees it right away. The click comes first, so it predicts that a treat is going to appear.

Work on sit until the kitten consistently walks over and sits in front of you quietly with all feet on the floor and then takes her treat without pawing at you. In this way, sit naturally progresses into "come when called." When the kitten is hungry, walk away from her and then make a distinct noise that the kitten will never hear in any other situation; a whistle works well. Immediately put the food down low so she can come and get it. Do this repeatedly until she always turns and runs to you right away when you give the cue to come. Then put the behavior on a variable rate of reinforcement, where you give her a food reward sometimes but not all the time.

20.10.2 Teaching targeting.

Targeting means to touch an object (such as a ball on the end of a pencil) with the nose. *(Video 4)* It is a game with many benefits.

1. It can be used to teach the kitten or an adult cat to go from one location to another. For instance, use targeting to teach a cat to go into the litter box if she's hesitant to use it, or to jump up and down from a pedestal.

2. It can be used as a game to divert attention from another animal or object, just as the toy was used during kitty kindergarten to divert the kitten from the dog she was afraid of. Targeting is especially useful with adult cats because they might not be as interested in playing with toys, making targeting a more successful method of diverting their attention. For instance, if one cat pesters another household cat, you can divert her attention from the other cat by playing the targeting game with her until she's no longer interested in the other pet. Over time, if performed consistently enough, this exercise will lead to a loss of interest in the other pet.

3. Targeting can also be used to train tricks such as spin, roll over and jump through a hoop.

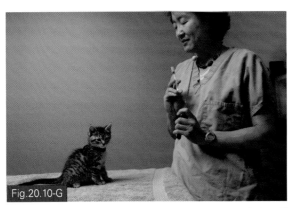 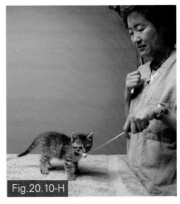

Fig.20.10-G, H, Step 1: Start with the target out of view. Then rapidly place it within an inch or so of the kitten so that it suddenly appears and gets her attention. Hold it completely still. She'll likely investigate it.

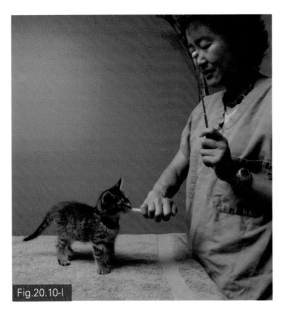

Fig.20.10-I, Step 2: When she investigates the target by touching it with her nose, immediately remove the target by holding it vertically again and place food in the kitten's mouth. Repeat this 5-10 times in row. Then increase the distance at which you present the target by 1-2 inches at a time, so the kitten has to move forward to touch it.

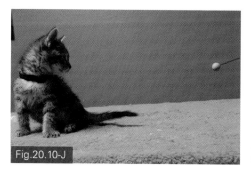

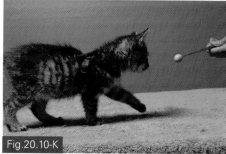

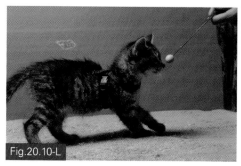

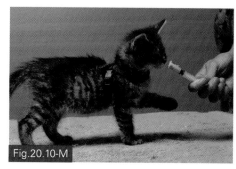

Fig.20.10-J to Fig.20.10-M: When the kitten consistently responds to visual presentation of the target by moving toward it and touching it with her nose, you can add a cue word. For the cat to learn the cue word quickly, it must predict a consequence; in this case the word "target" will predict the appearance of the target. To teach the cue word, say "target" in a distinct voice that stands out from other environmental sounds and words. Immediately follow by presenting the target crisply so that it gets the cat's attention right away. Now the kitten can go touch the target to earn a treat.

References

American Association of Feline Practitioners. 2004. *Feline Behavior Guidelines from the American Association of Feline Practitioners.* http://www.aafponline.org/resources/guidelines/ Feline_Behavior_Guidelines. pdf (Accessed June 1, 2008).

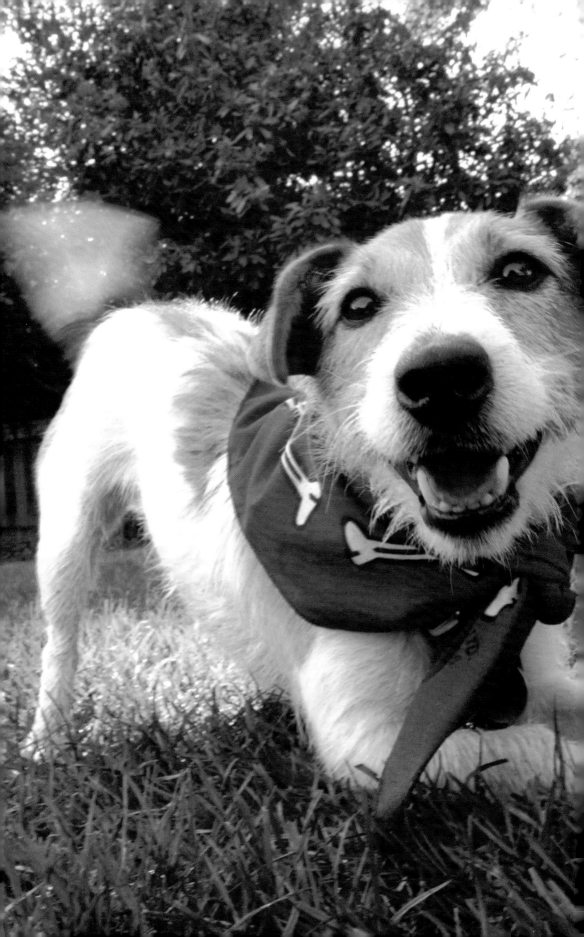

Appendix 1: DVD Table of Contents

Chapter 1: **Fear**

Video 1: Fear of Inanimate Objects
Video 2: The Body Language of Fear
Video 3: Counterconditioning to the Car
Video 4: Fear and Aggression
Video 5: How and How Not to Greet a Dog
Video 6: A Fearful Australian Cattle Dog

Chapter 2: **Dominance vs. Unruly Behavior**

Video 1: Dominance-Related Behavior or Something Else?
Video 2: Unruly Behavior Can Develop Into Aggression
Video 3: Teaching Dogs to Learn to Earn

Chapter 3: **Classical Conditioning (a.k.a. Associative Learning)**

Video 1: Kitten Classically Conditioned to the Sounds of a Can Opening

Chapter 4: **Operant Conditioning Basics (Learning by Trial and Error)**

Video 1: Operant Conditioning Demonstration: Shaping a Dog to Step Into a Box
Video 2: Shaping Demonstration: Teaching a Dog to Do a Somersault
Video 3: What's My Motivation?
Video 4: Communication: What Your Dog Cares About

Chapter 5: **Methods of Behavior Modification**

Video 1: Habituation to Captain Kirk
Video 2: Classical vs. Operant Counterconditioning
Video 3: Tips for Giving Treats
Video 4: Counterconditioning to Grooming (Crude Version)
Video 5: Counterconditioning: A More Refined Version
Video 6: Counterconditioning to Petting 1
Video 7: Counterconditioning to Petting 2
Video 8: Operant Counterconditioning a Dog-Aggressive Dog
Video 9: Flooding vs. Counterconditioning: Dog Who Is Fearful of Metal Grates
Video 10: Does Giving Treats Reward Aggression?

Chapter 6: Preparing Pets for the Hospital Visit

Video 1: Crate Training—Using Toys as Reinforcers

Chapter 7: Preparing the Environment for the Pet's Visit

Video 1: The Effect of Waiting Room Design

Chapter 8: Exam Room Tips

Video 1: A Cat Shows That He's More Comfortable in His Carrier
Video 2: When to Avoid Scruffing

Chapter 9: Moving Dogs Around the Facility

Video 1: Removing Dogs From Their Kennel
Video 2: Removing an Aggressive Cocker Spaniel From a Kennel

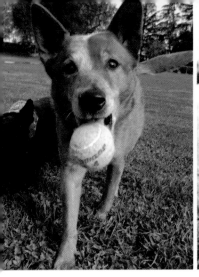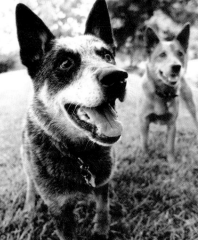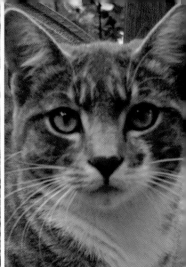

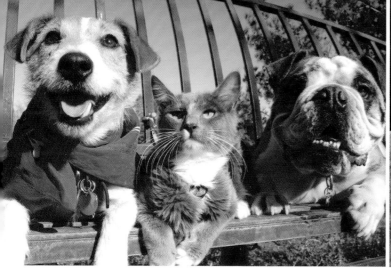
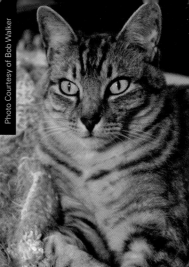

Photo Courtesy of Bob Walker

Chapter 13: **Restraining Dogs for Procedures**

Chapter 14: **Dealing with Difficult Dogs**

Chapter 15: **Restraint for Standard Positions in Cats**

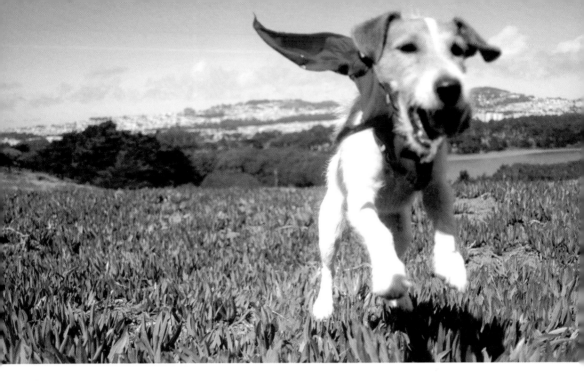

Appendix 2:

Other products by Dr. Sophia Yin

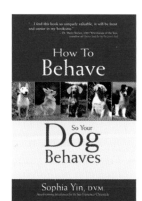

How to Behave So Your Dog Behaves

Pages: 256
Size: 9" x 6"
Type: Hardback
Retail price: $22.95
Publisher: TFH Publications
© 2004 Sophia Yin
Order through: amazon.com

Whether or not you're aware of it, every interaction you have with your dog is a training session. Whether your dog is learning something you want him to learn is another matter. If you want a well-behaved dog, you're going to have to modify your own behavior in order to modify his. The best way to achieve this is to understand how dogs think and learn. In this book readers learn:

- The simple strategy for modifying virtually all behaviors in dogs
- How their every move or action conveys something to their dog
- How to use all of their dog's motivators to their advantage in training.
- How they can quickly go from a person their dog likes sometimes to their dog's best friend by setting rules, communicating the rules with correct timing, and rewarding good behaviors consistently until they become a habit.

Praise for How to Behave So Your Dog Behaves

"Sophia Yin's approach to dog training is a perfect meshing of the scientific theory and practical application. What is most important is her introduction to trainers of the significance of the person's behavior and its effect on the dog's learning ability. Sophia has done this better than anyone else, emphasizing in a very readable fashion the lasting effects of people's actions on their dog's behaviors. This is an important book for anyone who wants to maximize correct interactions with the pet."

Dr. Raymond Coppinger, PhD, Professor of Biology, Hampshire College, author of Dogs, A New Understanding Of Canine Origin, Behavior and Evolution

"There are books that emphasize normal behavior and learning theory and there are books that teach your dog to obey obedience commands, but this book includes both in a logical easy-to-read fashion —AND tells you what to do to correct things if your training program isn't going exactly as planned—AND gives you real-life situations where knowing and using that particular command would be helpful. That is rare. Dr. Yin knows how—and why—to train, and how to convey the finer points to the average dog owner who wants a better relationship with their dogs."

Dr. Leslie Larson Cooper, DVM, Diplomate, American College of Veterinary Behaviorists.

"It's often said that the only thing two dog trainers can agree on is what a third dog trainer is doing wrong. Not so! Now we can all agree that Sophia Yin's How to Behave So Your Dog Behaves offers much worth considering. Because she provides the rationale behind her techniques [the book] provides a framework people can use to examine their dog's behavioral issues. For those who have tried and failed to fix their dog's behavior problems the first two sections especially… are worth their weight in gold."

Sergeant Steve White, police K9 trainer and consultant

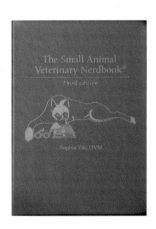

The Small Animal Veterinary Nerdbook® 3rd Edition

Pages: 450
Size: 5.5" x 7"
Type: In metal spiral binder with 21 tab dividers
Retail price: $89.00
www.nerdbook.com

First published in 1994, as a guide to help veterinary students survive clinics with more grace, poise, and knowledge than ever before, The Small Animal Veterinary Nerdbook® is now a classic for veterinary students in the U.S. and Canada. More than 20,000 veterinarians and veterinary students own this popular book. This pocket-sized reference gives you immediate access to accurate practical information on 21 subjects, with hand dividers and headers as well as sleek tables and charts.

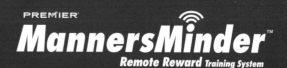

Training consists of 5 stages
Endless possible uses

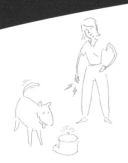

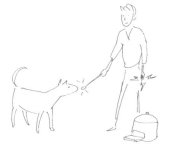

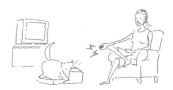

STAGE 1: Tone & Treat

Dogs learn that the tone means a treat is coming. The tone is then used to signal when a behavior has been performed correctly.

OTHER USES:

Agility: Go outs, directionals, contacts, teeter, dogwalk, weave poles, and improving speed on equipment.

Obedience: Go outs, directional retrieves.

Household: Crate training, rewarding quiet behavior when the dog is tethered away from the owner or is in a separate room.

STAGE 2: Targeting

Dogs learn to run to and touch a target with their nose in order to earn a treat.

OTHER USES:

Agility: Go outs, contacts, teeter, dog walk, weave poles, and improving speed on equipment.

Obedience: Go outs, directional retrieves, heeling.

Tricks: Spin, twist, somersault, training dogs to retrieve or put toys away.....

Household: To play with and exercise dogs. Like "Fetch!" but with a target.

STAGE 3: Down-stay

Dogs learn to stay lying down on a rug or bed for at least one minute.

OTHER USES:

Agility: Control and focus at the start line and on the pause table.

Obedience: Fast drop on recall.

Household: Training dogs to remain lying down while owners eat dinner.

Praise for the MannerMinder Dog Training System

"The MannersMinder is utterly amazing! We tried for months to get our dog to remain calm when visitors came to the door. But no matter what we did, she would jump on everyone from our mom to the mail man. Then we got MannersMinder. After just a few short training sessions, our dog's entire behavior changed when visitors arrived. Now she sits calmly in front of the machine, instead of wrecking havoc at the front door. It's like a little doggie babysitter. We cannot recommend this product highly enough, especially if you have an energetic dog in your life. Thank you!"

-C.C. USA

"I'm currently helping my son and his service dog make the transition into the school setting. My son is able to reward his dog without missing a beat. We love it!"

-Julie Shaw R.V.T.

"MannersMinder™ is a unique reward-based program that does more than help owners manage their dogs' barking and jumping. The program repairs the owner-pet relationship that barking and jumping behaviors damage and helps people and their dogs experience quality time together. Isn't that what having a dog is all about?"

-Nancy Peterson
The Humane Society of the United States

"This is one of the best pieces of training equipment brought to the public in the last 30+ years. Not only is the device designed so that the average public consumer can operate it effectively, the instructions that accompany the MannerdMinder are just outstandingly well presented. This product applies sound principles of learning and makes it clear."

-Dr. Marylee Nitschke,
Professor of psychology
Lifetime achievement award winner
Association of Pet Dog Trainers

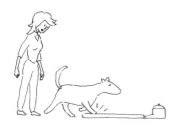
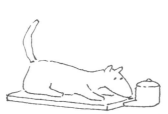
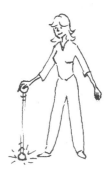

STAGE 4: Place

Dogs learn to run to the rug or bed and lie down on verbal cue.

OTHER USES:

Agility: Pause table, go outs, directionals, contacts, teeter, dogwalks and improving speed on equipment.

House hold: Separating dogs by sending them to lie down in their own locations.

STAGE 5: Down-stay With Distractions

Dogs learn to stay in a down-stay on the rug or bed even with big distractions such as the doorbell ringing, people knocking at the door, toys being tossed

OTHER USES:

Agility: Stronger down-stay on the pause table.

Obedience: Down-stay in and out of sight. The sit-stay can be rewarded by hand once the down-stay is trained.

Service Dogs: Train dogs to down-stay under tables, in vehicles, etc.

Household: Train dogs to lie in a down-stay while owners eat dinner, answer the door, work with other animals, manage the kids, or otherwise need their dog to lie calmly in the house. The training can also be transferred to outside the house and with rewards other than treats.

BEHAVIOR PROBLEMS:

Separation anxiety (high level): Manners-Minder™ allows owners to reward quiet, calm down-stays when they practice graduated departures from the house. Crate training (more difficult dog). Rewarding quiet behavior in anxious dogs.

Counter-condition to grooming, toenail trim, hair dryer, scary sounds, and fear-inducing objects that can be presented in a controlled manner.

My dog Barkley had an almost 8 year obsession with the lawnmower. Whenever I attempted to move it, even if it was just to get to something behind it in the garage, Barkley [would go] ballistic. He loved to bite the wheels, and attempted to herd it and jump over it while I was pushing it along. When I would shut him inside the house while I was mowing the lawn, I could hear him barking above the sound of the lawnmower.

Since Sunday we've been working on Stage 5 of the MannersMinder training protocol. Tonight I set him up under the pergola adjacent to the lawn area, which is fenced off from the lawn, and I managed to mow the entire lawn (approx 130 square meters) without a single bark. I honestly expected it to take weeks before I could achieve that, and I used less than one meal worth of kibble tonight. It was one of my best ever Christmas presents.

-Leandra Prior
Adelaide, South Australia

"More effective than any obedience school my dog has attended. You're really paying for the training material and DVD but for the results I got, I would have paid a grand. Some obedience schools run twice as much. The [Manners-Minder] is worth its weight in gold.

-David Novak: The Gadget Guy,
Indianapolis Star.

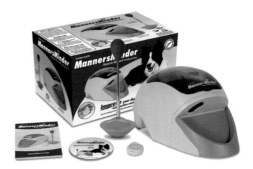